P9-AGU-395

Other books by the American Heart Association published by Times Books

American Heart Association Cookbook, 5th Edition

American Heart Association Low-Fat, Low-Cholesterol Cookbook

American Heart Association Low-Salt Cookbook

American Heart Association Kids' Cookbook

American Heart Association Family Guide to Stroke

American Heart Association Quick and Easy Cookbook

AMERICAN HEART ASSOCIATION BRAND NAME FAT AND CHOLESTEROL COUNTER

SECOND EDITION

American Heart Association[SM]

Fighting Heart Disease and Stroke

BRAND NAME

FAT AND CHOLESTEROL

COUNTER

SECOND EDITION

TIMES 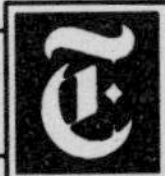 BOOKS

RANDOM HOUSE

Your contribution to the American Heart Association supports research that helps make publications like this possible. For more information, call 1-800-AHA-USA 1.

 Published in the United States by Times Books, a division of Random House, Inc., New York, and simultaneously in Canada by Random House of Canada Limited, Toronto.

Library of Congress Cataloging-in-Publication Data

Brand name fat and cholesterol counter / American Heart Association. — 2nd ed.

p. cm.

ISBN 0-8129-2367-7

1. Food—Cholesterol content—Tables. 2. Food—Fat content—Tables. 3. Food—Sodium content—Tables. I. American Heart Association.

TX553.C43B73 1995

641.1′4—dc20 95-7027

Manufactured in the United States of America

9 8 7 6 5 4 3

Design by Anistatia R. Miller

Inclusion in this book does not constitute an endorsement, implied or otherwise, by the American Heart Association. The AHA is not suggesting the nutritional superiority of any product listed in this guide over any product not listed in this guide.

Some of the company or product names in this book also may be registered as trademarks. It is not the intention of this book to present those trademarks in their registered format, but to provide information about those products.

ACKNOWLEDGMENTS

The dedication, talent, and untiring efforts of many people made this book a reality. Special thanks, however, go to the staff of the Diet Modification Center of Baylor College of Medicine, Houston, Texas, for compiling the database used for this publication. Lynne W. Scott, M.A., R.D./L.D., and her staff, especially Mary Carole McMann, M.P.H., R.D./L.D., were always available for consultation. Myrthala Miranda-Guzman entered all the information from food manufacturers into the computer, and Laura Frey coordinated correspondence with the manufacturers. Their expertise, cheerfully shared, is very much appreciated.

Jane Ruehl and Janice R. Moss edited and oversaw the production of this book, and Amy Lindsly helped with the proofreading. Word processors Gerre Gilford and Debra Bond never complained when asked to make one more change to the manuscript.

All of us hope that this book will serve three primary purposes: first and most important, to help you develop a more healthful eating plan; second, to show you the tremendous variety of foods you can choose from to make this plan as enjoyable as possible; and finally, to shorten and simplify your food-shopping trips.

Mary Winston, Ed.D., R.D.
Senior Science Consultant
Office of Scientific Affairs
American Heart Association
National Center

CONTENTS

FAT, CHOLESTEROL, AND YOUR HEART

Congratulations! You picked up this book.

That says you care about your health. Maybe you've been diagnosed with heart disease or have had a heart attack. Or you're healthy now and want to stay that way. You want to be one of the "lucky ones," the people who live long, healthy lives. You want to live free of the heart attacks and strokes that kill about 43 percent of all Americans.

As you probably know, luck has little to do with it. For the most part, the majority of people who escape heart disease do so because they know how to help make their hearts last a lifetime. They know that there are several factors that increase the risk of heart attack and stroke. Four of these are smoking, high blood cholesterol, high blood pressure, and physical inactivity. Therefore, they change their lives to reduce these risk factors.

People who want healthy hearts don't smoke. They keep their blood pressure under control, and they are physically active on a regular basis. To keep their blood cholesterol levels in the normal range, they also watch how much fat and cholesterol they eat. Those things are what this book is all about.

Eating Your Heart Out

Americans love to eat high-fat foods—rich desserts, cream sauces, fried foods, whole-milk dairy products. The trouble is, this habit is killing us.

Hundreds of scientific studies show that a diet high in total fat, saturated fat, and cholesterol can load the blood with fat. People who have high levels of fat in their blood are more likely to have a heart attack.

Atherosclerosis, a major cause of heart attack and stroke, is a disease process of the blood vessels. What happens is this: For reasons unknown (perhaps because an artery becomes damaged), fatty substances build up in the inner lining of the arteries. These substances are mostly cholesterol. The buildup gets worse and worse, until the artery is completely blocked. That stops the flow of blood. When this happens in an artery leading to the heart, that's a heart attack. When it happens in an artery leading to the brain, that's a stroke. You might think of a stroke as a "brain attack."

The cholesterol in your blood comes from two places. Your body produces it, and you get it from eating foods high in saturated fat and cholesterol. In a healthy person, the body produces all the cholesterol it needs. And it actually does need *some*. That's because cholesterol helps produce sex hormones and helps form cell membranes and protective sheaths around your nerves.

Down with High Cholesterol

What level of blood cholesterol is safe? Studies show clearly that the higher your cholesterol level rises above 200 mg/dl (milligrams per deciliter), the more likely you are to have a heart attack. People who keep their blood cholesterol levels *below 200 mg/dl* are least likely to have a heart attack.

The following blood cholesterol level guidelines were determined by the National Cholesterol Education Program, a program of the National Heart, Lung, and Blood Institute. These guidelines are based on measurements of total cholesterol and high-density lipoprotein (HDL) cholesterol. Many scientists think that HDL cholesterol carries harmful cholesterol away from the body's tissues. Therefore, HDL cholesterol is often called "good cholesterol."

Classification Based on Total Cholesterol and HDL Cholesterol

Total Cholesterol Level	Classification
Less than 200 mg/dl	Desirable
200–239 mg/dl	Borderline High Risk
240 mg/dl or greater	High Risk
HDL Cholesterol Level	
Less than 35 mg/dl	High Risk

Low HDL Cholesterol (and Other Risk Factors)

As the above guidelines show, a low HDL cholesterol level is also a risk factor for heart disease. Two other contributing factors are obesity and diabetes.

So, in addition to keeping your blood pressure and blood cholesterol levels normal, being physically active, and not smoking, it's important to stay at your best weight. It's also important to have your HDL cholesterol level, along with total cholesterol, checked regularly.

How Low Can You Go?

Some people have naturally low cholesterol levels, between 140 and 200 mg/dl. Many of us, however, have to work at it to stay at about 200 mg/dl.

In some people, the blood cholesterol levels are extremely low—below 140 mg/dl. Scientists have found that people with high blood cholesterol (200 mg/dl or greater) are at a higher risk of death from heart attack. Some people have low blood cholesterol (less than 140 mg/dl) and have a low risk of heart disease. These people may, however, be at greater risk of dying from a variety of other causes. Their death rates from trauma, cancer, stroke caused by blood clots, and respiratory and infectious diseases increase.

Scientists are not sure why ultralow cholesterol levels cause this increased death rate from other causes. They do know that people with such low levels often seem to be in poor overall health. While scientists do more research in this area, you should aim for a blood cholesterol level below 200 mg/dl. This will help you stay your healthiest.

THE STORY ON SALT

If you're like most other Americans, you eat between 2,500 and 5,000 mg of sodium a day. That's far more than your body needs.

Scientific studies have shown that reducing the amount of sodium you eat may reduce your blood pressure. This is true if you have high blood pressure, as well as if your blood pressure is normal.

Help Prevent High Blood Pressure

In fact, the latest studies are showing that low-salt diets actually help *prevent* high blood pressure. We also know that certain people are "salt sensitive." That is, they tend to develop high blood pressure if they eat a lot of salty foods. The trouble is, there's no way to know in advance who is salt sensitive and who isn't.

Stop at 3,000 mg a Day

For these reasons, the American Heart Association strongly recommends that you eat no more than 3,000 mg of sodium a day. This is the equivalent of about 2 teaspoons of salt.

It's easy to measure the salt used in cooking and on the table. You can even eliminate most of that by using spices and herbs instead of salt when you cook. And you can throw away your salt shaker. But it's hard to measure "hidden" salt—the sodium in prepared foods.

That's where this book comes in. It lists the sodium content of hundreds of popular name brand food items. It also teaches you to read food labels to find the amount of sodium in a serving of prepared foods. These two things will help you balance and monitor your sodium intake on a daily basis.

THE AMERICAN HEART ASSOCIATION DIET

The American Heart Association Diet is a simple eating plan that can help you protect your heart. It's low in total fat, saturated fat, cholesterol, and sodium but high in nutrition and taste. It is designed for all healthy Americans over the age of two.

Kicking the Cholesterol Habit

On the following pages, you'll learn how to change the amount and kind of fat you eat so that you can reduce your blood cholesterol level and protect your heart. You'll also learn to limit sodium to help keep your blood pressure in the normal range. And you'll learn that many types of food can fit into a heart-healthy eating plan.

In fact, the American Heart Association Diet is not only good for your heart, it can also help prevent some forms of cancer and help control diabetes. That's because it shares the same basic eating concept as the diet recommendations of the American Cancer Society, the American Diabetes Association, and the U.S. Department of Agriculture/Health and Human Services Dietary Guidelines. This basic concept is to follow an eating plan that is low fat, low saturated fat, low cholesterol, low sodium, moderate calorie, balanced, and nutritious. In short, it's an eating plan you can count on—for life.

Getting Down to Basics

The basic AHA Diet provides about 1,600 calories and gives you all the nutrients you need. If you need additional calories, choose more foods from any of the groups listed on pages xix to xxii except "Fats and Oils" and "Meat, Poultry, Seafood, Dried Beans and Peas, and Eggs" (you can have extra dried beans and peas from this group, if you like).

After you read the American Heart Association Diet, you'll want to evaluate each food as part of your overall eating plan. In fact, some foods may not be appropriate for you. For example, if you have cardiovascular disease and you're on a more restricted diet, your doctor may advise you to eat even less saturated fat and cholesterol than the AHA diet allows. If you're on a low-sodium diet, cut back further on foods high in sodium. If you're trying to lose weight, you'll want to avoid the high-calorie foods listed in the diet and to cut down on the amount of food you eat. Diabetes and allergies present other dietary challenges.

But at the American Heart Association, we know that when you permanently change your way of eating to low fat, low cholesterol, and moderate sodium, you're helping your heart stay its healthiest. And there's more good news: You can splurge once in a while with no ill effects! If you have an occasional dessert that's high in fat, simply reduce your fat intake for several days to compensate. If that's not convenient, try eating only a small serving or share the dessert with your dining partner.

The American Heart Association Diet is outlined on the following pages. You'll find it's an eating plan you can put your whole heart into.

THE AHA DIET GUIDELINES

The following basic guidelines are all you need to know to create an eating plan to protect your heart.

- Eat no more than 6 ounces of lean meat, fish, and poultry every day.
- Eat fish and poultry more often than lean meat.
- When choosing meat, look for lean cuts.
- Use meatless main dishes as entrées as often as possible, or cook "low-meat" entrées by combining small amounts of meat with rice, pasta, beans, or vegetables.
- Use only about 5 to 8 teaspoons of fat and oils a day. Be sure to count what you use in cooking, plus in salad dressings and spreads. Vary the amount slightly according to your caloric needs.
- Cook with little or no fat. Boil, broil, bake, roast, poach, microwave, or steam foods.
- Eat no more than 3 or 4 egg *yolks* per week, including those used in cooking and store-bought products. Egg *whites* contain no fat, so they aren't limited.
- Eat very few organ meats, such as livers, brains, chitterlings, kidneys, hearts, gizzards, sweetbreads, and pork maws.
- Eat at least 5 servings of fruits and vegetables every day.
- Eat 6 or more servings of cereals and grains every day.
- Choose skim or 1% milk, and use nonfat or low-fat dairy products for your other choices.
- Eat no more than 3,000 mg of sodium daily.

Meat, Poultry, Seafood, Dried Beans and Peas, and Eggs

Choices: Pick the leanest cuts of meat.
Eat poultry and fish more often than meat.
Trim all visible fat before cooking.
Remove the skin before cooking poultry, unless roasting.

Daily Servings: Eat no more than 6 ounces of cooked poultry, seafood, or lean meat, or 2 or more servings of dried beans and peas a day.
Eat no more than 3 or 4 egg *yolks* a week.
Eat all the egg *whites* you want.

Serving Size: 3 ounces cooked (or 4 ounces raw) meat, poultry, or fish.
(Three ounces of meat is about the size of a deck of cards; it's also equal to about half a chicken breast or a chicken leg and thigh, or about half a cup of cooked flaked fish.)
1 cup cooked beans, peas, or legumes.

Vegetables and Fruits

Choices: Pick any vegetables and fruits.
Count coconut, olives, and avocados as fats (see "Fats and Oils" below).
Oranges, grapefruit, melons, and strawberries are excellent sources of vitamin C.
Deep yellow fruits, such as apricots and cantaloupes, are high in vitamin A.

	Dark green vegetables, such as spinach and broccoli, provide vitamin C and, along with deep yellow vegetables, such as carrots, are excellent sources of vitamin A.
Daily Servings:	5 or more.
Serving Size:	1 medium-size piece of fruit. ½ cup fruit juice. ½ to 1 cup cooked or raw vegetables.

Breads, Cereals, Pasta, and Starchy Vegetables

Choices:	You have a number of choices in this category. Consider the following: Nonfat or low-fat breads, rolls, crackers, and snacks. Hot or cold cereals (except granola, which may be high in saturated fat). Homemade quick breads made with skim or 1% milk and fats or oils low in saturated fat. Rice. Pasta made without egg yolk. Starchy vegetables (potatoes, lima beans, etc.) Nonfat or low-fat soups.
Daily Servings:	6 or more.
Serving Size:	1 slice of bread. ¼ to 1 cup hot or cold cereals. 1 cup cooked rice or pasta. ¼ to ½ cup starchy vegetables. 1 cup nonfat or low-fat soup.

Milk Products

Choices:	The key here is to choose a nonfat or low-fat variety. Choose from the following selections:

Skim or 1% milk.
Nonfat or low-fat dairy products, such as cheese, yogurt, and frozen desserts, where available.

Daily Servings: 2 or more for adults over 24 and children 2–10.
3 to 4 for ages 11–24 and women who are pregnant or lactating.

Serving Size: 8 ounces skim or 1% milk.
8 ounces nonfat or low-fat yogurt.
1 ounce nonfat or low-fat cheese.
½ cup nonfat or low-fat cottage cheese.
½ cup nonfat or low-fat frozen dairy dessert.

Fats and Oils

Choices: Yes, you do need some fats and oils. Just be careful to select from the following choices:
Vegetable oils (canola, corn, olive, safflower, sesame, soybean, sunflower).
Tub margarines with liquid vegetable oil listed as the first ingredient and with no more than 2 grams of saturated fat per tablespoon. (Margarine is still better for you than butter is. See "The Butter-Margarine Controversy (Trans Fatty Acids)," page 188.)
Salad dressings and mayonnaise with no more than 1 gram of saturated fat per tablespoon.

Daily Servings: 5 to 8 teaspoons, depending on how many calories you need.

Serving Size: 1 teaspoon vegetable oil or regular margarine.
2 teaspoons diet margarine.
1 tablespoon salad dressing.
2 teaspoons mayonnaise or peanut butter.
3 teaspoons seeds and nuts.
⅛ medium avocado.
10 small or 5 large olives.
½ ounce dried coconut.

Desserts

Choices: Select desserts that are made with acceptable ingredients and are low in fat, cholesterol, and calories. You can make your own desserts using ingredients from the above lists.

Snacks

Choices: Look to other food groups for snacks, such as fruits, raw vegetables and dips, nutritious cookies, low-fat crackers and pretzels, seeds, and nuts. Nonfat varieties of some snack foods are available. But please note that they usually have the same number of calories as the low-fat versions.

Beverages

Choices: Select fruit and vegetable juices, coffee, tea, or mineral water.
If you drink alcohol, have no more than about 8 ounces of wine, 24 ounces of beer, or 2 ounces of 100-proof distilled spirits a day.
If you don't drink, don't start.

Now that you know what kind of foods to choose, it's time to determine how much fat and sodium you can eat every day. That's an important step in keeping your blood cholesterol and blood pressure levels safe.

Figuring Your Daily Fat Intake

To figure the amount of fat you can have every day, you should know how many calories you need to maintain your best weight. That's easy to do. First, find your ideal weight in the table on page xxv.

Best Body Weight Ranges*

Height (Without Shoes)	Weight (Without Shoes)	
(feet/inches)	Men (pounds)	Women (pounds)
4′10″	—	92–121
4′11″	—	95–124
5′ 0″	—	98–127
5′ 1″	105–134	101–130
5′ 2″	108–137	104–134
5′ 3″	111–141	107–138
5′ 4″	114–145	110–142
5′ 5″	117–149	114–146
5′ 6″	121–154	118–150
5′ 7″	125–159	122–154
5′ 8″	129–163	126–159
5′ 9″	133–167	130–164
5′10″	137–172	134–169
5′11″	141–177	—
6′ 0″	145–182	—
6′ 1″	149–187	—
6′ 2″	153–192	—
6′ 3″	157–197	—

*This table is adapted from the Desirable Weight Tables prepared in 1959 by the Metropolitan Life Insurance Company. It is based on weights associated with the lowest mortality. For women 18 to 25 years old, subtract one pound for each year under 25.

The 1983 revision of the Metropolitan Life Insurance Company's Height and Weight Tables allows increased weight for certain heights. However, because obesity is a contributing factor for heart disease, the American Heart Association did not adopt the 1983 version.

Next, to find out how many calories you need, multiply your ideal weight by 15 if you're moderately active or 20 if you're very active. Children and lactating women have special calorie needs, so ask your doctor to guide you in these cases.

Got the total? From that figure, subtract the following number of calories, according to your age:

Age 25 to 34, subtract 0 calories
Age 35 to 44, subtract 100 calories
Age 45 to 54, subtract 200 calories
Age 55 to 64, subtract 300 calories
Age 65 or greater, subtract 400 calories

Let's use an example. If you were a 45-year-old man whose ideal weight is 145 pounds and who is moderately active, you'd take 145 pounds and multiply by 15, to get 2,175 calories. Then you'd subtract 200 calories, for a total of 1,975. If you were a moderately active, 35-year-old woman with an ideal weight of 120 pounds, you'd figure it like this: 120 pounds × 15 calories = 1,800 − 100 calories = 1,700 calories.

When you know how many calories you need every day, you can determine how many of those calories can come from fat. At the American Heart Association, we suggest that you keep your total fat intake to less than 30 percent of your total daily calories. Keep saturated fat and cholesterol to less than 10 percent of those daily calories.

To find out how much fat you can eat, multiply your total daily calories by .30. That will give you the total number of daily calories you can have from fat. To find out how many grams of fat that is, divide that number by 9. For example, if you can have 2,000 total calories a day, the equation is 2,000 × .30 = 600 calories from fat. Next, divide by 9, getting 67 grams of fat a day (rounded from 66.6).

To figure your saturated fat intake, multiply your total daily calories by .10, then divide by 9. Using the example above, 2,000 total calories a day × .10 = 200 calories from fat ÷ 9 = 22 grams of saturated fat (rounded from 22.2). For a quick reference, the table below shows the maximum grams of total fat and saturated fat for a variety of calorie levels. When figuring your total fat consumption, remember that it includes saturated, monounsaturated, and polyunsaturated fats. (See "Important Definitions," page xlii.)

Suggested Daily Fat Consumption

Daily Calories	Maximum Grams of Total Fat	Maximum Grams of Saturated Fat
1,200	40	13
1,400	47	16
1,600	53	18
1,800	60	20
2,000	67	22
2,200	73	24
2,400	80	27
2,600	87	29
2,800	93	31
3,000	100	33

All you have to do is check the food listings in this guide or the labels on food packages to find the number of grams of fat in a single serving. (For information on how to read food labels, see page xxix.) Then just keep track of the number of grams of total fat and saturated fat you eat every day—keeping that amount within the guidelines for your calorie level.

Figuring Your Daily Sodium Intake

The American Heart Association doesn't have specific criteria for sodium, but we recommend that you eat no more than 3,000 mg of it a day. Most foods from the food groups listed in the AHA Diet don't contain much sodium. You get most of your sodium from the salt added in cooking, at the table, and in prepared foods.

That makes your game plan easy. First, don't add salt when you're cooking. Instead, add herbs, spices, mustards, and vinegars for flavor. Second, keep the salt shaker off the table. Then all you have to worry about is the salt in packaged foods.

This book will show you the sodium level of hundreds of name brand canned, frozen, and prepared foods. When buying packaged foods, whenever possible choose a low-salt version or one without added salt. Be on the lookout for ingredients with sodium in the name: sodium citrate, sodium bicarbonate, monosodium glutamate. Make sure that these ingredients are listed near the end of the ingredients list. On the following pages, you'll find low-salt versions of almost every kind of packaged food.

Until recently, reading food labels was a hassle. It seemed as if the average person needed a math degree to calculate the fat content of a product.

But the new food labels make shopping for low-fat packaged foods much simpler. First, the amounts of fat, cholesterol, and sodium in one serving of the food are listed right on the label. And you can trust what you read on the package. That's because foods making health claims such as "low cholesterol" and "fat free" must meet specific legal criteria set by the U.S. government (see "Food Labels You Can Trust," page xxxiii).

The "Nutrition Facts" Label

The new label is called Nutrition Facts. Let's take a look at the sample label below and go over it step-by-step.

SERVING SIZE

Under the Nutrition Facts heading, you'll find the serving size. It's the average amount most people eat at one sitting. The rest of the values on the label, such as calories and fat, are based on this serving size. If you eat twice the amount, you'll have to double these figures. If you eat half the amount, you'll have to cut these figures in half.

CALORIES

The label first lists the number of calories in one serving of the food. If you're overweight, you may want to watch your calories closely. If you haven't already, find out how

Nutrition Facts

Serving Size ½ cup (114g)
Servings Per Container 4

Amount Per Serving

Calories 90 Calories from Fat 30

	% Daily Value*
Total Fat 3g	**5%**
Saturated Fat 0g	**0%**
Cholesterol 0mg	**0%**
Sodium 300mg	**13%**
Total Carbohydrate 13g	**4%**
Dietary Fiber 3g	**12%**
Sugars 3g	
Protein 3g	

Vitamin A	80%	•	Vitamin C	60%
Calcium	4%	•	Iron	4%

* Percent Daily Values are based on a 2,000 calorie diet. Your daily values may be higher or lower depending on your calorie needs:

	Calories	2,000	2,500
Total Fat	Less than	65g	80g
Sat Fat	Less than	20g	25g
Cholesterol	Less than	300mg	300mg
Sodium	Less than	2,400mg	2,400mg
Total Carbohydrate		300g	375g
Fiber		25g	30g

Calories per gram:
Fat 9 • Carbohydrate 4 • Protein 4

many calories you need to maintain your best weight (see page xxiii). Then you can use this calorie listing to help plan your daily menu.

DAILY VALUES

The percentages listed along the right side of the label also can help you plan what to eat each day. They relate to the Daily Values listed at the bottom of the label. Daily Values show the amounts of various nutrients recommended for a 2,000-calorie diet and a 2,500-calorie diet. If you need more calories, your personal daily values would be higher. If you need fewer calories, your daily values would be lower. But as a quick reference guide, the "% Daily Value" column shows you the percentage of your daily requirements of the different nutrients one serving of the food provides. In general, look for a low percent of daily value for fat, saturated fat, cholesterol, and sodium. But try to reach 100 percent of your daily requirement for total carbohydrate, dietary fiber, vitamins, and minerals.

TOTAL FAT

To the right of the calorie listing is Calories from Fat. You can use that, along with the listing for Total Fat, to determine how much fat you're getting in your diet. If you haven't determined how many grams of fat you can eat every day and still keep your heart healthy, see page xxiii. When you know how many grams of fat you can have, simply add up the fat grams of everything you eat. If you're trying to cut down on fat, limit your calories from fat. Look for foods higher in carbohydrates and lower in fat.

SATURATED FAT

Under Total Fat, the label lists Saturated Fat. Since many foods contain saturated fat, you'll want to watch this figure carefully. Why? Because it's the chief culprit in raising blood cholesterol, a major risk factor for heart disease.

CHOLESTEROL

Here's another "bad guy," because dietary cholesterol raises blood cholesterol. You'll want to limit your cholesterol intake to fewer than 300 milligrams a day.

SODIUM

Sodium's most common form is salt, but it's also found in combination with other chemicals such as monosodium glutamate (MSG). Scientists know it as something that can contribute to high blood pressure in some people. They just don't know *which* people. So keep your sodium intake low—under 3,000 mg a day.

TOTAL CARBOHYDRATE

Carbohydrates are your good friends. Most of them give you nutrients and energy but very little fat. You'll find them in foods such as bread, cereals, potatoes, fruits, and vegetables. In general, eat foods low in fat and high in carbohydrates.

DIETARY FIBER

Your grandmother probably called it "roughage" and encouraged you to eat more of it. Good advice. For optimal health, you need both soluble and insoluble kinds of dietary fiber. The difference is that soluble fiber dissolves in water and insoluble fiber doesn't. You'll find fiber in abundance in fruits, vegetables, whole-grain foods, beans, and peas. A few examples of foods with soluble fiber are whole-wheat bread, wheat cereal, cabbage, and carrots. Some foods that contain insoluble fiber are oatmeal, beans, peas, and citrus fruits. Soluble fiber can help reduce your blood cholesterol level, a risk factor for heart disease. Fiber may also play a preventive role in some types of cancer.

PROTEIN

If you're like most other Americans, you eat more protein every day than you actually need. In general, where you find lots of animal protein, you find lots of fat and cholesterol, too. That means you should eat only small servings of lean meat, fish, and poultry. Choose skim or low-fat milk and nonfat or low-fat yogurt and cheese. For protein without the fat, try beans, grains, and cereals.

VITAMINS AND MINERALS

The label lists the percentage of each vitamin and mineral the product contains. You'll want to aim for 100 percent of each every day. Remember: You can't reach this goal by eating just one kind of food. To get a balanced diet, search out a variety of foods from each food group. Cover all the bases and you'll hit a home run.

Food Labels You Can Trust

When you see words such as "Fat Free," "Lite," and "Low Cholesterol" on packaged foods, you can now rest assured that these claims are true. Why? Because the U.S. Food and Drug Administration has set strict definitions for all key words and health claims used on food product labels. We've listed the key words below, along with exactly what they mean.

Key Words	What They Mean
Calorie Free	Fewer than 5 calories per serving
Light (Lite)	⅓ less calories or no more than ½ the fat of the higher-calorie, higher-fat version or no more than ½ the sodium of the higher-sodium version

Fat Free	Less than 0.5 gram of fat per serving
Low Fat	3 grams of fat (or less) per serving
Reduced Fat or Less Fat	At least 25% less fat per serving than the higher-fat version
Lean	Less than 10 grams of fat, 4 grams of saturated fat, and 95 milligrams of cholesterol per serving
Extra Lean	Less than 5 grams of fat, 2 grams of saturated fat, and 95 milligrams of cholesterol per serving
Low in Saturated Fat	1 gram of saturated fat (or less) per serving and not more than 15% of calories from saturated fat
Cholesterol Free	2 milligrams of cholesterol (or less) and 2 grams of saturated fat (or less) per serving
Low Cholesterol	20 milligrams of cholesterol (or less) and 2 grams of saturated fat (or less) per serving
Reduced Cholesterol	At least 25% less cholesterol than the higher-cholesterol version and 2 grams (or less) of saturated fat per serving
Sodium Free (No Sodium)	Less than 5 milligrams of sodium per serving and no sodium chloride (NaCl) in ingredients
Very Low Sodium	35 milligrams of sodium (or less) per serving
Low Sodium	140 milligrams of sodium (or less) per serving
Reduced or Less Sodium	At least 25% less sodium per serving than the higher-sodium version
Sugar Free	Less than 0.5 gram of sugar per serving

High Fiber	5 grams of fiber (or more) per serving
Good Source of Fiber	2.5 to 4.9 grams of fiber per serving

When making a specific health claim, the food must also meet specific standards. See a few key examples below.

To Make Health Claims About:	**The Food Must Be:**
Heart disease and fats	Low in fat, saturated fat, and cholesterol
Blood pressure and sodium	Low in sodium
Heart disease and fruits, vegetables, and grain products	A fruit, vegetable, or grain product low in fat, saturated fat, and cholesterol, that contains at least 0.6 gram of soluble fiber, without fortification, per serving

The American Heart Association prepared this *Brand Name Fat and Cholesterol Counter* to help you make healthful changes in your eating habits. You may have picked up this book because you want to cut the fat and cholesterol in your diet to reduce your risk factors for heart disease. Or your doctor may have prescribed the AHA Diet because you have cardiovascular disease. Or you may have high blood pressure and may need to watch your sodium also.

Whatever your reasons, you came to the right place. You can start by comparing the way you eat now with the AHA eating plan on page xviii. Perhaps you're not getting enough fruits and vegetables to give you many of the vitamins and minerals you need. Or you may be eating too many high-fat, high-cholesterol, or high-sodium foods.

After you understand how the AHA Diet works and determine how many calories and how much fat, cholesterol, and sodium you can eat every day, you can use this book to find foods that fit into a delicious, heart-healthy diet.

Just remember: Eat low-fat, low-cholesterol foods from all the food groups, not from just a few. Variety is the spice of life—and the key to a healthful and nutritious eating plan.

Reading the Food Tables

On the following pages, you'll find more than 4,000 foods. They were included in the guide because of their nutritional content. That is, they meet AHA criteria, or guidelines, for fat, saturated fat, and cholesterol.

AHA CRITERIA

In the introduction to each chapter, you'll find a chart showing the AHA criteria for total fat, saturated fat, and cholesterol in the food products listed in that chapter. Since manufacturers may change a product's composition after the AHA has reviewed it, you'll want to continue to read the nutrition labels of any product you buy or write directly to the manufacturer—just to make sure. Use these AHA criteria to find additional foods to make part of your eating plan.

ANNUAL REVISIONS

For each name brand product in this book, the manufacturers supplied the product name, serving size, and nutritional values. This information is listed exactly as submitted by the manufacturer. You may find minor variations between the listing in the book and on the package. The information may have changed slightly or the label may have been redesigned. We will revise this guide annually so that you'll have the most up-to-date information possible.

Food Products Made by Tobacco Companies

It's no secret that cigarette smoking is the number one preventable cause of death and disability in the United States. It contributes to heart disease, cancer, emphysema, and low birth weight in babies. Because of the enormous negative effect on public health caused by tobacco products and because of the activities of tobacco companies and their affiliates regarding regulation of these products, we have placed an asterisk (*) beside food products made by these companies or their corporate subsidiaries or parents. We identified these companies from lists compiled in 1994 by the Advocacy Institute, Washington, D.C. You may wish to consider this background, in addition to the nutritional content of a product, when choosing foods for yourself and your family.

NO ENDORSEMENTS

By policy, the AHA doesn't endorse any commercial product. We are not suggesting that the products listed in this guide are nutritionally superior to products not listed here. In each category, we tried to include all the food products that met AHA criteria for total fat, saturated fat, and cholesterol. If you are aware of any food products that meet our criteria but aren't listed, please let us know. We'll try to include them in future editions. (See "Foods We Didn't Include" on page xl.)

FOOD TABLE LISTINGS

You'll find that the listings are divided into 22 chapters by type of food product. Entries are alphabetized under various categories within each chapter. When the name of a product begins with a number, that entry is alphabetized as if the number were spelled out.

For each food, we've listed portion size, grams of total fat and saturated fat, milligrams of cholesterol and sodium, and number of calories. The values for each listing are for the product as sold unless otherwise indicated. Many of the numbers have been rounded off for your convenience. When you see parentheses around an amount in the listings, it means that specific information was not available for that item. Instead, the amount was estimated, either by analyzing the ingredients listed on the label or by gathering information from USDA Handbook No. 8 series.

ABBREVIATIONS

You'll find the following abbreviations in this book:

cal.	calorie(s)
chol.	cholesterol
diam	diameter
env	envelope
fl oz	fluid ounce(s)

g	gram(s)
in.	inch(es)
<	less than
lrg	large
med	medium
mg	milligram(s)
n/a	not available
oz	ounce(s)
pkg	package
pkt	packet
sat.	saturated
sml	small
sod.	sodium
tbsp	tablespoon(s)
tsp	teaspoon(s)
tot.	total
tr	trace
USDA	USDA Handbook No. 8 series

GENERIC LISTINGS

If most brands of a specific food contain about the same amounts of the nutrients we discuss, we list the food generically among the brand name entries. For example, listed with the brand name entries for canned fish, you'll see a generic entry for tuna packed in water. That's because many brands of water-packed tuna provide about the same amounts of total fat, saturated fat, cholesterol, sodium, and calories. Such generic entries for "most brands" are in bold type.

PRODUCTS THAT "DON'T FIT"

If a product, either generic or name brand, doesn't fit into a subcategory, we list it at the end of the category as "Other." For example, in the chapter "Breads and Bread Products," you'll find a miscellaneous subcategory called "Other Breads."

INTRODUCTORY TABLES

At the beginning of most chapters, you'll find two tables. The first lists the AHA criteria for maximum total fat, saturated fat, and cholesterol for products in that chapter (main dishes, salad dressings, crackers, etc.).* The second table lists a few foods in this category that we do not recommend eating often because they're so high in total fat, saturated fat, and/or cholesterol. We've listed them so that you can compare them with the more healthful, lower-fat items found in the listings that follow.

Foods We Didn't Include

Some of your favorite foods may not be listed in this guide. Often that's because they exceed at least one of the AHA criteria for fat, saturated fat, and cholesterol. Also, new products have been introduced since this book went to press. In some cases, the manufacturer did not supply the needed information about its products. And it's always possible that some foods are available that we simply aren't aware of.

If you know of foods that should be listed here, please help us include them in future editions. All we need is the following information:

- Exact name of the product;
- Name of the manufacturer (and address, if possible);
- Serving size; and
- Amount of fat, saturated fat, cholesterol, sodium, and calories the product contains per serving.

*The AHA criteria are, for the most part, consistent with FDA nutrient content claims for total fat, saturated fat, and cholesterol. The exception is for the "Fats and Oils" category. Although they are high in fat, the food products listed there are important to the AHA Diet. They can help lower blood cholesterol levels. Although the total fat content of these fats and oils is about the same, the amount of saturated fat varies considerably. Therefore, we determined the maximum amount of saturated fat that these types of products can contain and still be part of a heart-healthy diet.

Send this information to:

Diet Modification Clinic
6565 Fannin, F770
Houston, TX 77030

On the other hand, you may wonder why some foods that contain ingredients such as cream, egg yolks, butter, palm kernel oil, and coconut oil *are* listed. That's because these foods contain such tiny amounts of these high-fat, high-cholesterol ingredients that the foods still meet the AHA criteria.

IMPORTANT DEFINITIONS

Atherosclerosis A blood vessel disease in which fat, cholesterol, and other substances are deposited in the inner walls of the arteries, making the arteries thick, irregular, and hard. As these fatty deposits build up, the arteries become narrower and blood flow is greatly reduced.

Calorie A common measurement of the heat or energy supplied by food when it is broken down for use by the body. Carbohydrates, protein, fat, and alcohol supply calories.

Cholesterol A fatlike substance that is produced by your body and is contained in foods of animal origin only. A healthy body produces all the cholesterol it needs. The cholesterol you get from foods can increase your blood cholesterol level, which, in turn, increases your risk of heart disease. Cholesterol is found in egg yolks, organ meats, meats, fish, other seafood, poultry, and whole-milk dairy products.

Hydrogenated Fat The type of fat that results from a chemical process designed to change a liquid vegetable oil (naturally high in unsaturated fats) to a more solid (and more saturated) form. This process helps keep the fat in food products fresh longer. The greater the degree of hydrogenation, the more saturated the fat becomes. Hydrogenated tub margarines and spreads are acceptable if they list liquid vegetable oil as the first ingredient and contain no more than 2 grams of saturated fat per tablespoon.

Monounsaturated Fat A type of fat found in canola, olive, and peanut oils. It is also found in foods such as meats, nuts, and seeds. Monounsaturated fat tends to lower blood cholesterol, especially when it's used to replace the saturated fat in your diet.

Polyunsaturated Fat A type of fat found in safflower, sunflower, corn, and soybean oils. It's also found in nuts and seeds. Polyunsaturated fat tends to lower blood cholesterol when it is used as part of a low-saturated fat, low-cholesterol eating plan.

Saturated Fat The type of fat that's the main culprit in raising blood cholesterol. Saturated fat is found in both animal and plant foods. Animal foods containing large amounts of saturated fat include beef, veal, lamb, pork, butter, cream, whole milk, cheese, and other dairy products made from whole milk. The plant sources of saturated fat are coconut oil, cocoa butter, palm and palm kernel oil, and some shortenings and margarines. Many commercially baked goods are made with these oils.

Sodium An element that is essential to good health but that is needed in only a tiny amount each day. Most foods in their natural state contain small amounts of sodium. About 40 percent of ordinary table salt is sodium by weight. Most Americans consume far more sodium than their bodies need. In some people, this can contribute to high blood pressure.

AMERICAN HEART

FOOD TABLES

ASSOCIATION

BEVERAGES AND BEVERAGE MIXES

This chapter starts off with great news: Most beverages and beverage mixes contain very little or no fat. The few exceptions include flavored coffees. Many of those contain chocolate and/or creamer, both of which are high in fat and saturated fat. Therefore, we didn't include such flavored coffee mixes in this book.

We evaluated the beverages and beverage mixes the way you will drink them—as purchased, made according to package directions, or made with *skim milk*.

Like all the other entries in this book, the drinks and drink mixes entries that follow list sodium content. The AHA does not have criteria for sodium but recommends a total of no more than 3,000 mg a day.

Generic Listings

By far, most of the foods in this book are brand name products. However, if a product is listed without a brand name, it means that most brands of the product contain about the same amount of fat, saturated fat, and cholesterol and that these amounts are within the AHA criteria cited below.

If you find products that were introduced after this book went to press, use the generic listings and the following tables to help you evaluate them.

AHA Criteria for Beverages and Beverage Mixes*

	Tot. Fat (g)	Sat. Fat (g)	Chol. (mg)
Alcoholic, carbonated, and noncarbonated beverages; coffee and tea	<0.5	<0.5	<2
Mixes for cocoa, flavored milk beverages, and instant breakfasts, prepared	3	2	20

*Per serving.

Beverages You'll Want to Limit

Some beverages, like the example below, are too high in fat, saturated fat, and/or cholesterol to meet AHA criteria. Such products aren't included in this book, and we recommend that you don't drink them often.

Compare the amounts of fat, saturated fat, cholesterol, sodium, and calories in this example with the more healthful alternatives listed on the following pages.

Sample Beverage to Limit

	Tot. Fat (g)	Sat. Fat (g)	Chol. (mg)	Sod. (mg)	Cal.
Cappuccino-flavored instant coffee, sugar sweetened, made with 2 rounded tsp powder and 6 fl oz water	2.1*	1.8*	(0)	104	62

Adapted from USDA Handbook No. 8 series.

*These values exceed AHA criteria for beverages.

	Tot. Fat (g)	Sat. Fat (g)	Chol. (mg)	Sod. (mg)	Cal.
ALCOHOLIC BEVERAGES					
Beer, light (12 fl oz)					
Most brands (USDA)	0.0	0.0	0	10	100
Beer, regular (12 fl oz)					
Most brands (USDA)	0.0	0.0	0	19	146
Gin (1½ fl oz)					
Most brands (USDA)	0.0	0.0	0	1	110
Liqueur, coffee (1½ fl oz)					
Most brands (USDA)	0.1	0.1	0	4	174
Liqueur, crème de menthe (1½ fl oz)					
Most brands (USDA)	0.1	0.0	0	3	186
Rum (1½ fl oz)					
Most brands (USDA)	0.0	0.0	0	0	97
Vodka (1½ fl oz)					
Most brands (USDA)	0.0	0.0	0	0	97
Whiskey (1½ fl oz)					
Most brands (USDA)	0.0	0.0	0	0	105
Wine, dessert (2 fl oz)					
Most brands (USDA)	0.0	0.0	0	5	90
Wine, table (3½ fl oz)					
Most brands (USDA)	0.0	0.0	0	8	72
ALCOHOLIC BEVERAGE MIXERS					
DAIQUIRI MIXERS					
Strawberry Daiquiri Tropical Fruit Mixer (8 fl oz)					
Bacardi (Coca-Cola Foods)	0.0	0.0	0	0	140
MARGARITA MIXERS					
Margarita Tropical Fruit Mixer (8 fl oz)					
Bacardi (Coca-Cola Foods)	0.0	0.0	0	0	100
TROPICAL FRUIT MIXERS					
Rum Runner Tropical Fruit Mixer (8 fl oz)					
Bacardi (Coca-Cola Foods)	0.0	0.0	0	10	140

	Tot. Fat (g)	Sat. Fat (g)	Chol. (mg)	Sod. (mg)	Cal.
Piña Colada Mixers					
Piña Colada Tropical Fruit Mixer (8 fl oz)					
Bacardi (Coca-Cola Foods)	0.0	0.0	0	10	140
BEVERAGE SYRUPS—*see* "SWEET TOPPINGS AND SAUCES," BEVERAGE SYRUPS, page 374					
BREAKFAST AND MEAL-REPLACEMENT BEVERAGES					
Chocolate-Flavored Breakfast and Meal-Replacement Beverages					
Chocolate-Flavored Breakfast and Meal-Replacement Beverage Mixes					
Chocolate Fantasy Flavored Powder, made with 1½ cups skim milk (12 oz)					
Ultra Slim-Fast Plus (Slim-Fast Foods)	2.0	(1.2)	<15	330	250
Chocolate Flavored Powder, made with 1 cup skim milk (8 oz)					
Slim-Fast (Slim-Fast Foods)	1.0	(0.5)	9	210	190
Chocolate Instant Breakfast, made with 1 cup skim milk (1 cup)					
Pillsbury (Grand Metropolitan PLC)	1.5	1.0	10	320	220
Chocolate Malt Flavored Powder, made with 1 cup skim milk (8 oz)					
Slim-Fast (Slim-Fast Foods)	1.0	(0.5)	9	230	190
Chocolate Mocha Supreme, made with 1 cup skim milk (9 fl oz)					
Nestlé Sweet Success (Nestlé Food Company)	1.5	1.0	6	336	180
Chocolate Raspberry Truffle, made with 1 cup skim milk (9 fl oz)					
Nestlé (Nestlé Food Company)	2.0	1.0	6	360	180

	Tot. Fat (g)	Sat. Fat (g)	Chol. (mg)	Sod. (mg)	Cal.
Chocolate Royale Flavored Powder, made with 1 cup skim milk (8 oz) Ultra Slim-Fast (Slim-Fast Foods)	1.0	(0.5)	8	230	200
Classic Chocolate Malt Instant Breakfast, made with 1 cup skim milk (9 fl oz) Carnation (Nestlé Food Company)	1.5	0.8	6	240	220
Classic Chocolate Malt No Sugar Added Instant Breakfast, made with 1 cup skim milk (9 fl oz) Carnation (Nestlé Food Company)	2.0	0.8	6	240	160
Creamy Milk Chocolate Instant Breakfast, made with 1 cup skim milk (9 fl oz) Carnation (Nestlé Food Company)	1.3	0.8	6	240	220
Creamy Milk Chocolate, made with 1 cup skim milk (9 fl oz) Nestlé (Nestlé Food Company)	2.0	1.0	6	336	180
Creamy Milk Chocolate No Sugar Added Instant Breakfast, made with 1 cup skim milk (9 fl oz) Carnation (Nestlé Food Company)	1.3	0.8	6	216	160
Dark Chocolate Fudge, made with 1 cup skim milk (9 fl oz) Nestlé (Nestlé Food Company)	2.0	1.0	6	336	180
Dutch Chocolate Flavored Water Mixable Powder, made with 1 cup water (8 oz) Ultra Slim-Fast (Slim-Fast Foods)	<1.0	(0.0)	8	260	220
Rich Chocolate Almond, made with 1 cup skim milk (9 fl oz) Nestlé (Nestlé Food Company)	1.5	1.0	6	336	180

	Tot. Fat (g)	Sat. Fat (g)	Chol. (mg)	Sod. (mg)	Cal.
CHOCOLATE-FLAVORED BREAKFAST AND MEAL-REPLACEMENT BEVERAGES *(cont'd)*					
Prepared Chocolate-Flavored Breakfast and Meal-Replacement Beverages					
Chocolate Mocha Supreme (10 fl oz)					
Nestlé Sweet Success (Nestlé Food Company)	3.0	1.0	5	220	200
Chocolate Raspberry Truffle (10 fl oz)					
Nestlé Sweet Success (Nestlé Food Company)	3.0	1.0	5	220	200
Chocolate Royale (11 oz)					
Ultra Slim-Fast (Slim-Fast Foods)	3.0	(1.0)	10	220	230
Creamy Milk Chocolate (10 fl oz)					
Nestlé Sweet Success (Nestlé Food Company)	3.0	1.0	5	240	200
Creamy Milk Chocolate (12 fl oz)					
Nestlé Sweet Success (Nestlé Food Company)	1.5	1.0	<5	300	220
Creamy Milk Chocolate Instant Breakfast (10 fl oz)					
Carnation (Nestlé Food Company)	2.5	1.0	5	230	220
Dark Chocolate Fudge (10 fl oz)					
Nestlé Sweet Success (Nestlé Food Company)	3.0	1.0	5	220	200
Dark Chocolate Fudge (12 fl oz)					
Nestlé Sweet Success (Nestlé Food Company)	1.5	1.0	<5	310	220
Lite Chocolate (10 fl oz)					
Sego (Pet)	3.0	(1.6)	(4)	400	150
Lite Dutch Chocolate (10 fl oz)					
Sego (Pet)	3.0	(1.6)	(4)	400	150
Milk Chocolate (11 oz)					
Ultra Slim-Fast (Slim-Fast Foods)	3.0	(1.0)	5	180	200

	Tot. Fat (g)	Sat. Fat (g)	Chol. (mg)	Sod. (mg)	Cal.
Rich Chocolate Almond (10 fl oz) Nestlé Sweet Success (Nestlé Food Company)	3.0	1.0	5	240	200
Rich Chocolate Almond (12 fl oz) Nestlé Sweet Success (Nestlé Food Company)	1.5	1.0	<5	300	220
Very Chocolate (10 fl oz) Sego (Pet)	1.5	0.0	5	310	240
Very Chocolate Malt (10 fl oz) Sego (Pet)	1.5	0.0	5	310	240
COFFEE-FLAVORED BREAKFAST AND MEAL-REPLACEMENT BEVERAGES					
Coffee-Flavored Breakfast and Meal-Replacement Beverage Mixes					
Cafe Mocha Flavored Powder, made with 1 cup skim milk (8 oz) Ultra Slim-Fast (Slim-Fast Foods)	1.0	(0.3)	8	280	200
Cafe Mocha Instant Breakfast, made with 1 cup skim milk (9 fl oz) Carnation (Nestlé Food Company)	0.7	0.4	6	216	220
Prepared Coffee-Flavored Breakfast and Meal-Replacement Beverages					
Cafe Mocha Instant Breakfast (10 fl oz) Carnation (Nestlé Food Company)	2.5	0.5	5	210	220
Coffee (11 oz) Ultra Slim-Fast (Slim-Fast Foods)	3.0	(1.0)	10	150	200
FRUIT-JUICE-FLAVORED BREAKFAST AND MEAL-REPLACEMENT BEVERAGES					
Fruit-Juice-Flavored Breakfast and Meal-Replacement Beverage Mixes					
Fruit Juice Mixable Powder, made with 1 cup juice (8 oz) Ultra Slim-Fast (Slim-Fast Foods)	<1.0	(0.0)	<10	30	200

	Tot. Fat (g)	Sat. Fat (g)	Chol. (mg)	Sod. (mg)	Cal.
STRAWBERRY-FLAVORED BREAKFAST AND MEAL-REPLACEMENT BEVERAGES					
Prepared Strawberry-Flavored Breakfast and Meal-Replacement Beverages					
Strawberry Supreme (11 oz)					
Ultra Slim-Fast (Slim-Fast Foods)	3.0	(1.0)	5	220	210
Strawberry-Flavored Breakfast and Meal-Replacement Beverage Mixes					
Strawberry Creme Instant Breakfast, made with 1 cup skim milk (9 fl oz)					
Carnation (Nestlé Food Company)	0.7	0.4	6	288	220
Strawberry Creme No Sugar Added Instant Breakfast, made with 1 cup skim milk (9 fl oz)					
Carnation (Nestlé Food Company)	0.7	0.4	6	216	150
Strawberry Flavored Powder, made with 1 cup skim milk (8 oz)					
Slim-Fast (Slim-Fast Foods)	1.0	(0.3)	9	220	190
Strawberry Supreme Flavored Powder, made with 1 cup skim milk (8 oz)					
Ultra Slim-Fast (Slim-Fast Foods)	1.0	(0.3)	8	250	190
VANILLA-FLAVORED BREAKFAST AND MEAL-REPLACEMENT BEVERAGES					
Prepared Vanilla-Flavored Breakfast and Meal-Replacement Beverages					
Smooth Vanilla Creme (10 fl oz)					
Nestlé Sweet Success (Nestlé Food Company)	3.0	1.0	5	220	200
Vanilla-Flavored Breakfast and Meal-Replacement Beverage Mixes					
Creamy Vanilla Delight, made with 1 cup skim milk (9 fl oz)					
Nestlé Sweet Success (Nestlé Food Company)	0.7	0.6	6	312	180

	Tot. Fat (g)	Sat. Fat (g)	Chol. (mg)	Sod. (mg)	Cal.
French Vanilla Flavored Powder, made with 1 cup skim milk (8 oz) Ultra Slim-Fast (Slim-Fast Foods)	1.0	(0.3)	8	250	190
French Vanilla Instant Breakfast, made with 1 cup skim milk (9 fl oz) Carnation (Nestlé Food Company)	0.7	0.4	6	240	220
French Vanilla No Sugar Added Instant Breakfast, made with 1 cup skim milk (9 fl oz) Carnation (Nestlé Food Company)	0.7	0.4	6	216	150
Vanilla Flavored Powder, made with 1 cup skim milk (8 oz) Slim-Fast (Slim-Fast Foods)	1.0	(0.3)	6	220	190
OTHER BREAKFAST AND MEAL-REPLACEMENT BEVERAGES					
Other Breakfast and Meal-Replacement Beverage Mixes					
Variety Pack Instant Breakfast (made with 1 cup skim milk) (1 cup) Pillsbury (Grand Metropolitan PLC)	1.5	1.0	10	320	220
CARBONATED BEVERAGES					
CLUB SODAS					
Club soda (8 fl oz) **Most brands** (USDA)	**0.0**	**0.0**	**0**	**48**	**0**
COLAS					
Caffeine-Free Coca-Cola Classic (8 fl oz) Coca-Cola (Coca-Cola USA) . . .	0.0	0.0	0	9	97
Caffeine-Free Diet Coke (8 fl oz) Coca-Cola (Coca-Cola USA) . . .	0.0	0.0	0	4	1
Clear Cola (12 oz) Hansen (Hansen Beverage Co) .	0.0	0.0	0	0	140

	Tot. Fat (g)	Sat. Fat (g)	Chol. (mg)	Sod. (mg)	Cal.
Colas ***(cont'd)***					
Coca-Cola Classic (8 fl oz)					
Coca-Cola (Coca-Cola USA) . . .	0.0	0.0	0	9	97
Coke II (8 fl oz)					
Coca-Cola (Coca-Cola-USA) . . .	0.0	0.0	0	4	105
Cola (8 fl oz)					
Most brands (USDA)	**0.0**	**0.0**	**0**	**8**	**104**
Diet Cherry Coca-Cola (8 fl oz)					
Coca-Cola (Coca-Cola USA) . . .	0.0	0.0	0	4	1
Diet Coke (8 fl oz)					
Coca-Cola (Coca-Cola USA) . . .	0.0	0.0	0	4	1
Diet cola, sweetened with aspartame (8 fl oz)					
Most brands (USDA)	**0.0**	**0.0**	**0**	**16**	**0**
Diet Mr. Pibb (8 fl oz)					
Mr. Pibb (Coca-Cola USA)	0.0	0.0	0	2	1
Tab (8 fl oz)					
Coca-Cola (Coca-Cola USA) . . .	0.0	0.0	0	4	1
Flavored Colas					
Cherry Coca-Cola (8 fl oz)					
Coca-Cola (Coca-Cola USA) . . .	0.0	0.0	0	4	104
Mr. Pibb (8 fl oz)					
Mr. Pibb (Coca-Cola USA)	0.0	0.0	0	7	97
Cream Sodas					
Cream soda (8 fl oz)					
Most brands (USDA)	**0.0**	**0.0**	**0**	**32**	**128**
Fruit-Flavored Sodas					
Berry Sodas					
Berry Soda (8 fl oz)					
Minute Maid (Coca-Cola USA) . .	0.0	0.0	0	9	111
Wild Berry Soda (12 fl oz)					
Health Valley (Health Valley Foods)	0.0	0.0	0	0	160
Cherry Sodas—*see also* Flavored Colas, above					
Black Cherry Soda (8 fl oz)					
Minute Maid (Coca-Cola USA) . .	0.0	0.0	0	11	110

	Tot. Fat (g)	Sat. Fat (g)	Chol. (mg)	Sod. (mg)	Cal.
Cherry Soda (12 oz)					
Hansen (Hansen Beverage Co) .	0.0	0.0	0	0	130
Grape Sodas					
Grape Soda (8 fl oz)					
Most brands (USDA)	**0.0**	**0.0**	**0**	**40**	**104**
Fanta (Coca-Cola USA)	0.0	0.0	0	9	117
Minute Maid (Coca-Cola USA) ..	0.0	0.0	0	9	121
Grapefruit Sodas					
Grapefruit Soda					
Fresca (Coca-Cola USA) (8 fl oz)	0.0	0.0	0	1	3
Hansen (Hansen Beverage Co) (12 fl oz)	0.0	0.0	0	0	130
Minute Maid (Coca-Cola USA) (8 fl oz)	0.0	0.0	0	9	108
Lemon-Lime Sodas					
Diet Lemon-Lime Soda (8 fl oz)					
Mello Yello (Coca-Cola USA) ...	0.0	0.0	0	tr	4
Sprite (Coca-Cola USA)	0.0	0.0	0	0	3
Lemon-Lime Soda					
Most brands (USDA) (8 fl oz) ..	**0.0**	**0.0**	**0**	**24**	**96**
Hansen (Hansen Beverage Co) (12 fl oz)	0.0	0.0	0	0	130
Mello Yello (Coca-Cola USA) (8 fl oz)	0.0	0.0	0	9	119
Sprite (Coca-Cola USA) (8 fl oz) .	0.0	0.0	0	31	100
Orange Sodas					
Diet Orange Soda (8 fl oz)					
Minute Maid (Coca-Cola USA) ..	0.0	0.0	0	0	2
Orange Soda (8 fl oz)					
Most brands (USDA)	**0.0**	**0.0**	**0**	**32**	**120**
Fanta (Coca-Cola USA)	0.0	0.0	0	9	118
Minute Maid (Coca-Cola USA) ..	0.0	0.0	0	0	118
Peach Sodas					
Peach Soda					
Hansen (Hansen Beverage Co) (12 fl oz)	0.0	0.0	0	0	130
Minute Maid (Coca-Cola USA) (8 fl oz)	0.0	0.0	0	9	110

	Tot. Fat (g)	Sat. Fat (g)	Chol. (mg)	Sod. (mg)	Cal.
FRUIT-FLAVORED SODAS *(cont'd)*					
Pineapple Sodas					
Pineapple Soda (8 fl oz)					
Minute Maid (Coca-Cola USA) . .	0.0	0.0	0	9	109
Raspberry Sodas					
Raspberry Soda					
Hansen (Hansen Beverage Co) (12 fl oz)	0.0	0.0	0	0	130
Minute Maid (Coca-Cola USA) (8 fl oz)	0.0	0.0	0	9	111
Strawberry Sodas					
Strawberry Soda (8 fl oz)					
Minute Maid (Coca-Cola USA) . .	0.0	0.0	0	9	122
Other Fruit-Flavored Sodas					
Fruit Punch Soda (8 fl oz)					
Minute Maid (Coca-Cola USA) . .	0.0	0.0	0	10	117
Kiwi Strawberry Soda (12 oz)					
Hansen (Hansen Beverage Co) .	0.0	0.0	0	0	130
Mandarin Lime Soda (12 oz)					
Hansen (Hansen Beverage Co) .	0.0	0.0	0	0	130
GINGER ALES					
Ginger Ale					
Most brands (USDA) (8 fl oz) . .	**0.0**	**0.0**	**0**	**16**	**80**
Fanta (Coca-Cola USA) (8 fl oz) .	0.0	0.0	0	4	86
Health Valley (Health Valley Foods) (12 fl oz)	0.0	0.0	0	0	160
ROOT BEERS					
Clear Root Beer (12 oz)					
Hansen (Hansen Beverage Co) .	0.0	0.0	0	0	140
Old Fashioned Root Beer (12 fl oz)					
Health Valley (Health Valley Foods)	0.0	0.0	0	0	160
Root Beer (8 fl oz)					
Most brands (USDA)	**0.0**	**0.0**	**0**	**32**	**104**
Fanta (Coca-Cola USA)	0.0	0.0	0	4	111
Ramblin' (Coca-Cola USA)	0.0	0.0	0	4	120
Sarsaparilla Root Beer (12 fl oz)					
Health Valley (Health Valley Foods)	0.0	0.0	0	0	160

	Tot. Fat (g)	Sat. Fat (g)	Chol. (mg)	Sod. (mg)	Cal.
SPARKLING/SPRING WATERS					
Berry Sparkling/Spring Waters					
All Natural Wild Berry Flavored Beverage with Sparkling Water (8 fl oz) Royal Mistic (Joseph Victori Wines)	0.0	0.0	0	5	100
Cherry Sparkling/Spring Waters					
All Natural Black Cherry Flavored Beverage with Sparkling Water (8 fl oz) Royal Mistic (Joseph Victori Wines)	0.0	0.0	0	40	100
Wild Cherry Sparkling Mineral Water & Fruit Juice Flavor (8 fl oz) Koala Springs	0.0	0.0	0	25	100
Lemon Sparkling/Spring Waters					
Sparkling Mineral Water with Essence of Lemon (8 fl oz) Koala Springs	0.0	0.0	0	0	0
Lime Sparkling/Spring Waters					
Sparkling Mineral Water with Essence of Lime (8 fl oz) Koala Springs	0.0	0.0	0	0	0
Mixed Fruit Sparkling/Spring Waters					
All Natural Tropical Supreme Flavored Beverage with Sparkling Water (8 fl oz) Royal Mistic (Joseph Victori Wines)	0.0	0.0	0	10	100
Cranberry & Melon Sparkling Mineral Water & Fruit Juice Flavor (8 fl oz) Koala Springs	0.0	0.0	0	25	100
Kiwi, Lime & Grapefruit Sparkling Mineral Water & Fruit Juice Flavor (8 fl oz) Koala Springs	0.0	0.0	0	25	100

	Tot. Fat (g)	Sat. Fat (g)	Chol. (mg)	Sod. (mg)	Cal.
SPARKLING/SPRING WATERS *(cont'd)*					
Lemon, Lime & Orange Sparkling Mineral Water & Fruit Juice Flavor (8 fl oz) Koala Springs	0.0	0.0	0	25	100
Mandarin & Orange Sparkling Mineral Water & Fruit Juice Flavor (8 fl oz) Koala Springs	0.0	0.0	0	25	90
Orange & Mango Sparkling Mineral Water & Fruit Juice Flavor (8 fl oz) Koala Springs	0.0	0.0	0	25	100
Raspberry & Guava Sparkling Mineral Water & Fruit Juice Flavor (8 fl oz) Koala Springs	0.0	0.0	0	25	100
Strawberry & Peach Sparkling Mineral Water & Fruit Juice Flavor (8 fl oz) Koala Springs	0.0	0.0	0	25	100
Natural/Plain Sparkling/ Spring Waters					
America's Premium Mountain Valley Spring Water (8 fl oz) Mountain Valley Spring	0.0	0.0	0	0	0
Natural Sparkling Mineral Water (8 fl oz) Koala Springs	0.0	0.0	0	0	0
Natural Spring Water (8 fl oz) Royal Mistic (Joseph Victori Wines)	0.0	0.0	0	0	0
Orange Sparkling/Spring Waters					
All Natural Tangerine Orange Flavored Beverage with Sparkling Water (8 fl oz) Royal Mistic (Joseph Victori Wines)	0.0	0.0	0	10	100

	Tot. Fat (g)	Sat. Fat (g)	Chol. (mg)	Sod. (mg)	Cal.
Peach Sparkling/Spring Waters					
All Natural Peach Vanilla Flavored Beverage with Sparkling Water (8 fl oz)					
Royal Mistic (Joseph Victori Wines)	0.0	0.0	0	10	100
TONIC WATER					
Tonic water (8 fl oz)					
Most brands (USDA)	**0.0**	**0.0**	**0**	**8**	**80**
COCOA MIXES					
Cocoa Mix with Mini Marshmallows, made with water (6 oz)					
Swiss Miss (Hunt-Wesson)	1.0	0.4	5	170	110
Diet Cocoa Mix, made with water (6 oz)					
Swiss Miss (Hunt-Wesson)	<1.0	0.0	1	180	20
Double Rich Hot Cocoa Mix, made with water (6 oz)					
Swiss Miss (Hunt-Wesson)	1.0	0.5	0	150	110
Hot Cocoa Mix (1 env)					
Weight Watchers (H.J. Heinz)	0.0	0.0	0	160	70
Hot Cocoa Mix with Marshmallows (1 env)					
Weight Watchers (H.J. Heinz)	0.0	0.0	5	150	70
Lite Cocoa Mix, made with water (6 oz)					
Swiss Miss (Hunt-Wesson)	<1.0	0.0	1	160	70
Milk Chocolate Hot Cocoa Mix, made with water (6 oz)					
Swiss Miss (Hunt-Wesson)	1.0	0.4	5	125	110
Sugar Free Cocoa Mix with Sugar Free Marshmallows, made with water (6 oz)					
Swiss Miss (Hunt-Wesson)	<1.0	0.0	2	120	50
Sugar Free Cocoa Mix, made with water (6 oz)					
Swiss Miss (Hunt-Wesson)	<1.0	0.0	2	125	60

Beverages and Beverage Mixes

	Tot. Fat (g)	Sat. Fat (g)	Chol. (mg)	Sod. (mg)	Cal.
COFFEE SUBSTITUTES—*see also* COFFEES, below					
All Natural Coffee Substitute (1.5 g)					
Cafix (Cafix of North America)	0.0	0.0	0	3	6
Coffee Flavor Instant Hot Beverage, made with water (8 fl oz)					
Postum (Kraft General Foods)*	0.0	0.0	0	0	10
Instant Hot Beverage, made with water (8 fl oz)					
Postum (Kraft General Foods)*	0.0	0.0	0	0	10
COFFEES—*see also* COFFEE SUBSTITUTES, above					
BREWED COFFEES					
Coffee, brewed, decaffeinated, unsweetened (8 fl oz)					
Most brands (USDA)	**0.0**	**0.0**	**0**	**8**	**8**
Coffee, brewed, regular, unsweetened (8 fl oz)					
Most brands (USDA)	**0.0**	**0.0**	**0**	**8**	**8**
INSTANT COFFEES					
Coffee, instant, decaffeinated, made with water (8 fl oz)					
Most brands (USDA)	**0.0**	**0.0**	**0**	**8**	**5**
Coffee, instant, regular, made with water (8 fl oz)					
Most brands (USDA)	**0.0**	**0.0**	**0**	**8**	**5**
FLAVORED MILK BEVERAGES					
CHOCOLATE-FLAVORED MILK BEVERAGES					
Chocolate Caramel Flavored Drink (8 fl oz)					
Hershey's (Hershey Food Co)	2.5	0.0	<5	115	160
Chocolate Cherry Flavored Drink (8 fl oz)					
Hershey's (Hershey Food Co)	2.5	0.0	<5	115	160
Chocolate Fudge Shake Mix (0.75 oz)					
Weight Watchers (H.J. Heinz)	1.0	0.0	0	140	80

*Tobacco company, corporate subsidiary, or parent.

	Tot. Fat (g)	Sat. Fat (g)	Chol. (mg)	Sod. (mg)	Cal.
Chocolate Marshmallow Flavored Drink (8 fl oz)					
Hershey's (Hershey Food Co) . .	2.5	0.0	<5	115	160
Chocolate Milk Mix (2 tbsp dry)					
Hershey's (Hershey Food Co) . .	0.0	0.0	0	30	70
Chocolate Yogurt Shake (1 shake)					
Weight Watchers (H.J. Heinz) . .	1.0	0.0	5	140	220
Genuine Chocolate Flavored Drink (8 fl oz)					
Hershey's (Hershey Food Co) . .	2.5	0.0	<5	115	160
Instant Chocolate Flavored Malted Milk, made with skim milk (1 cup)					
Kraft (Kraft General Foods)*	1.4	0.3	4	166	166
FRUIT-FLAVORED MILK BEVERAGES					
Banana Split Flavored Drink (8 fl oz)					
Hershey's (Hershey Food Co) . .	2.5	0.0	<5	115	160
Orange Shake Mix (0.75 oz)					
Weight Watchers (H.J. Heinz) . .	0.0	0.0	0	210	70
Strawberry Drink (8 fl oz)					
Hershey's (Hershey Food Co) . .	2.0	0.0	0	90	140
OTHER FLAVORED MILK BEVERAGES					
Instant Natural Flavored Malted Milk, made with skim milk (1 cup)					
Kraft (Kraft General Foods)*	2.4	1.3	9	211	176
FRUIT-FLAVORED BEVERAGES (noncarbonated)					
POWDERED DRINK MIXES					
Cherry Powdered Drink Mixes					
Black Cherry Blowout Fruit Flavored Drink Mix, made with sugar and water (8 fl oz)					
Wyler's (T.J. Lipton)	0.0	0.0	0	20	100
Black Cherry Unsweetened Soft Drink Mix, made with sugar and water (8 fl oz)					
Kool-Aid (Kraft General Foods)* .	0.0	0.0	0	20	100

*Tobacco company, corporate subsidiary, or parent.

	Tot. Fat (g)	Sat. Fat (g)	Chol. (mg)	Sod. (mg)	Cal.
POWDERED DRINK MIXES *(cont'd)*					
Cherry Charger Fruit Flavored Drink Mix, made with sugar and water (8 fl oz)					
Wyler's (T.J. Lipton)	0.0	0.0	0	15	100
Cherry Sugar Free Low Calorie Soft Drink Mix, made with water (8 fl oz)					
Kool-Aid (Kraft General Foods)* .	0.0	0.0	0	5	5
Cherry Sugar Sweetened Soft Drink Mix, made with water (8 fl oz)					
Kool-Aid (Kraft General Foods)* .	0.0	0.0	0	0	60
Cherry Unsweetened Soft Drink Mix, made with sugar and water (8 fl oz)					
Kool-Aid (Kraft General Foods)* .	0.0	0.0	0	10	100
Citrus Powdered Drink Mixes					
Citrus Blend Low Calorie Soft Drink Mix, made with water (8 fl oz)					
Crystal Light (Kraft General Foods)*	0.0	0.0	0	0	5
Grape Powdered Drink Mixes					
Electric Grape Fruit Flavored Drink Mix, made with sugar and water (8 fl oz)					
Wyler's (T.J. Lipton)	0.0	0.0	0	10	100
Grape Sugar Free Low Calorie Soft Drink Mix, made with water (8 fl oz)					
Kool-Aid (Kraft General Foods)* .	0.0	0.0	0	0	5
Grape Sugar Sweetened Soft Drink Mix, made with water (8 fl oz)					
Kool-Aid (Kraft General Foods)* .	0.0	0.0	0	0	60
Grape Unsweetened Soft Drink Mix, made with sugar and water (8 fl oz)					
Kool-Aid (Kraft General Foods)* .	0.0	0.0	0	15	100

*Tobacco company, corporate subsidiary, or parent.

	Tot. Fat (g)	Sat. Fat (g)	Chol. (mg)	Sod. (mg)	Cal.
Lemonade Powdered Drink Mixes					
Lemon Landslide Fruit Flavored Drink Mix, made with sugar and water (8 fl oz)					
Wyler's (T.J. Lipton)	0.0	0.0	0	15	100
Lemonade Low Calorie Soft Drink Mix, made with water (8 fl oz)					
Crystal Light (Kraft General Foods)*	0.0	0.0	0	0	5
Lemonade Punch Sugar Sweetened Drink Mix, made with water (8 fl oz)					
Country Time (Kraft General Foods)*	0.0	0.0	0	10	70
Lemonade Sugar Free Low Calorie Drink Mix, made with water (8 fl oz)					
Country Time (Kraft General Foods)*	0.0	0.0	0	0	5
Lemonade Sugar Free Low Calorie Soft Drink Mix, made with water (8 fl oz)					
Kool-Aid (Kraft General Foods)* .	0.0	0.0	0	0	5
Lemonade Sugar Sweetened Drink Mix, made with water (8 fl oz)					
Country Time (Kraft General Foods)*	0.0	0.0	0	15	70
Lemonade Sugar Sweetened Soft Drink Mix, made with water (8 fl oz)					
Kool-Aid (Kraft General Foods)* .	0.0	0.0	0	0	70
Lemonade Unsweetened Soft Drink Mix, made with sugar and water (8 fl oz)					
Kool-Aid (Kraft General Foods)* .	0.0	0.0	0	15	100
Pink Lemonade Sugar Free Low Calorie Drink Mix, made with water (8 fl oz)					
Country Time (Kraft General Foods)*	0.0	0.0	0	0	5

*Tobacco company, corporate subsidiary, or parent.

	Tot. Fat (g)	Sat. Fat (g)	Chol. (mg)	Sod. (mg)	Cal.
Powdered Drink Mixes *(cont'd)*					
Pink Lemonade Sugar Sweetened Drink Mix, made with water (8 fl oz)					
Country Time (Kraft General Foods)*	0.0	0.0	0	15	70
Pink Lemonade Unsweetened Soft Drink Mix, made with sugar and water (8 fl oz)					
Kool-Aid (Kraft General Foods)*	0.0	0.0	0	15	100
Power Pink Lemonade Fruit Flavored Drink Mix, made with sugar and water (8 fl oz)					
Wyler's (T.J. Lipton)	0.0	0.0	0	15	100
Lemon-Lime Powdered Drink Mixes					
Lemon Lime Blitzer Fruit Flavored Drink Mix, made with sugar and water (8 fl oz)					
Wyler's (T.J. Lipton)	0.0	0.0	0	0	100
Lemon-Lime Low Calorie Soft Drink Mix, made with water (8 fl oz)					
Crystal Light (Kraft General Foods)*	0.0	0.0	0	0	5
Lemon-Lime Unsweetened Soft Drink Mix, made with sugar and water (8 fl oz)					
Kool-Aid (Kraft General Foods)*	0.0	0.0	0	10	100
Mixed Berry Powdered Drink Mixes					
Incrediberry Sugar Free Low Calorie Soft Drink Mix, made with water (8 fl oz)					
Kool-Aid (Kraft General Foods)*	0.0	0.0	0	0	5
Incrediberry Sugar Sweetened Soft Drink Mix, made with water (8 fl oz)					
Kool-Aid (Kraft General Foods)*	0.0	0.0	0	0	60
Incrediberry Unsweetened Soft Drink Mix, made with sugar and water (8 fl oz)					
Kool-Aid (Kraft General Foods)*	0.0	0.0	0	10	100

*Tobacco company, corporate subsidiary, or parent.

	Tot. Fat (g)	Sat. Fat (g)	Chol. (mg)	Sod. (mg)	Cal.
Megaberry Fruit Flavored Drink Mix, made with sugar and water (8 fl oz)					
Wyler's (T.J. Lipton)	0.0	0.0	0	30	100
Orange Powdered Drink Mixes					
Orange Flavored Drink Mix, made with water (8 fl oz)					
Tang (Kraft General Foods)*	0.0	0.0	0	0	100
Orange Flavored Sugar Free Low Calorie Drink Mix, made with water (8 fl oz)					
Tang (Kraft General Foods)*	0.0	0.0	0	0	5
Orange Sugar Sweetened Soft Drink Mix, made with water (8 fl oz)					
Kool-Aid (Kraft General Foods)* .	0.0	0.0	0	0	60
Orange Unsweetened Soft Drink Mix, made with sugar and water (8 fl oz)					
Kool-Aid (Kraft General Foods)* .	0.0	0.0	0	15	100
Outrageous Orange Fruit Flavored Drink Mix, made with sugar and water (8 fl oz)					
Wyler's (T.J. Lipton)	0.0	0.0	0	20	100
Punch Powdered Drink Mixes					
Fruit Punch Low Calorie Soft Drink Mix, made with water (8 fl oz)					
Crystal Light (Kraft General Foods)*	0.0	0.0	0	0	5
Tropical Punch Fruit Flavored Drink Mix, made with sugar and water (8 fl oz)					
Wyler's (T.J. Lipton)	0.0	0.0	0	0	100
Tropical Punch Sugar Free Low Calorie Soft Drink Mix, made with water (8 fl oz)					
Kool-Aid (Kraft General Foods)* .	0.0	0.0	0	10	5
Tropical Punch Sugar Sweetened Soft Drink Mix, made with water (8 fl oz)					
Kool-Aid (Kraft General Foods)* .	0.0	0.0	0	0	60

*Tobacco company, corporate subsidiary, or parent.

	Tot. Fat (g)	Sat. Fat (g)	Chol. (mg)	Sod. (mg)	Cal.
Powdered Drink Mixes *(cont'd)*					
Tropical Punch Unsweetened Soft Drink Mix, made with sugar and water (8 fl oz)					
Kool-Aid (Kraft General Foods)*	0.0	0.0	0	20	100
Tutti Fruity Fruit Flavored Drink Mix, made with sugar and water (8 fl oz)					
Wyler's (T.J. Lipton)	0.0	0.0	0	0	100
Raspberry Powdered Drink Mixes					
Radical Razzberry Fruit Flavored Drink Mix, made with sugar and water (8 fl oz)					
Wyler's (T.J. Lipton)	0.0	0.0	0	15	100
Raspberry Ice Low Calorie Soft Drink Mix, made with water (8 fl oz)					
Crystal Light (Kraft General Foods)*	0.0	0.0	0	0	5
Raspberry Sugar Sweetened Soft Drink Mix, made with water (8 fl oz)					
Kool-Aid (Kraft General Foods)*	0.0	0.0	0	0	60
Raspberry Unsweetened Soft Drink Mix, made with sugar and water (8 fl oz)					
Kool-Aid (Kraft General Foods)*	0.0	0.0	0	35	100
Strawberry Powdered Drink Mixes					
Slam Dunk Strawberry Fruit Flavored Drink Mix, made with sugar and water (8 fl oz)					
Wyler's (T.J. Lipton)	0.0	0.0	0	45	100
Strawberry Sugar Sweetened Soft Drink Mix, made with water (8 fl oz)					
Kool-Aid (Kraft General Foods)*	0.0	0.0	0	0	60
Strawberry Unsweetened Soft Drink Mix, made with sugar and water (8 fl oz)					
Kool-Aid (Kraft General Foods)*	0.0	0.0	0	35	100

*Tobacco company, corporate subsidiary, or parent.

	Tot. Fat (g)	Sat. Fat (g)	Chol. (mg)	Sod. (mg)	Cal.
Other Powdered Drink Mixes					
Blitzing Bananaberry Fruit Flavored Drink Mix, made with sugar and water (8 fl oz)					
Wyler's (T.J. Lipton)	0.0	0.0	0	25	100
Cranberry Breeze Low Calorie Soft Drink Mix, made with water (8 fl oz)					
Crystal Light (Kraft General Foods)*	0.0	0.0	0	0	5
Great Bluedini Sugar Free Low Calorie Soft Drink Mix, made with water (8 fl oz)					
Kool-Aid (Kraft General Foods)*	0.0	0.0	0	0	5
Great Bluedini Sugar Sweetened Soft Drink Mix, made with water (8 fl oz)					
Kool-Aid (Kraft General Foods)*	0.0	0.0	0	0	60
Great Bluedini Unsweetened Soft Drink Mix, made with sugar and water (8 fl oz)					
Kool-Aid (Kraft General Foods)*	0.0	0.0	0	10	100
Mango Flavored Drink Mix, made with water (8 fl oz)					
Tang (Kraft General Foods)*	0.0	0.0	0	0	100
Piña-Pineapple Sugar Sweetened Soft Drink Mix, made with water (8 fl oz)					
Kool-Aid (Kraft General Foods)*	0.0	0.0	0	0	60
Piña-Pineapple Unsweetened Soft Drink Mix, made with sugar and water (8 fl oz)					
Kool-Aid (Kraft General Foods)*	0.0	0.0	0	10	100
Pink Grapefruit Low Calorie Soft Drink Mix, made with water (8 fl oz)					
Crystal Light (Kraft General Foods)*	0.0	0.0	0	0	5
Pink Swimmingo Sugar Free Low Calorie Soft Drink Mix, made with water (8 fl oz)					
Kool-Aid (Kraft General Foods)*	0.0	0.0	0	0	5

*Tobacco company, corporate subsidiary, or parent.

	Tot. Fat (g)	Sat. Fat (g)	Chol. (mg)	Sod. (mg)	Cal.
Powdered Drink Mixes ***(cont'd)***					
Pink Swimmingo Sugar Sweetened Soft Drink Mix, made with water (8 fl oz)					
Kool-Aid (Kraft General Foods)* .	0.0	0.0	0	0	60
Pink Swimmingo Unsweetened Soft Drink Mix, made with sugar and water (8 fl oz)					
Kool-Aid (Kraft General Foods)* .	0.0	0.0	0	15	100
Purplesaurus Rex Sugar Free Low Calorie Soft Drink Mix, made with water (8 fl oz)					
Kool-Aid (Kraft General Foods)* .	0.0	0.0	0	5	5
Purplesaurus Rex Sugar Sweetened Soft Drink Mix, made with water (8 fl oz)					
Kool-Aid (Kraft General Foods)* .	0.0	0.0	0	0	60
Purplesaurus Rex Unsweetened Soft Drink Mix, made with sugar and water (8 fl oz)					
Kool-Aid (Kraft General Foods)* .	0.0	0.0	0	30	100
Rock-A-Dile Red Sugar Free Low Calorie Soft Drink Mix, made with water (8 fl oz)					
Kool-Aid (Kraft General Foods)* .	0.0	0.0	0	0	5
Rock-A-Dile Red Sugar Sweetened Soft Drink Mix, made with water (8 fl oz)					
Kool-Aid (Kraft General Foods)* .	0.0	0.0	0	0	60
Rock-A-Dile Red Unsweetened Soft Drink Mix, made with sugar and water (8 fl oz)					
Kool-Aid (Kraft General Foods)* .	0.0	0.0	0	30	100
Watermelon Wipeout Fruit Flavored Drink Mix, made with sugar and water (8 fl oz)					
Wyler's (T.J. Lipton)	0.0	0.0	0	0	100

*Tobacco company, corporate subsidiary, or parent.

	Tot. Fat (g)	Sat. Fat (g)	Chol. (mg)	Sod. (mg)	Cal.
READY-TO-DRINK BEVERAGES (NONCARBONATED)					
Apple Ready-to-Drink Beverages (noncarbonated)—*see also* Mixed Fruit Ready-to-Drink Beverages, page 30					
Jammin' Apple (8 fl oz)					
Hi-C (Coca-Cola Foods)	0.0	0.0	0	30	130
Cherry Ready-to-Drink Beverages (noncarbonated)					
Cherry (8 fl oz)					
Hi-C (Coca-Cola Foods)	0.0	0.0	0	30	130
Cherry Soft Drink (6.75 fl oz)					
Kool-Aid Bursts (Kraft General Foods)*	0.0	0.0	0	35	100
Chucklin' Cherry Squeezit (1 bottle)					
Betty Crocker (General Mills) ...	0.0	0.0	0	0	110
Wild Cherry All Natural Juice Drink (6.75 fl oz)					
Capri Sun (Kraft General Foods)*	0.0	0.0	0	20	110
Citrus Ready-to-Drink Beverages (noncarbonated)					
Citrus (8 fl oz)					
Five Alive (Coca-Cola Foods) ...	0.0	0.0	0	25	120
Citrus Consciousness (8 fl oz)					
Minute Maid Fruitopia (Coca-Cola Foods)	0.0	0.0	0	25	120
Citrus Punch (8 fl oz)					
Minute Maid (Coca-Cola Foods)	0.0	0.0	0	25	130
Tropical Citrus (8 fl oz)					
Five Alive (Coca-Cola Foods) ...	0.0	0.0	0	25	120
Cranberry Ready-to-Drink Beverages (noncarbonated)					
Cranberry Apple Cocktail (8 fl oz)					
Minute Maid (Coca-Cola Foods)	0.0	0.0	0	25	170
Cranberry Juice Cocktail (8 fl oz)					
Most brands	**0.0**	**0.0**	**0**	**8**	**144**
Ocean Spray (Ocean Spray Cranberries)	0.0	0.0	0	35	140

*Tobacco company, corporate subsidiary, or parent.

	Tot. Fat (g)	Sat. Fat (g)	Chol. (mg)	Sod. (mg)	Cal.
Ready-to-Drink Beverages (noncarbonated) ***(cont'd)***					
Lightstyle Low Calorie Cranberry Juice Cocktail (8 fl oz)					
Ocean Spray (Ocean Spray Cranberries)	0.0	0.0	0	35	40
Grape Ready-to-Drink Beverages (noncarbonated)					
Grape (8 fl oz)					
Hi-C (Coca-Cola Foods)	0.0	0.0	0	30	130
Grape All Natural Juice Drink (6.75 fl oz)					
Capri Sun (Kraft General Foods)*	0.0	0.0	0	20	110
Grape Beyond (8 fl oz)					
Minute Maid Fruitopia (Coca-Cola Foods)	0.0	0.0	0	25	130
Grape Punch (8 fl oz)					
Minute Maid (Coca-Cola Foods)	0.0	0.0	0	25	130
Grape Soft Drink (6.75 fl oz)					
Kool-Aid Bursts (Kraft General Foods)*	0.0	0.0	0	30	100
Grumpy Grape Squeezit (1 bottle)					
Betty Crocker (General Mills) . . .	0.0	0.0	0	0	110
Grapefruit Ready-to-Drink Beverages (noncarbonated)					
Lightstyle Low Calorie Pink Grapefruit Juice Cocktail (8 fl oz)					
Ocean Spray (Ocean Spray Cranberries)	0.0	0.0	0	35	40
Pink Grapefruit Juice Cocktail (8 fl oz)					
Minute Maid (Coca-Cola Foods)	0.0	0.0	0	25	110
Ocean Spray (Ocean Spray Cranberries)	0.0	0.0	0	35	110
Ruby Red & Tangerine Grapefruit Juice Drink (8 fl oz)					
Ocean Spray (Ocean Spray Cranberries)	0.0	0.0	0	35	130
Ruby Red Grapefruit Juice Drink (8 fl oz)					
Ocean Spray (Ocean Spray Cranberries)	0.0	0.0	0	35	130

*Tobacco company, corporate subsidiary, or parent.

	Tot. Fat (g)	Sat. Fat (g)	Chol. (mg)	Sod. (mg)	Cal.
Lemonade Ready-to-Drink Beverages (noncarbonated)					
All Natural Lemonade Limeade Flavored Beverage (8 fl oz)					
Royal Mistic (Joseph Victori Wines)	0.0	0.0	0	45	100
Cranberry Lemonade (8 fl oz)					
Minute Maid (Coca-Cola Foods)	0.0	0.0	0	25	120
Minute Maid Naturals (Coca-Cola Foods)	0.0	0.0	0	25	110
Cranberry Lemonade Meditation (8 fl oz)					
Minute Maid Fruitopia (Coca-Cola Foods)	0.0	0.0	0	25	110
Lemonade (8 fl oz)					
Minute Maid (Coca-Cola Foods)	0.0	0.0	0	0	110
Minute Maid Naturals (Coca-Cola Foods)	0.0	0.0	0	25	110
Newman's Own	0.0	0.0	0	40	110
Lemonade Fruit Flavored Drink (8 fl oz)					
Wyler's (T.J. Lipton)	0.0	0.0	0	30	110
Lemonade Fruit Juice Beverage (8 fl oz)					
Koala Springs	0.0	0.0	0	0	100
Lemonade Love (8 fl oz)					
Minute Maid Fruitopia (Coca-Cola Foods)	0.0	0.0	0	25	110
Old Fashioned Lemonade (8 oz)					
Hansen (Hansen Beverage Co)	0.0	0.0	0	15	100
Pink Lemonade (8 fl oz)					
Hansen (Hansen Beverage Co)	0.0	0.0	0	15	110
Minute Maid (Coca-Cola Foods)	0.0	0.0	0	25	110
Pink Lemonade Euphoria (8 fl oz)					
Minute Maid Fruitopia (Coca-Cola Foods)	0.0	0.0	0	25	120
Raspberry Lemonade (8 fl oz)					
Minute Maid (Coca-Cola Foods)	0.0	0.0	0	0	120
Minute Maid Naturals (Coca-Cola Foods)	0.0	0.0	0	25	120

	Tot. Fat (g)	Sat. Fat (g)	Chol. (mg)	Sod. (mg)	Cal.
READY-TO-DRINK BEVERAGES (NONCARBONATED) ***(cont'd)***					
Raspberry Psychic Lemonade (8 fl oz)					
Minute Maid Fruitopia (Coca-Cola Foods)	0.0	0.0	0	25	120
Strawberry Lemonade (8 oz)					
Hansen (Hansen Beverage Co)	0.0	0.0	0	15	100
Mixed Berry Ready-to-Drink Beverages (noncarbonated)					
Berry Punch (8 fl oz)					
Minute Maid (Coca-Cola Foods)	0.0	0.0	0	25	130
Boppin' Berry (8 fl oz)					
Hi-C (Coca-Cola Foods)	0.0	0.0	0	30	130
Incrediberry Soft Drink (6.75 fl oz)					
Kool-Aid Bursts (Kraft General Foods)*	0.0	0.0	0	30	100
Red Berry All Natural Juice Drink (6.75 fl oz)					
Capri Sun (Kraft General Foods)*	0.0	0.0	0	20	100
Wild Berry (8 fl oz)					
Hi-C (Coca-Cola Foods)	0.0	0.0	0	30	120
Yo Yogi Berry All Natural Juice Drink (6.75 fl oz)					
Capri Sun (Kraft General Foods)*	0.0	0.0	0	20	100
Mixed Fruit Ready-to-Drink Beverages (noncarbonated)					
All Natural Lime Tropical Flavored Beverage (8 fl oz)					
Royal Mistic (Joseph Victori Wines)	0.0	0.0	0	0	100
All Natural Raspberry Guava Flavored Beverage (8 fl oz)					
Royal Mistic (Joseph Victori Wines)	0.0	0.0	0	0	110
All Natural Watermelon Kiwi Flavored Beverage (8 fl oz)					
Royal Mistic (Joseph Victori Wines)	0.0	0.0	0	0	110

*Tobacco company, corporate subsidiary, or parent.

	Tot. Fat (g)	Sat. Fat (g)	Chol. (mg)	Sod. (mg)	Cal.
Apple Cranberry Medley (8 fl oz) Minute Maid Naturals (Coca-Cola Foods)	0.0	0.0	0	25	170
Citrus Cranberry Juice Drink (8 fl oz) Ocean Spray Refreshers (Ocean Spray Cranberries)	0.0	0.0	0	35	140
Citrus Peach Juice Drink (8 fl oz) Ocean Spray Refreshers (Ocean Spray Cranberries)	0.0	0.0	0	35	120
Cran-Blueberry Blueberry Cranberry Drink (8 fl oz) Ocean Spray (Ocean Spray Cranberries)	0.0	0.0	0	35	160
Cran-Cherry Cherry Cranberry Drink (8 fl oz) Ocean Spray (Ocean Spray Cranberries)	0.0	0.0	0	35	160
Cran-Grape Grape Cranberry Drink (8 fl oz) Ocean Spray (Ocean Spray Cranberries)	0.0	0.0	0	35	170
Cran-Raspberry Raspberry Cranberry Drink (8 fl oz) Ocean Spray (Ocean Spray Cranberries)	0.0	0.0	0	35	140
Cran-Strawberry Cranberry Strawberry Drink (8 fl oz) Ocean Spray (Ocean Spray Cranberries)	0.0	0.0	0	35	140
Cranapple Cranberry Apple Drink (8 fl oz) Ocean Spray (Ocean Spray Cranberries)	0.0	0.0	0	35	160
Cranicot Cranberry Apricot Drink (8 fl oz) Ocean Spray (Ocean Spray Cranberries)	0.0	0.0	0	35	160
Crantastic Fruit Punch (8 fl oz) Ocean Spray (Ocean Spray Cranberries)	0.0	0.0	0	35	150

	Tot. Fat (g)	Sat. Fat (g)	Chol. (mg)	Sod. (mg)	Cal.
READY-TO-DRINK BEVERAGES (NONCARBONATED) ***(cont'd)***					
Double Fruit Cooler (8 fl oz) Hi-C (Coca-Cola Foods)	0.0	0.0	0	30	130
Fruit Integration (8 fl oz) Minute Maid Fruitopia (Coca-Cola Foods)	0.0	0.0	0	25	120
Fruit Medley (8 fl oz) Minute Maid Naturals (Coca-Cola Foods)	0.0	0.0	0	25	120
Kiwi, Lime & Grapefruit Fruit Juice Beverage (8 fl oz) Koala Springs	0.0	0.0	0	0	110
Lightstyle Low Calorie Cran-Grape Grape-Cranberry Juice Drink (8 fl oz) Ocean Spray (Ocean Spray Cranberries)	0.0	0.0	0	35	40
Lightstyle Low Calorie Cran-Raspberry Raspberry Cranberry Juice Drink (8 fl oz) Ocean Spray (Ocean Spray Cranberries)	0.0	0.0	0	35	40
Mandarin & Orange Fruit Juice Beverage (8 fl oz) Koala Springs	0.0	0.0	0	0	110
Mauna La'i iMango-Mango! Mango & Hawaiian Guava Fruit Juice Drink (8 fl oz) Ocean Spray (Ocean Spray Cranberries)	0.0	0.0	0	35	130
Mauna La'i Paradise Passion Hawaiian Guava & Passion Fruit Flavored Juice Drink (8 fl oz) Ocean Spray (Ocean Spray Cranberries)	0.0	0.0	0	35	130
Orange Cranberry Juice Drink (8 fl oz) Ocean Spray Refreshers (Ocean Spray Cranberries)	0.0	0.0	0	35	130

	Tot. Fat (g)	Sat. Fat (g)	Chol. (mg)	Sod. (mg)	Cal.
Orange Grape Blend (8 fl oz) Minute Maid Naturals (Coca-Cola Foods)	0.0	0.0	0	35	120
Raspberry & Guava Fruit Juice Beverage (8 fl oz) Koala Springs	0.0	0.0	0	0	120
Stompin' Banana Berry (8 fl oz) Hi-C (Coca-Cola Foods)	0.0	0.0	0	30	130
Strawberry & Peach Fruit Juice Beverage (8 fl oz) Koala Springs	0.0	0.0	0	0	120
Strawberry Kiwi Melon Juice Cocktail (8 oz) Hansen (Hansen Beverage Co)	0.0	0.0	0	15	100
Tangerine Pineapple Passion Fruit Juice Cocktail (8 oz) Hansen (Hansen Beverage Co)	0.0	0.0	0	15	120
Tropical Medley (8 fl oz) Minute Maid Naturals (Coca-Cola Foods)	0.0	0.0	0	25	120
Orange Ready-to-Drink Beverages (noncarbonated)					
Orange (8 fl oz) Hi-C (Coca-Cola Foods)	0.0	0.0	0	25	130
Orange All Natural Juice Drink (6.75 fl oz) Capri Sun (Kraft General Foods)*	0.0	0.0	0	25	100
Orange Beverage (8 fl oz) Bright & Early (Coca-Cola Foods)	0.0	0.0	0	30	120
Orange Punch (8.45 fl oz) Minute Maid (Coca-Cola Foods)	0.0	0.0	0	0	130
Orange Punch Soft Drink (6.75 fl oz) Kool-Aid Bursts (Kraft General Foods)*	0.0	0.0	0	30	100
Smarty Arty Orange Squeezit (1 bottle) Betty Crocker (General Mills)	0.0	0.0	0	45	110

*Tobacco company, corporate subsidiary, or parent.

	Tot. Fat (g)	Sat. Fat (g)	Chol. (mg)	Sod. (mg)	Cal.
READY-TO-DRINK BEVERAGES (NONCARBONATED) *(cont'd)*					
Punch Ready-to-Drink Beverages (noncarbonated)					
All Natural Frozen Fruit Punch (8 fl oz)					
Just Pik't (The Fresh Juice Company)	0.0	0.0	0	30	125
California Paradise Punch Juice Cocktail (8 oz)					
Hansen (Hansen Beverage Co)	0.0	0.0	0	15	120
Concord Punch (8 fl oz)					
Minute Maid (Coca-Cola Foods)	0.0	0.0	0	25	130
Fruit Punch (8 fl oz)					
Hi-C (Coca-Cola Foods)	0.0	0.0	0	30	130
Minute Maid (Coca-Cola Foods)	0.0	0.0	0	25	120
Minute Maid (Coca-Cola USA)	0.0	0.0	0	5	119
Fruit Punch All Natural Juice Drink (6.75 fl oz)					
Capri Sun (Kraft General Foods)*	0.0	0.0	0	20	100
Fruit Punch Fruit Flavored Drink (8 fl oz)					
Wyler's (T.J. Lipton)	0.0	0.0	0	5	130
Hula Punch (8 fl oz)					
Hi-C (Coca-Cola Foods)	0.0	0.0	0	30	120
Maui Punch All Natural Juice Drink (6.75 fl oz)					
Capri Sun (Kraft General Foods)*	0.0	0.0	0	20	110
Mean Green Punch Squeezit (1 bottle)					
Betty Crocker (General Mills)	0.0	0.0	0	0	110
Red Punch Squeezit (1 bottle)					
Betty Crocker (General Mills)	0.0	0.0	0	0	110
Safari Punch All Natural Juice Drink (6.75 fl oz)					
Capri Sun (Kraft General Foods)*	0.0	0.0	0	20	100
Tropical Punch (8 fl oz)					
Minute Maid (Coca-Cola Foods)	0.0	0.0	0	5	120
Tropical Punch Soft Drink (6.75 fl oz)					
Kool-Aid Bursts (Kraft General Foods)*	0.0	0.0	0	30	100

*Tobacco company, corporate subsidiary, or parent.

	Tot. Fat (g)	Sat. Fat (g)	Chol. (mg)	Sod. (mg)	Cal.
Strawberry Ready-to-Drink Beverages (noncarbonated)					
Silly Billy Strawberry (1 bottle) Betty Crocker (General Mills) . . .	0.0	0.0	0	0	110
Strawberry Cooler All Natural Juice Drink (6.75 fl oz) Capri Sun (Kraft General Foods)*	0.0	0.0	0	20	100
Strawberry Passion Awareness (8 fl oz) Minute Maid Fruitopia (Coca-Cola Foods)	0.0	0.0	0	30	120
Other Ready-to-Drink Beverages (noncarbonated)					
All Natural Mango Mania (8 fl oz) Mega Mistic (Joseph Victori Wines)	0.0	0.0	0	0	110
Concord Medley (8 fl oz) Minute Maid Naturals (Coca-Cola Foods)	0.0	0.0	0	25	130
Ecto Cooler (8 fl oz) Hi-C (Coca-Cola Foods)	0.0	0.0	0	25	130
Fruity Bubble Gum (8 fl oz) Hi-C (Coca-Cola Foods)	0.0	0.0	0	25	120
Great Bluedini Soft Drink (6.75 fl oz) Kool-Aid Bursts (Kraft General Foods)*	0.0	0.0	0	30	100
Mauna La'i Island Guava Hawaiian Guava Fruit Juice Drink (8 fl oz) Ocean Spray (Ocean Spray Cranberries)	0.0	0.0	0	35	130
Mountain Cooler All Natural Juice Drink (6.75 fl oz) Capri Sun (Kraft General Foods)*	0.0	0.0	0	20	100
Pacific Cooler All Natural Juice Drink (6.75 fl oz) Capri Sun (Kraft General Foods)*	0.0	0.0	0	20	110
Pink Swimmingo Soft Drink (6.75 fl oz) Kool-Aid Bursts (Kraft General Foods)*	0.0	0.0	0	30	100

*Tobacco company, corporate subsidiary, or parent.

	Tot. Fat (g)	Sat. Fat (g)	Chol. (mg)	Sod. (mg)	Cal.
READY-TO-DRINK BEVERAGES (NONCARBONATED) ***(cont'd)***					
Rock-A-Dile Red Soft Drink (6.75 fl oz)					
Kool-Aid Bursts (Kraft General Foods)*	0.0	0.0	0	30	100
Surfer Cooler All Natural Juice Drink (6.75 fl oz)					
Capri Sun (Kraft General Foods)*	0.0	0.0	0	20	100
Wildberry Squeezit (1 bottle)					
Betty Crocker (General Mills)	0.0	0.0	0	0	110
RECONSTITUTED FROM FROZEN BEVERAGES					
Apple Reconstituted from Frozen Beverages					
Apple Beverage (8 fl oz)					
Bright & Early (Coca-Cola Foods)	0.0	0.0	0	10	120
Citrus Reconstituted from Frozen Beverages					
Citrus (8 fl oz)					
Five Alive (Coca-Cola Foods)	0.0	0.0	0	25	120
Citrus fruit juice drink (8 fl oz)					
Most brands (USDA)	**0.0**	**0.0**	**0**	**8**	**112**
Citrus Punch (8 fl oz)					
Minute Maid (Coca-Cola Foods)	0.0	0.0	0	25	120
Cranberry Reconstituted from Frozen Beverages					
All Natural Frozen Cranberry Juice Cocktail (8 fl oz)					
Just Pik't (The Fresh Juice Company)	0.0	0.0	0	0	135
Reduced Calorie Cranberry Juice Cocktail (8 fl oz)					
Ocean Spray (Ocean Spray Cranberries)	0.0	0.0	0	35	50
Grape Reconstituted from Frozen Beverages					
Grape (8 fl oz)					
Bright & Early (Coca-Cola Foods)	0.0	0.0	0	5	140

*Tobacco company, corporate subsidiary, or parent.

	Tot. Fat (g)	Sat. Fat (g)	Chol. (mg)	Sod. (mg)	Cal.
Grape Juice Cocktail (8 fl oz)					
America's Choice (A & P)	0.0	0.0	0	10	130
Grape Punch (8 fl oz)					
Minute Maid (Coca-Cola Foods)	0.0	0.0	0	5	130
Lemonade Reconstituted from Frozen Beverages					
All Natural Frozen Lemonade (8 fl oz)					
Just Pik't (The Fresh Juice Company)	0.0	0.0	0	0	110
Country Style Lemonade (8 fl oz)					
Minute Maid (Coca-Cola Foods)	0.0	0.0	0	0	120
Cranberry Lemonade (8 fl oz)					
Minute Maid (Coca-Cola Foods)	0.0	0.0	0	0	120
Lemonade (8 fl oz)					
Minute Maid (Coca-Cola Foods)	0.0	0.0	0	0	110
Ocean Spray (Ocean Spray Cranberries)	0.0	0.0	0	35	110
Lemonade Beverage (8 fl oz)					
Bright & Early (Coca-Cola Foods)	0.0	0.0	0	5	120
Pink Lemonade (8 fl oz)					
Minute Maid (Coca-Cola Foods)	0.0	0.0	0	0	120
Raspberry Lemonade (8 fl oz)					
Minute Maid (Coca-Cola Foods)	0.0	0.0	0	0	120
Mixed Fruit Reconstituted from Frozen Beverages					
Berry Citrus (8 fl oz)					
Five Alive (Coca-Cola Foods) . . .	0.0	0.0	0	0	120
Berry Punch (8 fl oz)					
Minute Maid (Coca-Cola Foods)	0.0	0.0	0	35	130
Lemonade with Cranberry Juice (8 fl oz)					
Ocean Spray (Ocean Spray Cranberries)	0.0	0.0	0	35	110
Lemonade with Raspberry Juice (8 fl oz)					
Ocean Spray (Ocean Spray Cranberries)	0.0	0.0	0	35	110

	Tot. Fat (g)	Sat. Fat (g)	Chol. (mg)	Sod. (mg)	Cal.
Reconstituted from Frozen Beverages ***(cont'd)***					
Reduced Calorie Cran-Apple Apple Cranberry Drink (8 fl oz)					
Ocean Spray (Ocean Spray Cranberries)	0.0	0.0	0	35	50
Reduced Calorie Cran-Raspberry Raspberry Cranberry Drink (8 fl oz)					
Ocean Spray (Ocean Spray Cranberries)	0.0	0.0	0	35	50
Orange Reconstituted from Frozen Beverages					
Orange Beverage (8 fl oz)					
Bright & Early (Coca-Cola Foods)	0.0	0.0	0	30	120
Punch Reconstituted from Frozen Beverages					
Fruit Punch (8 fl oz)					
Minute Maid (Coca-Cola Foods)	0.0	0.0	0	5	120
Ocean Spray (Ocean Spray Cranberries)	0.0	0.0	0	35	130
Fruit Punch Beverage (8 fl oz)					
Bright & Early (Coca-Cola Foods)	0.0	0.0	0	5	130
Tropical Punch (8 fl oz)					
Minute Maid (Coca-Cola Foods)	0.0	0.0	0	0	120
Other Reconstituted from Frozen Beverages					
Limeade (8 fl oz)					
Minute Maid (Coca-Cola Foods)	0.0	0.0	0	0	100
SPORTS DRINKS					
Fruit Punch (8 fl oz)					
PowerAde (Coca-Cola USA)	0.0	0.0	0	28	72
Grape (8 fl oz)					
PowerAde (Coca-Cola USA)	0.0	0.0	0	28	73
Lemon-Lime (8 fl oz)					
PowerAde (Coca-Cola USA)	0.0	0.0	0	28	72
Orange (8 fl oz)					
PowerAde (Coca-Cola USA)	0.0	0.0	0	28	72

	Tot. Fat (g)	Sat. Fat (g)	Chol. (mg)	Sod. (mg)	Cal.
TEAS					
Flavored Teas					
Brewed Flavored Teas					
Various flavors (1 tea bag) Lipton (T.J. Lipton)	0.0	0.0	0	0	0
Herbal tea, brewed, unsweetened (8 fl oz) **Most brands** (USDA)	**0.0**	**0.0**	**0**	**2**	**3**
Instant Flavored Teas					
Cinnamon Apple Instant Herbals (1 env) Lipton (T.J. Lipton)	0.0	0.0	0	0	20
Cran Raspberry Sugar Free Iced Herbal Tea Mix (8 fl oz) Lipton (T.J. Lipton)	0.0	0.0	0	0	10
Lemon Cooler Sugar Free Iced Herbal Tea Mix (8 fl oz) Lipton (T.J. Lipton)	0.0	0.0	0	0	10
Lemon Flavored Instant Tea (2 tsp) Lipton (T.J. Lipton)	0.0	0.0	0	0	5
Orange Instant Herbals (1 env) Lipton (T.J. Lipton)	0.0	0.0	0	0	20
Ready-to-Drink Flavored Teas					
All Natural Peach Flavored Iced Tea (8 fl oz) Royal Mistic (Joseph Victori Wines)	0.0	0.0	0	5	90
All Natural Raspberry Flavored Iced Tea (8 fl oz) Royal Mistic (Joseph Victori Wines)	0.0	0.0	0	25	90
Diet Iced Tea Natural Lemon Flavored (8 fl oz) Royal Mistic (Joseph Victori Wines)	0.0	0.0	0	25	5
Natural Iced Tea Naturally Lemon Flavored (8 fl oz) Royal Mistic (Joseph Victori Wines)	0.0	0.0	0	20	90

	Tot. Fat (g)	Sat. Fat (g)	Chol. (mg)	Sod. (mg)	Cal.
FLAVORED TEAS *(cont'd)*					
Natural Lemon Flavor Frozen Iced Tea (8 fl oz)					
Just Pik't (The Fresh Juice Company)	0.0	0.0	0	0	75
Original Tea with Lemon (8 oz)					
Hansen (Hansen Beverage Co)	0.0	0.0	0	15	70
Red Herbal Strawberry Naturally Flavored Iced Tea (8 fl oz)					
Royal Mistic (Joseph Victori Wines)	0.0	0.0	0	0	100
Tangerine Tea (8 oz)					
Hansen (Hansen Beverage Co)	0.0	0.0	0	15	70
Tropical Tea (8 oz)					
Hansen (Hansen Beverage Co)	0.0	0.0	0	15	70
Wildberry Tea (8 oz)					
Hansen (Hansen Beverage Co)	0.0	0.0	0	15	70
REGULAR TEAS					
Brewed Regular Teas					
Tea, brewed, unsweetened (8 fl oz)					
Most brands (USDA)	**0.0**	**0.0**	**0**	**8**	**3**
Instant Regular Teas					
Calorie Free Decaffeinated Iced Tea Mix (1 tsp)					
Lipton (T.J. Lipton)	0.0	0.0	0	0	0
Calorie Free Iced Tea Mix (1 tsp)					
Lipton (T.J. Lipton)	0.0	0.0	0	0	0
Decaffeinated Iced Tea Low Calorie Soft Drink Mix, made with water (8 fl oz)					
Crystal Light (Kraft General Foods)*	0.0	0.0	0	0	5
Decaffeinated Instant Tea Mix (1 tsp)					
Lipton (T.J. Lipton)	0.0	0.0	0	0	0
Iced Tea Low Calorie Soft Drink Mix, made with water (8 fl oz)					
Crystal Light (Kraft General Foods)*	0.0	0.0	0	0	5

*Tobacco company, corporate subsidiary, or parent.

	Tot. Fat (g)	Sat. Fat (g)	Chol. (mg)	Sod. (mg)	Cal.
Iced Tea Mix with NutraSweet (1 tbsp)					
Lipton (T.J. Lipton)	0.0	0.0	0	0	5
Iced Tea Sugar Sweetened Drink Mix, made with water (8 fl oz)					
Country Time (Kraft General Foods)*	0.0	0.0	0	0	70
Instant Tea (1 heaping tsp)					
Lipton (T.J. Lipton)	0.0	0.0	0	0	0
Instant tea, decaffeinated, presweetened with sugar, made with water (8 fl oz)					
Most brands (USDA)	**0.0**	**0.0**	**0**	**0**	**87**
Instant tea, regular, presweetened with sugar, made with water (8 fl oz)					
Most brands (USDA)	**0.0**	**0.0**	**0**	**0**	**87**
Instant tea, unsweetened, made with water (8 fl oz)					
Most brands (USDA)	**0.0**	**0.0**	**0**	**8**	**3**
Low Calorie Iced Tea Mix (1 tsp)					
Lipton (T.J. Lipton)	0.0	0.0	0	0	0
Sugar Free No Lemon Iced Tea Mix (1 tbsp)					
Lipton (T.J. Lipton)	0.0	0.0	0	0	0
Sugar No Lemon Iced Tea Mix (1 tbsp)					
Lipton (T.J. Lipton)	0.0	0.0	0	0	80

*Tobacco company, corporate subsidiary, or parent.

BREADS AND BREAD PRODUCTS

From crusty French bread to soft corn tortillas, we've combed the country for the tastiest nonfat and low-fat breads. In this chapter, you'll find biscuits, cinnamon raisin bagels, and English muffins. You'll even find pancakes low in total fat, saturated fat, and cholesterol—if you make them according to package directions.

Like all the other entries in this book, the breads and bread products entries that follow list sodium content. The AHA does not have criteria for sodium but recommends a total of no more than 3,000 mg a day.

Mixes

"Complete" biscuit, pancake, and waffle mixes already contain fat. All you do is add water. Sometimes the result is low in fat. A few of these mixes are listed on the following pages. Other complete mixes, however, may be high in fat. Just be sure to read the labels.

There are also "incomplete" mixes, where you add the fat. Manufacturers of these mixes usually recommend adding eggs, whole milk, and butter or oil. If prepared this way, the mixes won't meet AHA criteria. To make sure you are getting a low-fat product, use egg whites or egg substitute, skim milk, and less oil or margarine.

Generic Listings

By far, most of the foods in this book are brand name products. However, if a product is listed without a brand name, it means that most brands of that product contain about the same amount of fat, saturated fat, and cholesterol and that these amounts are within the AHA criteria cited below.

If you find products that were introduced after this book went to press, use the generic listings and the following tables to help you evaluate them.

AHA Criteria for Breads and Bread Products*

	Tot. Fat (g)	Sat. Fat (g)	Chol. (mg)
Bagels, biscuits, breads, corn bread, English muffins, French toast, hamburger and hot dog buns, pancakes, pita bread, rolls, soft breadsticks, stuffing mixes (prepared), tortillas, and waffles	3	1	<2
Batter mixes, bread crumbs, croutons, and hard breadsticks	3	<0.5	<2
Quick-type sweet breads, such as sweet rolls and coffee cake	3	1	<2

*Per serving.

Breads and Bread Products You'll Want to Limit

Some breads and bread products, like the examples below, are too high in fat, saturated fat, and/or cholesterol to meet AHA criteria. Such products aren't included in this book, and we recommend that you don't eat them often.

Compare the amounts of fat, saturated fat, cholesterol, sodium, and calories in these examples with the more healthful alternatives listed on the following pages.

Sample Breads and Bread Products to Limit

	Tot. Fat (g)	Sat. Fat (g)	Chol. (mg)	Sod. (mg)	Cal.
Almond Danish pastry (2 oz, or about 3⅞″ in diam)	14.2*	3.1*	26*	206	244
Biscuit, made from mix with 2% milk (3″-diam biscuit)	6.9*	1.6*	(2)	544	191
Buttermilk pancakes, made from mix with egg, oil, and 2% milk (3 4″-diam pancakes)	8.7*	2.3*	81*	576	249
Cheese croissant (1 medium)	11.9*	5.5*	(27)*	316	236
Corn bread, made from mix with egg and 2% milk (3¾″ x 2½″ x ¾″)	6.0*	1.6*	37*	467	189
Corn-bread stuffing, made from mix with stick margarine (½ cup)	8.8*	1.8*	0	455	179
Crescent roll, made from refrigerated dough (2 2½″ in diam, or about 2 oz)	8.0*	2.0*	0	648	186

Adapted from USDA Handbook No. 8 series.

*These values exceed AHA criteria for breads and bread products.

	Tot. Fat (g)	Sat. Fat (g)	Chol. (mg)	Sod. (mg)	Cal.
BAGELS					
PLAIN BAGELS					
Plain Bagels (3½" bagel)					
Most brands (USDA)	**1.1**	**0.2**	**0**	**379**	**195**
S.B. Thomas (Best Foods Baking Group)	2.0	0.0	0	220	170
Original Bagels (1 bagel)					
Wolferman's	1.0	0.0	0	550	230
OTHER BAGELS					
Cinnamon Raisin Bagels (1 bagel)					
Wolferman's	1.0	0.0	0	230	230
Onion Bagels (1 bagel)					
S.B. Thomas (Best Foods Baking Group)	2.0	0.0	0	200	160
Wolferman's	1.0	0.0	0	660	230
BATTER MIXES—see COATING MIXES, page 55; PANCAKES/ WAFFLES, page 62					
BISCUITS—see also BREAD MIXES/ROLL MIXES, page 46					
Ballard Extra Lights Ovenready Biscuits (3 biscuits = 2¼ oz)					
Pillsbury (Grand Metropolitan PLC)	2.0	0.0	0	490	150
Ballard Extra Lights Ovenready Buttermilk Biscuits (3 biscuits = 2¼ oz)					
Pillsbury (Grand Metropolitan PLC)	2.0	0.0	0	490	150
Butter Biscuits (3 biscuits = 2¼ oz)					
Pillsbury (Grand Metropolitan PLC)	2.5	0.0	0	490	150
Buttermilk Biscuits (3 biscuits = 2¼ oz)					
Pillsbury (Grand Metropolitan PLC)	2.5	0.0	0	490	150
Country Biscuits (3 biscuits = 2¼ oz)					
Pillsbury (Grand Metropolitan PLC)	2.5	0.0	0	490	150

	Tot. Fat (g)	Sat. Fat (g)	Chol. (mg)	Sod. (mg)	Cal.
BISCUITS *(cont'd)*					
Toaster Biscuits (1 biscuit)					
Dunberry (Continental Baking Co)	3.0	1.0	0	310	150
BREAD CRUMBS/CRACKER CRUMBS					
Bread Crumbs (⅓ cup)					
Contadina (Nestlé Food Company)	1.5	0.0	0	700	100
Fat Free Cracker Crumbs (¼ cup)					
Nabisco Premium (Nabisco Foods)*	0.0	0.0	0	0	100
Graham Cracker Crumbs					
Most brands (USDA) (⅓ cup)	**2.7**	**0.8**	**0**	**190**	**109**
Nabisco Honey Maid (Nabisco Foods)* (⅛ of 9″ pieshell; ½ oz)	1.5	0.0	0	90	70
Italian Style Bread Crumbs (¼ cup)					
Progresso (Pet)	1.5	0.0	0	430	110
Plain Bread Crumbs (¼ cup)					
Progresso (Pet)	1.5	0.0	0	210	100
BREAD MIXES/ROLL MIXES					
Easy Breads Mix (¼ cup)					
Bisquick (General Mills)	<1.0	0.0	0	220	130
Reduced Fat Baking Mix (⅓ cup)					
Bisquick (General Mills)	2.5	0.5	0	460	150
BREADS—see also BREAD MIXES/ROLL MIXES, above					
Bran Breads					
Bran'nola Original Bread (1 slice)					
Arnold (Best Foods Baking Group)	2.0	0.0	0	125	90
Light Honey Bran Bread (2 slices)					
Wonder (Continental Baking Co)	0.5	0.0	0	190	80
Natural Whole Bran Bread (1 slice)					
Brownberry (Best Foods Baking Group)	1.0	0.0	0	140	60

*Tobacco company, corporate subsidiary, or parent.

	Tot. Fat (g)	Sat. Fat (g)	Chol. (mg)	Sod. (mg)	Cal.
Wheat bran bread (1 slice)					
Most brands (USDA)	**1.2**	**0.3**	**0**	**175**	**89**
DIET BREADS—*see SPECIFIC TYPE OF BREAD*					
FRENCH BREADS					
Crusty French Loaf (⅕ of loaf)					
Pillsbury (Grand Metropolitan PLC)	1.0	0.0	0	370	150
French Bread					
Most brands (USDA) (2 slices)	**1.1**	**0.3**	**0**	**304**	**138**
Bread du Jour (Continental Baking Co) (2 oz)	1.0	0.0	0	300	130
Wonder (Continental Baking Co) (1 slice)	1.5	0.0	0	160	80
Light French Bread (2 slices)					
Wonder (Continental Baking Co)	1.0	0.0	0	210	80
Parisian French Bread (2 slices)					
Dicarlo's (Continental Baking Co)	1.0	0.0	0	150	70
FRUIT BREADS/VEGETABLE BREADS					
Apple Strudel Toasting Bread (1 slice)					
Wolferman's	1.0	0.0	0	150	80
Blueberry Toasting Bread (1 slice)					
Wolferman's	0.0	0.0	0	230	210
Carrot & Raisin Sprouted Grain Loaf (1 slice)					
Lifestream Natural Foods Essene	0.0	0.0	0	15	130
Date & Cinnamon Sprouted Grain Loaf (1 slice)					
Lifestream Natural Foods Essene	0.0	0.0	0	15	140
Fruit & Nut Sprouted Grain Loaf (1 slice)					
Lifestream Natural Foods Essene	1.5	0.0	0	10	150
ITALIAN BREADS					
Family Italian Bread (1 slice)					
Wonder (Continental Baking Co)	1.0	0.0	0	170	70
Italian Bread (1 slice)					
Most brands (USDA)	**1.1**	**0.3**	**0**	**175**	**81**
Wonder (Continental Baking Co)	1.0	0.0	0	190	80
Light Italian Bread (2 slices)					
Wonder (Continental Baking Co)	1.0	0.0	0	230	80

	Tot. Fat (g)	Sat. Fat (g)	Chol. (mg)	Sod. (mg)	Cal.
LIGHT BREADS—*see SPECIFIC TYPE OF BREAD*					
MULTIGRAIN BREADS					
European Style Whole Grain Bread (1 slice)					
Rubschlager	0.5	0.0	0	135	70
5 Seed Sprouted Grain Loaf (1 slice)					
Lifestream Natural Foods Essene	0.0	0.0	0	10	130
Granola Bread (2 slices)					
Wonder (Continental Baking Co)	1.5	0.0	0	210	100
Hearty Seven Grain Multi Grain Bread (1 slice)					
Home Pride (Continental Baking Co)	2.0	0.0	0	200	100
Light Nine Grain Bread (2 slices)					
Wonder (Continental Baking Co)	1.0	0.0	0	230	80
Multigrain bread (2 slices)					
Most brands (USDA)	**2.0**	**0.4**	**0**	**254**	**130**
Multigrain Sprouted Grain Loaf (1 slice)					
Lifestream Natural Foods Essene	0.0	0.0	0	15	140
Seven Grain Bread (1 slice)					
Home Pride (Continental Baking Co)	1.0	0.0	0	130	60
OAT BREADS					
Bakery Light Oatmeal (2 slices)					
Arnold (Best Foods Baking Group)	1.0	0.0	0	140	80
Bran'nola Country Oat Bread (1 slice)					
Arnold (Best Foods Baking Group)	2.5	0.5	0	115	90
Hearty Honey Oats & Cracked Wheat Bread (1 slice)					
Home Pride (Continental Baking Co)	1.5	0.0	0	210	100
Light Oatmeal Bread (2 slices)					
Wonder (Continental Baking Co)	1.0	0.0	0	230	90
Natural Oatmeal Bread (1 slice)					
Brownberry (Best Foods Baking Group)	1.0	0.0	0	135	70

	Tot. Fat (g)	Sat. Fat (g)	Chol. (mg)	Sod. (mg)	Cal.
Oatmeal Cinnamon Toasting Bread (1 slice)					
Wolferman's	0.0	0.0	0	160	120
PUMPERNICKEL BREADS					
Danish Style Pumpernickel Bread (1 slice)					
Rubschlager	0.5	0.0	0	135	70
Natural Pumpernickel Rye Bread (1 slice)					
Brownberry (Best Foods Baking Group)	0.5	0.0	0	150	70
Pumpernickel Bread (1 slice)					
Most brands (USDA)	**1.0**	**0.1**	**0**	**215**	**80**
Beefsteak (Continental Baking Co)	1.0	0.0	0	180	70
Rubschlager	1.5	0.0	0	210	90
Pumpernickel Cocktail Bread (3 slices)					
Rubschlager	1.0	0.0	0	180	80
RAISIN BREADS					
Cinnamon & Raisin Toasting Bread (1 slice)					
Wolferman's	1.0	0.0	0	150	120
Cinnamon Raisin Bread (1 slice)					
Wonder (Continental Baking Co)	0.5	0.0	0	100	70
Raisin bread (2 slices)					
Most brands (USDA)	**2.2**	**0.6**	**0**	**202**	**142**
Raisin Brown Bread (½" slice)					
B&M (Pet)	0.5	0.0	0	360	130
Friend's (Pet)	0.5	0.0	0	360	130
Raisin Cinnamon Bread (1 slice)					
Arnold (Best Foods Baking Group)	1.0	0.0	0	90	70
Raisin Pumpernickel Bread (2 slices)					
Rubschlager	1.5	0.0	0	200	110
Raisin Sprouted Grain Loaf (1 slice)					
Lifestream Natural Foods Essene	0.0	0.0	0	10	130
RYE BREADS					
Cocktail Rye Breads					
Rye Cocktail Bread (3 slices)					
Rubschlager	1.5	0.0	0	180	80

	Tot. Fat (g)	Sat. Fat (g)	Chol. (mg)	Sod. (mg)	Cal.
RYE BREADS *(cont'd)*					
Sandwich Rye Breads					
Hearty Rye Bread (1 slice)					
Beefsteak (Continental Baking Co)	1.0	0.0	0	170	70
Jewish Style Deli Rye Bread (1 slice)					
Rubschlager	1.0	0.0	0	135	70
Light Rye Bread (2 slices)					
Beefsteak (Continental Baking Co)	1.0	0.0	0	250	70
Wonder (Continental Baking Co)	1.0	0.0	0	220	70
Marble Rye Bread (2 slices)					
Rubschlager	1.5	0.0	0	200	110
Mild Rye Bread (2 slices)					
Beefsteak (Continental Baking Co)	1.0	0.0	0	240	90
Natural Caraway Rye Bread (1 slice)					
Brownberry (Best Foods Baking Group)	1.0	0.0	0	160	70
Rye Bread (1 slice)					
Most brands (USDA)	**1.1**	**0.2**	**0**	**211**	**83**
Rubschlager	1.5	0.0	0	210	90
Wonder (Continental Baking Co)	1.0	0.0	0	170	70
Soft Rye Bread (1 slice)					
Beefsteak (Continental Baking Co)	1.0	0.0	0	180	70
Whole Rye Sprouted Grain Loaf (1 slice)					
Lifestream Natural Foods Essene	0.0	0.0	0	10	140
SOURDOUGH BREADS					
Light Sourdough Bread (2 slices)					
Wonder (Continental Baking Co)	1.0	0.0	0	250	80
Sourdough Bread					
Most brands (USDA) (2 slices)	**1.1**	**0.3**	**0**	**304**	**138**
Wonder (Continental Baking Co) (1 slice)	1.5	0.0	0	180	90
Sourdough Toasting Bread (1 slice)					
Wolferman's	0.0	0.0	0	205	80

	Tot. Fat (g)	Sat. Fat (g)	Chol. (mg)	Sod. (mg)	Cal.
Wheat Breads					
Austrian Wheat Bread (2 oz)					
Bread du Jour (Continental Baking Co)	1.5	0.0	0	280	130
Bakery Light Wheat Bread (2 slices)					
Arnold (Best Foods Baking Group)	1.0	0.0	0	120	80
Brick Oven Wheat Bread (2 slices)					
Arnold (Best Foods Baking Group)	3.0	0.0	0	170	110
Country Wheat Bread (1 slice)					
Arnold (Best Foods Baking Group)	1.5	0.0	0	170	90
Cracked Wheat Bread (1 slice)					
Wonder (Continental Baking Co)	1.0	0.0	0	150	70
Family Wheat Bread (1 slice)					
Wonder (Continental Baking Co)	1.0	0.0	0	150	70
Hearth Wheat Bread (1 slice)					
Brownberry (Best Foods Baking Group)	1.0	0.0	0	190	90
Heartland Harvest Toasting Bread (1 slice)					
Wolferman's	0.0	0.0	0	230	80
Hearty Golden Honey Wheat Bread (1 slice)					
Home Pride (Continental Baking Co)	1.5	0.0	0	210	90
Hearty 100% Stoneground Whole Wheat Bread (1 slice)					
Home Pride (Continental Baking Co)	1.5	0.0	0	250	90
Hearty Wheat Bread (1 slice)					
Beefsteak (Continental Baking Co)	1.0	0.0	0	160	70
Honey Wheat Bread (1 slice)					
Home Pride (Continental Baking Co)	1.0	0.0	0	150	70

	Tot. Fat (g)	Sat. Fat (g)	Chol. (mg)	Sod. (mg)	Cal.
WHEAT BREADS *(cont'd)*					
Light Wheat Bread					
Home Pride (Continental Baking Co) (3 slices)	1.5	0.0	0	300	110
Wonder (Continental Baking Co) (2 slices)	0.5	0.0	0	230	80
Light Wheat Calcium Bread (2 slices)					
Wonder (Continental Baking Co)	0.5	0.0	0	240	80
Natural Wheat Bread (2 slices)					
Brownberry (Best Foods Baking Group)	1.0	0.0	0	200	80
100% Soft Whole Wheat Bread (2 slices)					
Wonder (Continental Baking Co)	1.5	0.0	0	240	110
100% Stone-Ground Honey Whole Wheat Bread (1 slice)					
Rubschlager	1.0	0.0	0	135	70
100% Stoneground Whole Wheat Bread (1 slice)					
Wonder (Continental Baking Co)	1.5	0.0	0	190	80
100% Whole Wheat Bread (1 slice)					
Wonder (Continental Baking Co)	1.0	0.0	0	180	70
Soft Wheat Bread (1 slice)					
Beefsteak (Continental Baking Co)	1.0	0.0	0	150	70
Stone-Ground Honey Wheat Bread (1 slice)					
Rubschlager	1.5	0.0	0	180	90
Stoneground 100% Whole Wheat Bread (2 slices)					
Arnold (Best Foods Baking Group)	1.5	0.0	0	170	100
Wheat Bread (1 slice)					
Home Pride (Continental Baking Co)	1.0	0.0	0	160	70
Wheat Golden Country Style Bread (2 slices)					
Wonder (Continental Baking Co)	1.5	0.0	0	220	100
Wheat Toasting Bread (1 slice)					
Wolferman's	0.0	0.0	0	230	210

	Tot. Fat (g)	Sat. Fat (g)	Chol. (mg)	Sod. (mg)	Cal.
Whole wheat bread (1 slice)					
Most brands (USDA)	**1.2**	**0.3**	**(1)**	**149**	**70**
Whole Wheat Sprouted Grain Loaf (1 slice)					
Lifestream Natural Foods Essene	0.0	0.0	0	10	130
White Breads					
Brick Oven White Bread (2 slices)					
Arnold (Best Foods Baking Group)	2.5	0.0	0	230	130
Country White Bread (1 slice)					
Arnold (Best Foods Baking Group)	1.5	0.0	0	190	100
Diet white bread (2 slices)					
Most brands (USDA)	**1.2**	**0.3**	**0**	**208**	**96**
Hearty Buttermilk & Biscuit White Bread (1 slice)					
Home Pride (Continental Baking Co)	2.0	0.0	0	280	100
Iron Kids Bread (1 slice)					
Wonder (Continental Baking Co)	1.0	0.0	0	130	60
Light White Bread					
Home Pride (Continental Baking Co) (3 slices)	1.5	0.0	0	320	110
Wonder (Continental Baking Co) (2 slices)	1.0	0.0	0	230	80
Light White Calcium Bread (2 slices)					
Wonder (Continental Baking Co)	1.0	0.0	0	260	80
Natural White Bread (2 slices)					
Brownberry (Best Foods Baking Group)	1.5	0.0	0	160	120
Original Toasting Bread (1 slice)					
Wolferman's	0.0	0.0	0	166	80
Pipin' Hot Loaf (1/6 of loaf)					
Pillsbury (Grand Metropolitan PLC)	0.5	0.0	0	350	110
Robust White Bread (1 slice)					
Beefsteak (Continental Baking Co)	1.0	0.0	0	140	70
Vienna Bread (1 slice)					
Wonder (Continental Baking Co)	1.0	0.0	0	170	70

	Tot. Fat (g)	Sat. Fat (g)	Chol. (mg)	Sod. (mg)	Cal.
WHITE BREADS *(cont'd)*					
White Bread					
Most brands (USDA) (2 slices)	**1.8**	**0.4**	**0**	**270**	**134**
Home Pride (Continental Baking Co) (1 slice)	1.0	0.0	0	160	70
Wonder (Continental Baking Co) (1 slice)	1.0	0.0	0	150	70
White Calcium Bread (2 slices)					
Wonder (Continental Baking Co)	1.0	0.0	0	240	100
White Grain Bread (1 slice)					
Home Pride (Continental Baking Co)	1.0	0.0	0	140	60
White with Buttermilk Bread (1 slice)					
Wonder (Continental Baking Co)	1.0	0.0	0	180	80
OTHER BREADS					
Bagel Bread (1 slice)					
Rubschlager	2.0	0.0	0	180	90
German Style Kommissbrot Bread (1 slice)					
Rubschlager	1.0	0.0	0	150	70
Hearth Grain Bread (1 slice)					
Brownberry (Best Foods Baking Group)	1.5	0.0	0	190	90
Honey Wheat Berry Bread (1 slice)					
Arnold (Best Foods Baking Group)	1.0	0.0	0	160	70
Honey Whole Grain Cocktail Bread (3 slices)					
Rubschlager	1.0	0.0	0	180	80
Plain Brown Bread (½″ slice)					
B&M (Pet)	0.5	0.0	0	390	130
Friend's (Pet)	0.5	0.0	0	390	130
Swedish Style Limpa Bread (2 slices)					
Rubschlager	1.5	0.0	0	200	110
Westphalian Style Bread (1 slice)					
Rubschlager	0.5	0.0	0	135	70
BREADSTICKS					
READY-TO-COOK BREADSTICKS					
Garlic Poppyseed Breadsticks (1 breadstick)					
Wolferman's	2.0	0.0	0	280	130

	Tot. Fat (g)	Sat. Fat (g)	Chol. (mg)	Sod. (mg)	Cal.
Italian Breadsticks (1 breadstick)					
Bread du Jour (Continental Baking Co)	1.0	0.0	0	280	130
Sourdough Breadsticks (1 breadstick)					
Bread du Jour (Continental Baking Co)	1.0	0.0	0	280	130
READY-TO-EAT BREADSTICKS					
Cheese Breadsticks					
Delicious (Delicious Cookie Co) (1 breadstick)	0.5	0.0	0	85	40
Lance (4 breadsticks)	1.0	0.0	0	120	50
Garlic Breadsticks					
Delicious (Delicious Cookie Co) (1 breadstick)	0.0	0.0	0	60	35
Lance (4 breadsticks)	1.0	0.0	0	180	50
Italian Breadsticks (1 breadstick)					
Delicious (Delicious Cookie Co)	0.0	0	0	65	35
Plain Breadsticks (4 breadsticks)					
Lance	1.0	0.0	0	130	50
Sesame Breadsticks (1 breadstick)					
Delicious (Delicious Cookie Co)	0.5	0.0	0	60	35
Whole Wheat Sesame Breadsticks (1 breadstick)					
Delicious (Delicious Cookie Co)	0.0	0.0	0	50	30
COATING MIXES—*see also* BREAD CRUMBS/CRACKER CRUMBS, page 46					
Barbecue Chicken Seasoning & Coating Mixture Glaze (1/8 pkt)					
Shake'n Bake (Kraft General Foods)*	1.0	0.0	0	410	45
Barbecue Pork Seasoning & Coating Mixture Glaze (1/8 pkt)					
Shake'n Bake (Kraft General Foods)*	0.0	0.0	0	250	35
Extra Crispy Recipe for Chicken (1/8 pkt)					
Oven Fry (Kraft General Foods)*	1.0	0.0	0	420	60
Extra Crispy Recipe for Pork (1/8 pkt)					
Oven Fry (Kraft General Foods)*	1.5	0.0	0	340	60

*Tobacco company, corporate subsidiary, or parent.

	Tot. Fat (g)	Sat. Fat (g)	Chol. (mg)	Sod. (mg)	Cal.
COATING MIXES *(cont'd)*					
Herb & Garlic Seasoning Mix for Fresh Potatoes (1/6 pkt) Shake'n Bake Perfect Potatoes (Kraft General Foods)*	0.0	0.0	0	370	20
Home Style Flour Recipe for Chicken (1/8 pkt) Oven Fry (Kraft General Foods)*	1.0	0.0	0	470	40
Honey Mustard Seasoning & Coating Mixture Glaze (1/8 pkt) Shake'n Bake (Kraft General Foods)*	1.0	0.0	0	290	45
Hot & Spicy Chicken Seasoning & Coating Mixture (1/8 pkt) Shake'n Bake (Kraft General Foods)*	1.0	0.0	0	190	40
Hot & Spicy Pork Seasoning & Coating Mixture (1/8 pkt) Shake'n Bake (Kraft General Foods)*	0.5	0.0	0	220	45
Italian Herb Recipe Seasoning & Coating Mixture (1/8 pkt) Shake'n Bake (Kraft General Foods)*	0.5	0.0	0	300	40
Original Recipe for Chicken Seasoning & Coating Mixture (1/8 pkt) Shake'n Bake (Kraft General Foods)*	1.0	0.0	0	230	40
Original Recipe for Fish Seasoning & Coating Mixture (1/4 pkt) Shake'n Bake (Kraft General Foods)*	1.5	0.0	0	420	70
Original Recipe for Pork Seasoning & Coating Mixture (1/8 pkt) Shake'n Bake (Kraft General Foods)*	0.0	0.0	0	320	40
Tangy Honey Seasoning & Coating Mixture Glaze (1/8 pkt) Shake'n Bake (Kraft General Foods)*	1.0	0.0	0	280	45

*Tobacco company, corporate subsidiary, or parent.

	Tot. Fat (g)	Sat. Fat (g)	Chol. (mg)	Sod. (mg)	Cal.
COFFEE CAKES/DANISHES/ SWEET ROLLS—*see also* BREAD MIXES/ROLL MIXES, page 46					
Apple Buns (1 bun)					
Entenmann's (Kraft General Foods)*	0.0	0.0	0	140	150
Apricot Danish Twist (1/8 danish)					
Entenmann's (Kraft General Foods)*	0.0	0.0	0	110	150
Black Forest Pastry (1/9 danish)					
Entenmann's (Kraft General Foods)*	0.0	0.0	0	115	130
Blueberry Cheese Buns (1 bun)					
Entenmann's (Kraft General Foods)*	0.0	0.0	0	150	140
Cinnamon Apple Coffee Cake (1/9 cake)					
Entenmann's (Kraft General Foods)*	0.0	0.0	0	110	130
Cinnamon Apple Twist (1/8 danish)					
Entenmann's (Kraft General Foods)*	0.0	0.0	0	110	150
Cinnamon Raisin Buns (1 bun)					
Entenmann's (Kraft General Foods)*	0.0	0.0	0	125	160
Crumb Cake Light (2 cakes)					
Hostess (Continental Baking Co)	1.0	0.0	0	190	150
Lemon Twist (1/8 danish)					
Entenmann's (Kraft General Foods)*	0.0	0.0	0	140	130
Pineapple Cheese Buns (1 bun)					
Entenmann's (Kraft General Foods)*	0.0	0.0	0	150	140
Raspberry Cheese Buns (1 bun)					
Entenmann's (Kraft General Foods)*	0.0	0.0	0	135	160
Raspberry Cheese Pastry (1/9 danish)					
Entenmann's (Kraft General Foods)*	0.0	0.0	0	110	140

*Tobacco company, corporate subsidiary, or parent.

	Tot. Fat (g)	Sat. Fat (g)	Chol. (mg)	Sod. (mg)	Cal.
COFFEE CAKES/DANISHES/ SWEET ROLLS *(cont'd)*					
Raspberry Twist (1/8 danish) Entenmann's (Kraft General Foods)*	0.0	0.0	0	125	140
CRACKER CRUMBS—*see* BREAD CRUMBS/CRACKER CRUMBS, page 46					
CRUMPETS—see ENGLISH MUFFINS, below					
DANISHES—see COFFEE CAKES/DANISHES/SWEET ROLLS, page 57					
ENGLISH MUFFINS					
CINNAMON RAISIN/RAISIN ENGLISH MUFFINS					
Cinnamon & Raisin Mini English Muffins (1 mini muffin) Wolferman's	0.5	0.0	0	100	80
Cinnamon Raisin Deluxe English Muffins (1 muffin) Wolferman's	2.0	1.0	0	310	240
Golden Raisin Deluxe Bran English Muffins (1 muffin) Wolferman's	1.5	(0.3)	0	540	250
Raisin Cinnamon English Muffin Slices (1 slice) Amana (Amana Society Bakery)	0.0	0.0	0	120	80
Raisin English Muffins with Cinnamon (1 muffin) S.B. Thomas (Best Foods Baking Group)	1.0	0.0	0	170	140
Raisin Rounds (1 muffin) Wonder (Continental Baking Co)	2.0	0.0	0	240	150

*Tobacco company, corporate subsidiary, or parent.

	Tot. Fat (g)	Sat. Fat (g)	Chol. (mg)	Sod. (mg)	Cal.
CRUMPETS					
Blueberry Crumpets (1 crumpet)					
Wolferman's	0.5	0.0	0	250	100
Brown Sugar Cinnamon Crumpets (1 crumpet)					
Wolferman's	1.5	0.0	0	270	100
Buttermilk Crumpets (1 crumpet)					
Wolferman's	0.5	0.0	0	260	90
Lemon Poppy Seed Crumpets (1 crumpet)					
Wolferman's	0.5	0.0	0	280	90
Original Crumpets (1 crumpet)					
Wolferman's	0.5	0.0	0	260	90
Whole Grain Crumpets (1 crumpet)					
Wolferman's	1.0	0.0	0	310	100
FRUIT ENGLISH MUFFINS					
Apple Strudel Deluxe English Muffins (1 muffin)					
Wolferman's	5.0	1.0	0	370	250
Apple Strudel Mini English Muffins (1 mini muffin)					
Wolferman's	1.0	0.0	0	150	80
Apple-Cinnamon English Muffin Slices (1 slice)					
Amana (Amana Society Bakery)	0.0	0.0	0	120	80
Banana English Muffin Slices (1 slice)					
Amana (Amana Society Bakery)	0.0	0.0	0	80	70
Blueberry Deluxe English Muffins (1 muffin)					
Wolferman's	1.0	0.5	0	300	220
Blueberry English Muffin Slices (1 slice)					
Amana (Amana Society Bakery)	0.0	0.0	0	125	80
Blueberry Mini English Muffins (1 mini muffin)					
Wolferman's	<1.0	0.0	0	170	80
Cranberry Deluxe English Muffins (1 muffin)					
Wolferman's	1.0	0.5	0	340	240

	Tot. Fat (g)	Sat. Fat (g)	Chol. (mg)	Sod. (mg)	Cal.
FRUIT ENGLISH MUFFINS *(cont'd)*					
Cranberry Mini English Muffins (1 mini muffin)					
Wolferman's	0.0	0.0	0	135	70
Cranberry-Apple English Muffin Slices (1 slice)					
Amana (Amana Society Bakery)	0.0	0.0	0	90	80
Spicy Apple Deluxe English Muffins (1 muffin)					
Wolferman's	1.0	0.5	0	550	220
PLAIN/REGULAR ENGLISH MUFFINS					
Colossal English Muffins (1 muffin)					
Dunberry (Continental Baking Co)	1.0	0.0	0	350	190
English Muffins (1 muffin)					
Wonder (Continental Baking Co)	1.0	0.0	0	290	120
Low Sodium Deluxe English Muffins (1 muffin)					
Wolferman's	1.0	0.5	0	430	220
Original Deluxe English Muffins (1 muffin)					
Wolferman's	1.0	0.0	0	410	220
Original Mini English Muffins (1 mini muffin)					
Wolferman's	0.0	0.0	0	135	70
Plain English muffins (1 muffin)					
Most brands (USDA)	**1.0**	**0.1**	**0**	**265**	**134**
Regular English Muffin Slices (1 slice)					
Amana (Amana Society Bakery)	0.0	0.0	0	125	80
Regular English Muffins (1 muffin)					
S.B. Thomas (Best Foods Baking Group)	1.0	0.0	0	200	120
RAISIN ENGLISH MUFFINS—*see* CINNAMON RAISIN/RAISIN ENGLISH MUFFINS, page 58					
REGULAR ENGLISH MUFFINS—*see* PLAIN/REGULAR ENGLISH MUFFINS, above					

	Tot. Fat (g)	Sat. Fat (g)	Chol. (mg)	Sod. (mg)	Cal.
Sourdough English Muffins					
Sourdough English Muffin Slices (1 slice)					
Amana (Amana Society Bakery)	0.0	0.0	0	120	80
Sourdough English Muffins (1 muffin)					
Wonder (Continental Baking Co)	1.0	0.0	0	290	120
Sourdough Mini English Muffins (1 mini muffin)					
Wolferman's	0.0	0.0	0	140	70
Wheat English Muffins					
Honey Wheat English Muffin Slices (1 slice)					
Amana (Amana Society Bakery)	0.0	0.0	0	120	80
Honey Wheat English Muffins (1 muffin)					
S.B. Thomas (Best Foods Baking Group)	1.0	0.0	0	190	110
Wheat Deluxe English Muffins (1 muffin)					
Wolferman's	1.0	0.0	0	470	210
Other English Muffins					
Almond Poppyseed English Muffin Slices (1 slice)					
Amana (Amana Society Bakery)	1.0	0.0	0	90	70
Heartland Harvest Deluxe English Muffins (1 muffin)					
Wolferman's	1.0	0.5	0	460	230
Honey Nut Deluxe English Muffins (1 muffin)					
Wolferman's	2.5	0.0	0	510	240
Oatmeal Cinnamon Deluxe English Muffins (1 muffin)					
Wolferman's	1.0	1.0	0	330	250
FOCACCIA					
Focaccia (1/8 slice)					
Dicarlo's (Continental Baking Co)	1.5	0.0	0	260	130
HAMBURGER/HOT DOG BUNS					
Enriched Hamburger Buns (1 bun)					
Wonder (Continental Baking Co)	2.0	0.0	0	250	110

	Tot. Fat (g)	Sat. Fat (g)	Chol. (mg)	Sod. (mg)	Cal.
HAMBURGER/HOT DOG BUNS *(cont'd)*					
Enriched Hot Dog Buns (1 bun)					
Wonder (Continental Baking Co)	2.0	0.0	0	250	110
Hamburger buns, small (1 bun)					
Most brands (USDA)	**2.2**	**0.5**	**(1)**	**241**	**123**
Hot dog buns, small (1 bun)					
Most brands (USDA)	**2.2**	**0.5**	**(1)**	**241**	**123**
Light Hamburger Buns (1 bun)					
Wonder (Continental Baking Co)	1.5	0.0	0	210	80
Light Hot Dog Buns (1 bun)					
Wonder (Continental Baking Co)	1.5	0.0	0	210	80
Potato Rolls Hamburger Buns (1 bun)					
Home Pride (Continental Baking Co)	1.5	0.0	0	270	130
Potato Rolls Hot Dog Buns (1 bun)					
Home Pride (Continental Baking Co)	1.5	0.0	0	270	130
Wheat Sandwich Buns (1 bun)					
Brownberry (Best Foods Baking Group)	2.0	0.0	0	210	130
HOT DOG BUNS—*see* HAMBURGER/HOT DOG BUNS, above					
MUFFINS—*see* "DESSERTS," MUFFINS, page 174					
PANCAKES/WAFFLES—*see also* BREAD MIXES/ROLL MIXES, page 46					
PANCAKE/WAFFLE MIXES					
Extra Lights Complete Pancake Mix, made with water (3 4″-diam pancakes)					
Pillsbury Hungry Jack (Grand Metropolitan PLC)	2.0	0.5	0	600	150
Shake 'N Pour Buttermilk Pancake Mix (3 4″-diam pancakes)					
Gold Medal (General Mills)	3.0	1.0	0	680	200

	Tot. Fat (g)	Sat. Fat (g)	Chol. (mg)	Sod. (mg)	Cal.
Prepared Pancakes/Waffles					
Apple Cinnamon Crisp & Healthy Waffles (2 waffles) Downyflake (Pet)	1.5	0.5	0	350	160
Frozen Low Fat Waffles (2 waffles) Aunt Jemima (Quaker Oats Company)	1.5	0.0	0	330	160
Frozen Low Fat Pancakes (3 pancakes) Aunt Jemima (Quaker Oats Company)	1.5	0.0	0	580	130
Plain Crisp & Healthy Waffles (2 waffles) Downyflake (Pet)	1.5	0.5	0	350	160
PITA BREADS					
Mini Pita Breads					
White pita, mini (1 4″-diam pita) **Most brands** (USDA)	**0.4**	**0.0**	**0**	**152**	**78**
Whole wheat pita, mini (1 4″-diam pita) **Most brands** (USDA)	**0.7**	**0.1**	**0**	**151**	**76**
Regular-Size Pita Breads					
Sahara Regular Oat Bran Pita Bread (1 loaf) S.B. Thomas (Best Foods Baking Group)	1.0	0.0	0	300	130
Sahara Regular White Pita Bread (1 loaf) S.B. Thomas (Best Foods Baking Group)	1.0	0.0	0	290	150
Sahara Regular Whole Wheat Pita Bread (1 loaf) S.B. Thomas (Best Foods Baking Group)	1.0	0.0	0	310	130
White pita (1 6½″-diam pita) **Most brands** (USDA)	**0.7**	**0.1**	**0**	**322**	**165**
Whole wheat pita (1 6½″-diam pita) **Most brands** (USDA)	**1.7**	**0.3**	**0**	**340**	**170**

	Tot. Fat (g)	Sat. Fat (g)	Chol. (mg)	Sod. (mg)	Cal.
PIZZA CRUSTS					
All Ready Pizza Crust (¼ crust)					
Pillsbury (Grand Metropolitan PLC)	2.5	0.5	0	390	180
Pizza Crust Mix (¼ crust)					
Robin Hood (General Mills)	2.0	<0.5	0	340	160
Pizza Crust Mix, dry (⅓ cup)					
Ragú (Van den Bergh Foods)	1.0	0.0	0	270	130
Regular Crust Pizza Mix (⅓ pizza)					
Appian Way (Dial Corp)	3.0	1.0	0	740	250
ROLLS—*see also* BREAD MIXES/ROLL MIXES, page 46					
FRENCH ROLLS					
French Petite Roll (1 roll)					
Bread du Jour (Continental Baking Co)	2.0	0.0	0	530	230
French Rolls (1 roll)					
Dicarlo's (Continental Baking Co)	1.0	0.0	0	150	70
HARD ROLLS					
Hard rolls (1 3½"-diam roll)					
Most brands (USDA)	**2.4**	**0.3**	**0**	**310**	**167**
WHEAT ROLLS					
Ready-to-Cook Wheat Rolls					
Wheat Brown 'N Serve Rolls (1 roll)					
Wonder (Continental Baking Co)	0.5	0.0	0	135	70
Ready-to-Eat Wheat Rolls					
Bavarian Cracked Wheat Rolls (1 roll)					
Bread du Jour (Continental Baking Co)	1.0	0.0	0	190	90
WHITE ROLLS					
Ready-to-Cook White Rolls					
White Brown 'N Serve Rolls (1 roll)					
Wonder (Continental Baking Co)	0.5	0.0	0	135	70
Ready-to-Eat White Rolls					
Crusty Italian Rolls (1 roll)					
Bread du Jour (Continental Baking Co)	0.5	0.0	0	190	80

	Tot. Fat (g)	Sat. Fat (g)	Chol. (mg)	Sod. (mg)	Cal.
Extra Sourdough Rolls (1 roll)					
Dicarlo's (Continental Baking Co)	1.0	0.0	0	230	100
Light White Dinner Rolls (1 roll)					
Wonder (Continental Baking Co)	1.0	0.0	0	150	60
Potato Dinner Rolls (2 rolls)					
Arnold (Best Foods Baking Group)	1.5	0.0	0	125	110
Sourdough Rolls (1 roll)					
Bread du Jour (Continental Baking Co)	1.5	0.0	0	230	140
White Tea Dinner Rolls (1 roll)					
Wonder (Continental Baking Co)	1.0	0.0	0	210	80
OTHER ROLLS					
Ready-to-Eat Rolls					
Four Grain Roll (1 Sweden Crisp)					
Olof Sweden Crisp (Andre Prost)	<1.0	0.0	0	35	43
Oat Bran Roll (1 Sweden Crisp)					
Olof Sweden Crisp (Andre Prost)	1.2	0.2	0	32	44
Rye Rolls (1 roll)					
Bread du Jour (Continental Baking Co)	1.5	0.0	0	230	90
Whole Grain Roll (1 Sweden Crisp)					
Olof Sweden Crisp (Andre Prost)	<1.0	0.0	0	75	42
SCONES					
Blueberry Flavored Scones (1 scone)					
Dunberry (Continental Baking Co)	3.0	1.0	0	280	160
Cinnamon Raisin Flavored Scones (1 scone)					
Dunberry (Continental Baking Co)	3.0	1.0	0	300	150
SWEET ROLLS—*see* COFFEE CAKES/DANISHES/SWEET ROLLS, page 57					
TORTILLAS					
Corn tortillas (2 tortillas)					
Most brands (USDA)	**1.2**	**0.2**	**0**	**80**	**112**

	Tot. Fat (g)	Sat. Fat (g)	Chol. (mg)	Sod. (mg)	Cal.
TORTILLAS *(cont'd)*					
Honey Wheat Tortillas (1 tortilla)					
Soft Wraps (Continental Baking Co)	1.5	0.0	0	280	120
Original Tortillas (1 tortilla)					
Soft Wraps (Continental Baking Co)	1.5	0.0	0	280	110
Wraps (1 slice)					
Valley (Valley Bakery)	1.0	1.0	0	125	100

WAFFLES—*see* PANCAKES/ WAFFLES, page 62

CEREALS

Whole-grain cereals start out healthful and delicious. They naturally contain just a small amount of fat, but manufacturers often make them higher in fat in two ways:

1. They add nuts, coconut, or seeds; and/or
2. They spray the cereal with fat-based coatings that help retain crispness.

Crispness is fine; fat isn't. First, choose a cereal, such as the ones listed on the following tables, without a lot of added fat. Then use skim milk or 1% milk.

Like all the other entries in this book, the cereals entries that follow list sodium content. The AHA does not have criteria for sodium but recommends a total of no more than 3,000 mg a day.

Generic Listings

By far, most of the foods in this book are brand name products. However, if a product is listed without a brand name, it means that most brands of that product contain about the same amount of fat, saturated fat, and cholesterol and that these amounts are within the criteria cited below.

If you find products that were introduced after this book went to press, use the generic listings and the following tables to help you evaluate them.

AHA Criteria for Cereals*

	Tot. Fat (g)	Sat. Fat (g)	Chol. (mg)
All cooked and ready-to-eat cereals	3	<0.5	<2

*Per serving.

Cereals You'll Want to Limit

Some cereals, like the example below, are too high in fat, saturated fat, and/or cholesterol to meet AHA criteria. They aren't included in this book, and we recommend that you don't eat them often.

Compare the amounts of fat, saturated fat, cholesterol, sodium, and calories in this example with the more healthful alternatives listed on the following pages.

Sample Cereal to Limit

	Tot. Fat (g)	Sat. Fat (g)	Chol. (mg)	Sod. (mg)	Cal.
100% natural cereal (granola), plain (¼ cup)	6.1*	4.1*	(0)	12	133

Adapted from USDA Handbook No. 8 series.

*These values exceed AHA criteria for cereals.

	Tot. Fat (g)	Sat. Fat (g)	Chol. (mg)	Sod. (mg)	Cal.
COOKED CEREALS					
Bran Cereals, Cooked					
Organically Produced Oat Bran (⅓ cup dry)					
Arrowhead Mills	2.5	0.0	0	0	150
Organically Produced Wheat Bran (¼ cup dry)					
Arrowhead Mills	0.5	0.0	0	0	30
Farina—*see* Wheat Cereals, Cooked, Instant/Quick Wheat Cereals, Cooked, page 70; Regular Wheat Cereals, Cooked, page 71					
Grits					
Instant Grits					
Hominy Quick Grits (¼ cup dry)					
Alber's (Nestlé Food Company)	0.5	0.0	0	0	140
Instant Grits Original Flavor (1 pkt)					
Quaker (Quaker Oats Co)	0.0	0.0	0	300	100
Instant Grits with Bacon Bits (1 pkt)					
Quaker (Quaker Oats Co)	0.5	0.0	0	340	100
Instant Grits with Butter Flavor (1 pkt)					
Quaker (Quaker Oats Co)	1.5	0.0	0	320	100
Instant Grits with Red Eye Gravy and Ham (1 pkt)					
Quaker (Quaker Oats Co)	0.5	0.0	0	530	90
Instant Grits with Sausage Bits (1 pkt)					
Quaker (Quaker Oats Co)	1.0	0.0	0	480	100
Regular Grits					
Corn grits (1 cup cooked)					
Most brands (USDA)	**0.5**	**0.1**	**0**	**0**	**146**
Multigrain Cereals, Cooked					
Multigrain Hot Cereal					
Mother's (Quaker Oats Co) (½ cup dry)	1.5	0.0	0	10	130
Pritikin (Quaker Oats Co) (1 pkt)	1.5	0.0	0	0	160
Organically Produced 7 Grain Cereal (⅓ cup dry)					
Arrowhead Mills	1.5	0.0	0	0	140

	Tot. Fat (g)	Sat. Fat (g)	Chol. (mg)	Sod. (mg)	Cal.
OAT BRAN CEREALS, COOKED					
Oat Bran, Cooked					
Most brands (USDA) (1 cup cooked)	**1.9**	**0.4**	**0**	**2**	**87**
Mother's (Quaker Oats Co) (½ cup dry)	3.0	1.0	0	0	150
Quaker (Quaker Oats Co) (½ cup dry)	3.0	1.0	0	0	150
OATMEAL					
Instant/Quick Oatmeal					
Cinnamon Toast Flavor Instant Oatmeal (1 pkt)					
Quaker (Quaker Oats Co)	2.0	0.0	0	160	130
Cinnamon-Spice Instant Oatmeal (1 pkt)					
Quaker (Quaker Oats Co)	2.0	0.0	0	290	170
Instant/Quick Oatmeal (1 cup cooked)					
Most brands (USDA)	**2.4**	**0.4**	**0**	**1**	**145**
Regular Oatmeal					
Oatmeal (1 cup cooked)					
Most brands (USDA)	**2.4**	**0.4**	**0**	**1**	**145**
RICE CEREALS, COOKED					
Brown Rice Cream (¼ cup dry)					
Erewhon (U.S. Mills)	1.0	0.0	0	30	170
Cream of Rice (¼ cup dry)					
Nabisco (Nabisco Foods)*	0.0	0.0	0	0	170
WHEAT CEREALS, COOKED					
Instant/Quick Wheat Cereals, Cooked					
Farina, made with water and salt (⅔ cup)					
Pillsbury (Grand Metropolitan PLC)	0.0	0.0	0	270	80
Instant Cream of Wheat (3 tbsp dry)					
Nabisco (Nabisco Foods)*	0.0	0.0	0	85	120
Instant Cream of Wheat Hot Cereal Cinnamon Toast (1 pkt)					
Nabisco (Nabisco Foods)*	0.0	0.0	0	170	130
Instant Cream of Wheat Hot Cereal Fruit Variety Pack (1 pkt)					
Nabisco (Nabisco Foods)*	0.0	0.0	0	170	130

*Tobacco company, corporate subsidiary, or parent.

	Tot. Fat (g)	Sat. Fat (g)	Chol. (mg)	Sod. (mg)	Cal.
Instant Cream of Wheat Hot Cereal with real Apple 'n Cinnamon (1 pkt)					
Nabisco (Nabisco Foods)*	0.0	0.0	0	300	130
Instant Cream of Wheat Hot Cereal with real Brown Sugar Cinnamon (1 pkt)					
Nabisco (Nabisco Foods)*	0.0	0.0	0	220	130
Instant Cream of Wheat Original Hot Cereal (1 pkt)					
Nabisco (Nabisco Foods)*	0.0	0.0	0	260	100
Quick Cream of Wheat (3 tbsp dry)					
Nabisco (Nabisco Foods)*	0.0	0.0	0	85	120
Wheat Hearts (¼ cup dry)					
General Mills	1.0	0.0	0	0	130
Whole Wheat Natural Cereal (½ cup dry)					
Mother's (Quaker Oats Co)	1.0	0.0	0	0	130
Regular Wheat Cereals, Cooked					
Bear Mush (¼ cup dry)					
Arrowhead Mills	1.0	0.0	0	0	160
Farina (1 cup cooked)					
Most brands (USDA)	**0.2**	**0.0**	**0**	**1**	**116**
Organically Produced Cracked Wheat Cereal (¼ cup dry)					
Arrowhead Mills	0.5	0.0	0	0	140
Regular Cream of Wheat (3 tbsp dry)					
Nabisco (Nabisco Foods)*	0.0	0.0	0	0	120
Other Cooked Cereals					
Barley Plus (¼ cup dry)					
Erewhon (U.S. Mills)	1.0	0.0	0	0	170
READY-TO-EAT CEREALS					
Bran/Fiber Cereals, Ready to Eat					
All-Bran (½ cup)					
Kellogg's	1.0	0.0	0	280	80
All-Bran with Extra Fiber (½ cup)					
Kellogg's	1.0	0.0	0	150	50
Bran Buds (⅓ cup)					
Kellogg's	0.5	0.0	0	210	70

*Tobacco company, corporate subsidiary, or parent.

	Tot. Fat (g)	Sat. Fat (g)	Chol. (mg)	Sod. (mg)	Cal.
Bran/Fiber Cereals, Ready to Eat *(cont'd)*					
Bran Flakes (⅔ cup)					
Post (Kraft General Foods)*	0.5	0.0	0	210	90
Ralston (Ralston Foods)	1.0	0.0	0	220	110
Complete Bran Flakes (1 cup)					
Kellogg's	0.5	0.0	0	230	100
Crunchy Bran (¾ cup)					
Quaker (Quaker Oats Co)	1.0	0.0	0	250	90
Fat Free Healthy Fiber Flakes (¾ cup)					
Health Valley (Health Valley Foods)	0.0	0.0	0	10	100
Fiber One (½ cup)					
General Mills	1.0	0.0	0	140	60
Fiber 7 Flakes (¾ cup)					
Health Valley (Health Valley Foods)	0.0	0.0	0	10	100
Frosted Bran (¾ cup)					
Kellogg's	0.0	0.0	0	200	100
Fruit & Fibre Dates, Raisins & Walnuts Cereal (1 cup)					
Post (Kraft General Foods)*	3.0	0.5	0	260	210
Fruit & Fibre Peaches, Raisins & Almonds Cereal (1 cup)					
Post (Kraft General Foods)*	3.0	0.5	0	270	210
Multi-Bran Chex (1¼ cups)					
Ralston (Ralston Foods)	2.0	0.0	0	320	220
Oat Bran O's Cereal (¾ cup)					
Health Valley (Health Valley Foods)	0.0	0.0	0	10	110
Oat Bran with Toasted Wheat Germ (⅓ cup)					
Erewhon (U.S. Mills)	2.5	0.5	0	0	170
100% Bran Cereal (⅓ cup)					
Nabisco (Kraft General Foods)*	0.5	0.0	0	120	80
Organic Bran Cereal with Apples and Cinnamon (¾ cup)					
Health Valley (Health Valley Foods)	0.0	0.0	0	10	170

*Tobacco company, corporate subsidiary, or parent.

	Tot. Fat (g)	Sat. Fat (g)	Chol. (mg)	Sod. (mg)	Cal.
Organic Bran Cereal with Raisins (¾ cup)					
Health Valley (Health Valley Foods)	0.0	0.0	0	10	190
Ripple Crisp Honey Bran (1¼ cups)					
General Mills	1.0	0.0	0	410	190
10 Bran Apple Cinnamon Cereal (¾ cup)					
Health Valley (Health Valley Foods)	0.0	0.0	0	10	110
Toasted Wheat Bran (¼ cup)					
Quaker (Quaker Oats Co)	1.0	0.0	0	0	30
Unprocessed Bran (⅓ cup)					
Quaker (Quaker Oats Co)	0.0	0.0	0	190	30
CORN CEREALS, READY TO EAT					
Corn Flakes					
Blue Corn Flakes (¾ cup)					
Health Valley (Health Valley Foods)	0.0	0.0	0	10	90
Corn Flakes					
Erewhon (U.S. Mills) (1¼ cups)	2.5	0.0	0	100	210
Kellogg's (1 cup)	0.0	0.0	0	330	110
Malt-O-Meal (1 cup)	0.0	0.0	0	280	100
Ralston (Ralston Foods) (1¼ cups)	0.0	0.0	0	280	120
Country Corn Flakes (1 cup)					
General Mills	0.5	0.0	0	290	120
Frosted Flakes (¾ cup)					
Kellogg's	0.0	0.0	0	200	120
Malt-O-Meal	0.0	0.0	0	190	110
Ralston (Ralston Foods)	0.0	0.0	0	180	120
Kids Favorites Sugar Frosted Flakes (¾ cup)					
Quaker (Quaker Oats Co)	0.0	0.0	0	250	110
Post Toasties Cereal (1 cup)					
Post (Kraft General Foods)*	0.0	0.0	0	270	100
Total Corn Flakes (1⅓ cups)					
General Mills	0.5	0.0	0	210	110
Corn Puffs					
Berry Berry Kix (¾ cup)					
General Mills	1.5	0.0	0	180	120

*Tobacco company, corporate subsidiary, or parent.

	Tot. Fat (g)	Sat. Fat (g)	Chol. (mg)	Sod. (mg)	Cal.
Corn Cereals, Ready to Eat *(cont'd)*					
Body Buddies, Natural Fruit Flavor (1 cup)					
General Mills	1.0	0.0	0	290	110
Cocoa Puffs (1 cup)					
General Mills	1.0	0.0	0	190	120
Corn Pops (1 cup)					
Kellogg's	0.0	0.0	0	95	110
Count Chocula (1 cup)					
General Mills	1.0	0.0	0	190	120
Honey Crisp Corn (1 cup)					
Erewhon (U.S. Mills)	2.5	0.0	0	100	210
Kix (1⅓ cups)					
General Mills	1.0	0.0	0	270	120
Popeye Jeepers Crispy Corn Puffs Cereal (1⅓ cups)					
Quaker (Quaker Oats Co)	0.5	0.0	0	150	110
Puffed Corn Cereal (1 cup)					
Health Valley (Health Valley Foods)	0.0	0.0	0	0	80
Trix (1 cup)					
General Mills	1.5	0.0	0	140	120
Other Corn Cereals, Ready to Eat					
Boo Berry (1 cup)					
General Mills	1.0	0.0	0	200	120
Cap'N Crunch (25 g)					
Quaker (Quaker Oats Co)	1.5	0.0	0	190	100
Cap'N Crunch with Crunchberries (¾ cup)					
Quaker (Quaker Oats Co)	1.5	0.0	0	190	100
Cap'N Crunch's Christmas Crunch (¾ cup)					
Quaker (Quaker Oats Co)	1.5	0.0	0	190	100
Cap'N Crunch's Deep Sea Crunch (25 g)					
Quaker (Quaker Oats Co)	1.5	0.0	0	120	100
Coco-Roos (¾ cup)					
Malt-O-Meal	1.0	0.0	0	190	120

	Tot. Fat (g)	Sat. Fat (g)	Chol. (mg)	Sod. (mg)	Cal.
Cocoa Crunchies (¾ cup)					
Ralston (Ralston Foods)	1.0	0.0	0	170	120
Corn Chex (1¼ cups)					
Ralston (Ralston Foods)	0.0	0.0	0	270	110
Crisp Crunch (¾ cup)					
Ralston (Ralston Foods)	1.0	0.0	0	240	120
Frankenberry (1 cup)					
General Mills	1.0	0.0	0	200	120
King Vitamin (1½ cups)					
Quaker (Quaker Oats Co)	1.0	0.0	0	260	120
Nut & Honey Crunch (⅔ cup)					
Kellogg's	2.0	0.0	0	200	120
Popeye Jeepers Cereal (1⅓ cups)					
Quaker (Quaker Oats Co)	1.0	0.0	0	140	110
Ripple Crisp Honey Corn (¾ cup)					
General Mills	0.5	0.0	0	290	110
Sprinkle Spangles (1 cup)					
General Mills	1.5	0.0	0	125	120
FIBER CEREALS, READY TO EAT—*see* BRAN/FIBER CEREALS, READY TO EAT, page 71					
FRUIT CEREALS, READY TO EAT—*see also* RAISIN BRAN, READY TO EAT, page 81					
Apple Raisin Crisp (1 cup)					
Kellogg's	0.0	0.0	0	340	180
Blueberry Fruit Wheats Cereal (¾ cup)					
Nabisco (Kraft General Foods)* .	0.5	0.0	0	15	170
Blueberry Squares (1 cup)					
Kellogg's	1.0	0.0	0	15	180
Cranberry Muesli (¾ cup)					
Ralston (Ralston Foods)	3.0	0.0	0	180	200
Fruitful Bran (1¼ cups)					
Kellogg's	0.5	0.0	0	330	170
Fruit'n Wheat (¾ cup)					
Erewhon (U.S. Mills)	1.5	0.0	0	105	170
Just Right Fruit & Nut (1 cup)					
Kellogg's	2.0	0.0	0	250	200

*Tobacco company, corporate subsidiary, or parent.

	Tot. Fat (g)	Sat. Fat (g)	Chol. (mg)	Sod. (mg)	Cal.
FRUIT CEREALS, READY TO EAT *(cont'd)*					
Mueslix Crispy Blend (⅔ cup)					
Kellogg's	3.0	0.0	0	190	200
Nutri-Grain Almond Raisin (1¼ cups)					
Kellogg's	3.0	0.0	0	330	200
Peach Muesli (¾ cup)					
Ralston (Ralston Foods)	3.0	0.0	0	170	200
Raisin Squares (¾ cup)					
Kellogg's	1.0	0.0	0	0	180
Raspberry Fruit Wheats Cereal (¾ cup)					
Nabisco (Kraft General Foods)*	0.5	0.0	0	15	160
Raspberry Muesli (¾ cup)					
Ralston (Ralston Foods)	3.0	0.0	0	170	220
Strawberry Fruit Wheats Cereal (¾ cup)					
Nabisco (Kraft General Foods)*	0.5	0.0	0	15	170
Strawberry Squares (1 cup)					
Kellogg's	1.0	0.0	0	10	180
GRANOLA CEREALS, READY TO EAT					
Cinnamon & Raisins Low Fat Granola (½ cup)					
General Mills	2.5	0.0	0	210	210
Fat-Free Almond Granola O's Cereal (¾ cup)					
Health Valley (Health Valley Foods)	0.0	0.0	0	10	120
Fat-Free Apples and Cinnamon Granola O's Cereal (¾ cup)					
Health Valley (Health Valley Foods)	0.0	0.0	0	10	120
Fat-Free Date and Almond Granola (⅔ cup)					
Health Valley (Health Valley Foods)	0.0	0.0	0	25	180
Fat-Free Honey Crunch Granola O's Cereal (¾ cup)					
Health Valley (Health Valley Foods)	0.0	0.0	0	10	120

*Tobacco company, corporate subsidiary, or parent.

	Tot. Fat (g)	Sat. Fat (g)	Chol. (mg)	Sod. (mg)	Cal.
Fat-Free Raisin Cinnamon Granola (⅔ cup) Health Valley (Health Valley Foods)	0.0	0.0	0	25	180
Fat-Free Tropical Fruit Granola (⅔ cup) Health Valley (Health Valley Foods)	0.0	0.0	0	25	180
Low Fat Granola (½ cup) Kellogg's	3.0	0.0	0	70	210
Low Fat Granola with Raisins (⅔ cup) Kellogg's	3.0	0.0	0	65	210
Multigrain Cereals, Ready to Eat					
Amaranth Flakes (¾ cup) Health Valley (Health Valley Foods)	0.0	0.0	0	10	100
Apple Jacks (1 cup) Kellogg's	0.0	0.0	0	135	110
Apple Stroodles (¾ cup) Erewhon (U.S. Mills)	0.5	0.0	0	15	110
Aztec (1 cup) Erewhon (U.S. Mills)	0.0	0.0	0	70	110
Basic 4 (1 cup) General Mills	3.0	0.0	0	310	210
Cinnamon Mini Buns (¾ cup) Kellogg's	0.5	0.0	0	210	120
Cookie Crisp (1 cup) Ralston (Ralston Foods)	1.5	0.0	0	110	120
Crispix (1 cup) Kellogg's	0.0	0.0	0	230	110
Double Chex (1¼ cups) Ralston (Ralston Foods)	0.0	0.0	0	230	120
Double Dip Crunch (¾ cup) Kellogg's	0.0	0.0	0	160	110
8 Grain Flakes (1 cup) Lifestream Natural Foods	0.0	0.0	0	20	210
Froot Loops (1 cup) Kellogg's	1.0	0.0	0	125	120
Fruit Rings (¾ cup) Ralston (Ralston Foods)	1.0	0.0	0	115	100

	Tot. Fat (g)	Sat. Fat (g)	Chol. (mg)	Sod. (mg)	Cal.
MULTIGRAIN CEREALS, READY TO EAT *(cont'd)*					
Golden Grahams (¾ cup) General Mills	1.0	0.0	0	280	120
Graham Chex (1 cup) Ralston (Ralston Foods)	1.5	0	0	340	210
Grape-Nuts Cereal (½ cup) Post (Kraft General Foods)*	1.0	0.0	0	350	200
Grape-Nuts Flakes (¾ cup) Post (Kraft General Foods)*	1.0	0.0	0	140	100
Healthy Choice Multi-Grain Flakes (1 cup) Kellogg's	0.0	0.0	0	210	100
Healthy Choice Multi-Grain Squares (1¼ cups) Kellogg's	1.0	0.0	0	0	190
Healthy Choice Multi-Grains, Raisins, Oat Clusters & Almonds (1¼ cups) Kellogg's	2.0	0.0	0	250	200
Honey Puffed Kashi Seven Whole Grains and Sesame (1 cup) Kashi (Kashi Company)	1.0	0.0	0	6	120
Honeycomb Cereal (1⅓ cups) Post (Kraft General Foods)*	0.0	0.0	0	190	110
Just Right with Crunchy Nuggets (1 cup) Kellogg's	1.5	0.0	0	330	200
Kamut Flakes (⅔ cup) Erewhon (U.S. Mills)	0.0	0.0	0	75	110
Kashi Seven Whole Grains and Sesame Medley (½ cup) Kashi (Kashi Company)	1.0	0.0	0	50	100
Life (¾ cup) Quaker (Quaker Oats Co)	1.5	0.0	0	170	120
Multi Grain Cheerios (1 cup) General Mills	1.0	0.0	0	240	110
Multigrain Honey Puffs (¾ cup) Lifestream Natural Foods	3.0	0.0	0	15	130

*Tobacco company, corporate subsidiary, or parent.

	Tot. Fat (g)	Sat. Fat (g)	Chol. (mg)	Sod. (mg)	Cal.
Nutri-Grain Golden Wheat & Raisins (1¼ cups) Kellogg's	1.0	0.0	0	310	180
Organically Produced Kamut Flakes (⅓ cup) Arrowhead Mills	1.0	0.0	0	0	130
Popeye Fruit Curls (1 cup) Quaker (Quaker Oats Co)	1.0	0.0	0	170	120
Product 19 (1 cup) Kellogg's	1.0	0.0	0	610	200
Puffed Kashi (1 cup) Kashi (Kashi Company)	<1.0	0.0	0	0	70
Team Flakes (1¼ cups) Nabisco (Kraft General Foods)*	0.0	0.0	0	360	220
Tootie Fruities (1 cup) Malt-O-Meal	1.0	0.0	0	130	110
Triples (1 cup) General Mills	1.0	0.0	0	190	120
OAT BRAN CEREALS, READY TO EAT					
Oat Bran Cereal (1¼ cups) Quaker (Quaker Oats Co)	3.0	0.5	0	210	210
Oat Bran Flakes (¾ cup) Health Valley (Health Valley Foods)	0.0	0.0	0	10	100
Oat Bran Flakes with Raisins (¾ cup) Health Valley (Health Valley Foods)	0.0	0.0	0	10	100
OAT CEREALS, READY TO EAT					
Alpha Bits Cereal (1 cup) Post (Kraft General Foods)*	1.0	0.0	0	210	130
Apple Cinnamon O's (¾ cup) Lifestream Natural Foods	0.0	0.0	0	10	120
Apple-Cinnamon Tasteeos (1 cup) Ralston (Ralston Foods)	1.5	0.0	0	150	130
Apple Cinnamon Toasty O's (¾ cup) Malt-O-Meal	2.0	0.0	0	170	110
Banana-O's (¾ cup) Erewhon (U.S. Mills)	0.0	0.0	0	15	110
Cinnamon Oat Squares (1 cup) Quaker (Quaker Oats Co)	2.5	0.5	0	260	230

*Tobacco company, corporate subsidiary, or parent.

	Tot. Fat (g)	Sat. Fat (g)	Chol. (mg)	Sod. (mg)	Cal.
OAT CEREALS, READY TO EAT *(cont'd)*					
Honey & Nut Toasty O's (¾ cup) Malt-O-Meal	1.0	0.0	0	170	100
Honey Bunches of Oats with Almonds Cereal (¾ cup) Post (Kraft General Foods)*	3.0	0.5	0	180	130
Honey Graham Oh!s (¾ cup) Quaker (Quaker Oats Co)	2.0	0.5	0	180	110
Honey Nut Cheerios (1 cup) General Mills	1.5	0.0	0	270	120
Honey Nut Tasteeos (1 cup) Ralston (Ralston Foods)	1.5	0.0	0	250	130
Lucky Charms (1 cup) General Mills	1.0	0.0	0	210	120
Magic Stars (¾ cup) Ralston (Ralston Foods)	1.0	0.0	0	160	120
Marshmallow Alpha-Bits Cereal (1 cup) Post (Kraft General Foods)*	1.0	0.0	0	160	120
Marshmallow Mateys (1 cup) Malt-O-Meal	1.0	0.0	0	170	100
Nut & Honey Crunch O's (¾ cup) Kellogg's	2.5	0.0	0	200	120
Oat Cinnamon Life (1 cup) Quaker (Quaker Oats Co)	2.0	0.0	0	220	190
Oat Squares (1 cup) Quaker (Quaker Oats Co)	3.0	0.5	0	260	220
Oatmeal Crisp with Apples (1 cup) General Mills	2.5	0.0	0	350	210
Oatmeal Crisp with Raisins (1 cup) General Mills	3.0	0.0	0	260	210
Organically Produced Nature O's (1 cup) Arrowhead Mills	2.0	0.5	0	5	130
Organically Produced Oat Flakes (⅓ cup) Arrowhead Mills	2.5	0.5	0	0	130
Popeye Oat'MMMS Toasted Oat Cereal (1 cup) Quaker (Quaker Oats Co)	1.5	0.0	0	160	110

*Tobacco company, corporate subsidiary, or parent.

	Tot. Fat (g)	Sat. Fat (g)	Chol. (mg)	Sod. (mg)	Cal.
Super-O's (⅔ cup)					
Erewhon (U.S. Mills)	0.0	0.0	0	60	110
Tasteeos (1¼ cups)					
Ralston (Ralston Foods)	2.5	0.0	0	260	130
Toasted Oatmeal (1 pouch)					
Quaker (Quaker Oats Co)	0.5	0.0	0	140	80
Toasty O's (1 cup)					
Malt-O-Meal	2.0	0.0	0	220	100
RAISIN BRAN, READY TO EAT					
Raisin Bran Cereal					
Erewhon (U.S. Mills) (1 cup)	0.5	0.0	0	100	160
Health Valley (Health Valley Foods) (1¼ cups)	0.0	0.0	0	20	200
Kellogg's (1 cup)	1.0	0.0	0	300	170
Malt-O-Meal (1¼ cups)	1.0	0.0	0	290	200
Post (Kraft General Foods)* (1 cup)	1.0	0.0	0	300	190
Ralston (Ralston Foods) (¾ cup)	1.0	0.0	0	290	190
Total Raisin Bran (1 cup)					
General Mills	1.0	0.0	0	240	180
RICE CEREALS, READY TO EAT					
All Natural Nutty Rice Original Cereal (½ cup)					
Pacific Grain Products	1.5	0.0	0	110	210
Apple Cinnamon Rice Krispies (¾ cup)					
Kellogg's	0.0	0.0	0	220	110
Cocoa Crispy Rice (1 cup)					
Ralston (Ralston Foods)	1.0	0.0	0	340	200
Cocoa Krispies (¾ cup)					
Kellogg's	0.5	0.0	0	190	120
Crisp Rice (1¼ cups)					
Ralston (Ralston Foods)	0.0	0.0	0	330	130
Crispy Brown Rice (1 cup)					
Erewhon (U.S. Mills)	0.0	0.0	0	180	110
Health Valley (Health Valley Foods)	0.0	0.0	0	0	110
Crispy Rice (1 cup)					
Malt-O-Meal	0.0	0.0	0	250	120
Frosted Krispies (¾ cup)					
Kellogg's	0.0	0.0	0	230	110

*Tobacco company, corporate subsidiary, or parent.

	Tot. Fat (g)	Sat. Fat (g)	Chol. (mg)	Sod. (mg)	Cal.
RICE CEREALS, READY TO EAT *(cont'd)*					
Fruity Marshmallow Krispies (¾ cup)					
Kellogg's	0.0	0.0	0	180	110
Kenmei Rice Bran (¾ cup)					
Kellogg's	1.0	0.0	0	250	110
No Salt Added Crispy Brown Rice (1 cup)					
Erewhon (U.S. Mills)	0.0	0.0	0	10	110
Poppets (1 cup)					
Erewhon (U.S. Mills)	1.0	0.0	0	10	120
Puffed Rice					
Malt-O-Meal (1 cup)	0.0	0.0	0	0	60
Quaker (Quaker Oats Co) (1 g)	0.0	0.0	0	0	40
Rice Chex (1 cup)					
Ralston (Ralston Foods)	0.0	0.0	0	230	120
Rice Krispies (1¼ cups)					
Kellogg's	0.0	0.0	0	360	110
Rice Krispies Treats Cereal (¾ cup)					
Kellogg's	1.5	0.0	0	170	120
Special K (1 cup)					
Kellogg's	0.0	0.0	0	250	110
WHEAT CEREALS, READY TO EAT					
Shredded Wheat					
Apple Cinnamon Squares (¾ cup)					
Kellogg's	1.0	0.0	0	15	180
Frosted Mini-Wheats (1 cup)					
Kellogg's	1.0	0.0	0	0	190
Frosted Mini-Wheats Bite Size (1 cup)					
Kellogg's	1.0	0.0	0	0	190
Frosted Wheat Bites Cereal (1 cup)					
Nabisco (Kraft General Foods)*	1.0	0.0	0	10	190
Shredded Wheat Cereal					
Nabisco (Kraft General Foods)* (2 biscuits)	0.5	0.0	0	0	160
Quaker (Quaker Oats Co) (3 biscuits)	1.5	0.5	0	0	110

*Tobacco company, corporate subsidiary, or parent.

	Tot. Fat (g)	Sat. Fat (g)	Chol. (mg)	Sod. (mg)	Cal.
Shredded Wheat'N Bran Cereal (1¼ cups)					
Nabisco (Kraft General Foods)* .	1.0	0.0	0	0	200
Spoon Size Shredded Wheat Cereal (1 cup)					
Nabisco (Kraft General Foods)* .	0.5	0.0	0	0	170
Wheat Flakes					
Crispy Wheats 'n Raisins (1 cup)					
General Mills	1.0	0.0	0	270	190
Multi-Vitamin Whole Grain Flakes (1 cup)					
Ralston (Ralston Foods)	1.0	0.0	0	300	120
Organically Produced Wheat Flakes (⅓ cup)					
Arrowhead Mills	0.5	0.0	0	0	110
Wheat Flakes (1 cup)					
Erewhon (U.S. Mills)	0.5	0.0	0	135	180
Wheaties Honey Gold (¾ cup)					
General Mills	0.5	0.0	0	200	110
Wheat Germ					
Honey Crunch Wheat Germ (1⅔ tbsp)					
Quaker (Quaker Oats Co)	1.0	0.0	0	0	50
Toasted wheat germ (⅛ cup)					
Most brands (USDA)	**1.5**	**0.3**	**0**	**1**	**54**
Wheat Germ					
Arrowhead Mills (3 tbsp)	0.5	0.0	0	0	50
Quaker (Quaker Oats Co) (2 tbsp)	1.0	0.0	0	0	50
Wheat Puffs					
Golden Crisp Cereal (¾ cup)					
Post (Kraft General Foods)*	0.0	0.0	0	40	110
Golden Sugar Puffs (¾ cup)					
Malt-O-Meal	0.0	0.0	0	25	100
Puffed Wheat					
Malt-O-Meal (1 cup)	0.0	0.0	0	0	50
Quaker (Quaker Oats Co) (1 g) .	0.0	0.0	0	0	35
Smacks (¾ cup)					
Kellogg's	0.5	0.0	0	75	110

*Tobacco company, corporate subsidiary, or parent.

	Tot. Fat (g)	Sat. Fat (g)	Chol. (mg)	Sod. (mg)	Cal.
WHEAT CEREALS, READY TO EAT *(cont'd)*					
Sweet Puffs (1 cup)					
Quaker (Quaker Oats Co)	0.5	0.0	0	80	130
Other Wheat Cereals, Ready to Eat					
Almond Delight (1 cup)					
Ralston (Ralston Foods)	3.0	0.0	0	410	210
Nutri-Grain Golden Wheat (¾ cup)					
Kellogg's	0.5	0.0	0	240	100
Nutty Nuggets (½ cup)					
Ralston (Ralston Foods)	1.5	0.0	0	220	180
Wheat Chex (1¼ cups)					
Ralston (Ralston Foods)	1.0	0.0	0	390	190
OTHER READY-TO-EAT CEREALS					
Almond Flavor Honey Clusters and Flakes Cereal (¾ cup)					
Health Valley (Health Valley Foods)	0.0	0.0	0	20	130
Apple Cinnamon Honey Clusters and Flakes Cereal (¾ cup)					
Health Valley (Health Valley Foods)	0.0	0.0	0	20	130
Galaxy Grahams (¾ cup)					
Erewhon (U.S. Mills)	0.5	0.0	0	60	100
Honey Crunch Honey Clusters and Flakes Cereal (¾ cup)					
Health Valley (Health Valley Foods)	0.0	0.0	0	20	130
Kaboom (1¼ cups)					
General Mills	1.5	0.0	0	280	120
Organically Produced Barley Flakes (⅓ cup)					
Arrowhead Mills	1.0	0.0	0	0	110
Organically Produced Rye Flakes (⅓ cup)					
Arrowhead Mills	0.5	0.0	0	0	110
Raisin Grahams (1 cup)					
Erewhon (U.S. Mills)	1.0	0.0	0	105	190

CONDIMENTS

What would Mexican food be without chili peppers? Or Chinese food without hot mustard? The simple truth is, condiments lift ordinary foods to new heights.

Fortunately, most condiments are low in calories and contain little or no fat and cholesterol. Olives are an exception. They do contain fat, so we've listed them in the "Fats and Oils" chapter on page 197.

Like all the other entries in this book, the condiments entries that follow list sodium content. The AHA does not have criteria for sodium but recommends a total of no more than 3,000 mg a day.

Generic Listings

By far, most of the foods in this book are brand name products. However, if a product is listed without a brand name, it means that most brands of that product contain about the same amount of fat, saturated fat, and cholesterol and that these amounts are within the criteria cited below.

If you find products that were introduced after this book went to press, use the generic listings and the following tables to help you evaluate them.

AHA Criteria for Condiments*

	Tot. Fat (g)	Sat. Fat (g)	Chol. (mg)
Horseradish, hot sauce, ketchup, marinade, mustard, soy sauce, steak sauce, teriyaki sauce	<0.5	<0.5	<2
Pickle relishes and pickles	3	1	20

*Per serving.

Condiments You'll Want to Limit

The condiments listed in this book are all low in fat. Higher-fat foods that are sometimes considered condiments are listed elsewhere in this book. For example, mayonnaise is listed with "Salad Dressings and Sandwich Spreads," and sour cream is listed with "Dairy Products and Dairy Substitutes."

	Tot. Fat (g)	Sat. Fat (g)	Chol. (mg)	Sod. (mg)	Cal.
CAPERS					
Capers, drained (1 tsp)					
Progresso (Pet)	0.0	0.0	0	105	0
CHILI/PICANTE/SALSA/TACO SAUCES—*see also* "GRAVIES AND SAUCES," ENCHILADA SAUCES, page 251					
CHILI SAUCES					
Chili Sauce (1 tbsp)					
Del Monte	0.0	0.0	0	480	20
Red Chile Sauce (¼ cup)					
Las Palmas (Pet)	0.5	0.0	0	310	15
PICANTE SAUCES					
Hot Picante Sauces					
Hot Picante (2 tbsp)					
Chi-Chi's (Hormel)	0.0	0.0	0	270	10
Hot Picante Salsa (2 tbsp)					
Old El Paso (Pet)	0.0	0.0	0	230	10
Hot Salsa Picante (2 tbsp)					
Clemente Jacques (Van den Bergh Foods)	0.0	0.0	0	270	10
Hot Thick 'n Chunky Picante (2 tbsp)					
Old El Paso (Pet)	0.0	0.0	0	160	10
Medium Picante Sauces					
Medium Picante (2 tbsp)					
Chi-Chi's (Hormel)	0.0	0.0	0	200	10
Medium Salsa Picante (2 tbsp)					
Clemente Jacques (Van den Bergh Foods)	0.0	0.0	0	270	10
Medium Thick 'n Chunky Picante (2 tbsp)					
Old El Paso (Pet)	0.0	0.0	0	140	10
Mild Picante Sauces					
Mild Picante (2 tbsp)					
Chi-Chi's (Hormel)	0.0	0.0	0	210	10
Mild Salsa Picante (2 tbsp)					
Clemente Jacques (Van den Bergh Foods)	0.0	0.0	0	270	10
Mild Thick 'n Chunky Picante (2 tbsp)					
Old El Paso (Pet)	0.0	0.0	0	130	10

	Tot. Fat (g)	Sat. Fat (g)	Chol. (mg)	Sod. (mg)	Cal.
SALSAS					
Hot Salsas					
Hot Italian Salsa (2 tbsp)					
Progresso (Pet)	0.0	0.0	0	170	10
Hot Pico de Gallo Salsa (2 tbsp)					
Old El Paso (Pet)	0.0	0.0	0	260	5
Hot Salsa (2 tbsp)					
Chi-Chi's (Hormel)	0.0	0.0	0	160	10
Newman's Own	0.0	0.0	0	150	10
The Fat Free Gourmet (Harry's Premium Snacks)	0.0	0.0	0	88	15
Tostitos (Frito-Lay)	0.0	0.0	0	260	15
Hot Salsa Mexicana (2 tbsp)					
Las Palmas (Pet)	0.0	0.0	0	75	10
Thick & Chunky Hot Salsa					
Ortega (Nabisco Foods)* (2 tbsp)	0.0	0.0	0	370	10
Smart Temptations (American Specialty Brands) (1 tbsp)	0.0	0.0	0	130	8
Thick 'n Chunky Hot Salsa (2 tbsp)					
Old El Paso (Pet)	0.0	0.0	0	130	10
Medium Salsas					
Garden Style Medium Salsa (2 tbsp)					
Ortega (Nabisco Foods)*	0.0	0.0	0	420	10
Medium Green Chili Salsa (2 tbsp)					
Old El Paso (Pet)	0.0	0.0	0	110	10
Medium Homestyle Salsa (2 tbsp)					
Old El Paso (Pet)	0.0	0.0	0	110	5
Medium Italian Salsa (2 tbsp)					
Progresso (Pet)	0.0	0.0	0	170	10
Medium Picante Salsa (2 tbsp)					
Old El Paso (Pet)	0.0	0.0	0	230	10
Medium Pico de Gallo Salsa (2 tbsp)					
Old El Paso (Pet)	0.0	0.0	0	260	5
Medium Salsa (2 tbsp)					
Chi-Chi's (Hormel)	0.0	0.0	0	140	10
Newman's Own	0.0	0.0	0	105	10
Tostitos (Frito-Lay)	0.0	0.0	0	260	15

*Tobacco company, corporate subsidiary, or parent.

	Tot. Fat (g)	Sat. Fat (g)	Chol. (mg)	Sod. (mg)	Cal.
Medium Salsa Mexicana (2 tbsp)					
Las Palmas (Pet)	0.0	0.0	0	85	10
Medium Salsa Verde (2 tbsp)					
Chi-Chi's (Hormel)	0.0	0.0	0	180	15
Old El Paso (Pet)	0.0	0.0	0	95	10
Medium Thick & Chunky Salsa					
Ortega (Nabisco Foods)* (2 tbsp)	0.0	0.0	0	320	10
Smart Temptations (American Specialty Brands) (1 tbsp)	0.0	0.0	0	130	8
Medium Thick 'n Chunky Salsa (2 tbsp)					
Old El Paso (Pet)	0.0	0.0	0	140	10
Mexican Homestyle Salsa (2 tbsp)					
Clemente Jacques (Van den Bergh Foods)	0.0	0.0	0	240	10
Organic Fat Free Salsa (2 tbsp)					
Muir Glen	0.0	0.0	0	75	15
Pico De Gallo (2 tbsp)					
Chi-Chi's (Hormel)	0.0	0.0	0	170	10
Mild Salsas					
Mild Garden Style Salsa (2 tbsp)					
Ortega (Nabisco Foods)*	0.0	0.0	0	420	10
Mild Homestyle Salsa (2 tbsp)					
Old El Paso (Pet)	0.0	0.0	0	110	5
Mild Italian Salsa (2 tbsp)					
Progresso (Pet)	0.0	0.0	0	170	10
Mild Picante Salsa (2 tbsp)					
Old El Paso (Pet)	0.0	0.0	0	230	10
Mild Salsa (2 tbsp)					
Chi-Chi's (Hormel)	0.0	0.0	0	150	10
Newman's Own	0.0	0.0	0	105	10
The Fat Free Gourmet (Harry's Premium Snacks)	0.0	0.0	0	74	15
Tostitos (Frito-Lay)	0.0	0.0	0	230	15
Mild Salsa Mexicana (2 tbsp)					
Las Palmas (Pet)	0.0	0.0	0	90	10
Mild Salsa Verde (2 tbsp)					
Chi-Chi's (Hormel)	0.0	0.0	0	180	15

*Tobacco company, corporate subsidiary, or parent.

	Tot. Fat (g)	Sat. Fat (g)	Chol. (mg)	Sod. (mg)	Cal.
SALSAS *(cont'd)*					
Mild Thick 'n Chunky Salsa (2 tbsp)					
Old El Paso (Pet)	0.0	0.0	0	140	10
Salsa Verde (2 tbsp)					
Clemente Jacques (Van den Bergh Foods)	0.0	0.0	0	270	10
Thick & Chunky Salsa (Mild)					
Ortega (Nabisco Foods)* (2 tbsp)	0.0	0.0	0	320	10
Smart Temptations (American Specialty Brands) (1 tbsp)	0.0	0.0	0	130	8
TACO SAUCES					
Hot Taco Sauces					
Hot Taco Sauce (1 tbsp)					
Old El Paso (Pet)	0.0	0.0	0	90	5
Hot Thick & Smooth Taco Sauce (1 tbsp)					
Ortega (Nabisco Foods)*	0.0	0.0	0	120	10
Medium Taco Sauces					
Chunky Taco Sauce (2 tbsp)					
Lawry's (Lawry's Foods)	0.0	0.0	0	250	10
Medium Extra Chunky Taco Sauce (1 tbsp)					
Old El Paso (Pet)	0.0	0.0	0	80	5
Medium Taco Sauce (1 tbsp)					
Old El Paso (Pet)	0.0	0.0	0	70	5
Medium Thick & Smooth Taco Sauce (1 tbsp)					
Ortega (Nabisco Foods)*	0.0	0.0	0	125	10
Taco Sauce (1 tbsp)					
Old El Paso (Pet)	0.0	0.0	0	85	5
Taco Sauce N Seasoner (2 tbsp)					
Lawry's (Lawry's Foods)	0.0	0.0	0	320	15
Thick & Chunky Taco Sauce (1 tbsp)					
Chi-Chi's (Hormel)	0.0	0.0	0	75	10
Mild Taco Sauces					
Mild Extra Chunky Taco Sauce (1 tbsp)					
Old El Paso (Pet)	0.0	0.0	0	80	5

*Tobacco company, corporate subsidiary, or parent.

	Tot. Fat (g)	Sat. Fat (g)	Chol. (mg)	Sod. (mg)	Cal.
Mild Taco Sauce					
Old El Paso (Pet) (1 tbsp)	0.0	0.0	0	85	5
Pancho Villa (Pet) (2 tbsp)	0.0	0.0	0	170	15
Mild Thick & Smooth Taco Sauce (1 tbsp)					
Ortega (Nabisco Foods)*	0.0	0.0	0	125	10
CHUTNEY—*see* RELISHES, OTHER RELISHES, page 102					
COCKTAIL SAUCES					
Cocktail Sauce (¼ cup)					
Kraft Sauceworks (Kraft General Foods)*	0.5	0.0	0	800	60
Silver Spring (Silver Spring Gardens)	0.0	0.0	0	690	55
Hot Seafood Cocktail Sauce (2 tbsp)					
Chelten House (Chelten House Products)	0.0	0.0	0	130	15
Dockside (Chelten House Products)	0.0	0.0	0	130	15
Seafood Cocktail Sauce					
Chelten House (Chelten House Products) (2 tbsp)	0.0	0.0	0	130	15
Del Monte (1 tbsp)	0.0	0.0	0	210	25
Dockside (Chelten House Products) (2 tbsp)	0.0	0.0	0	130	15
HORSERADISH					
Beet Style Horseradish (1 tsp)					
Silver Spring (Silver Spring Gardens)	0.0	0.0	0	40	0
Cream Style Horseradish (1 tsp)					
Kraft (Kraft General Foods)*	0.0	0.0	0	50	0
Silver Spring (Silver Spring Gardens)	0.0	0.0	0	10	0
Horseradish (1 tsp)					
Most brands (USDA)	**0.0**	**0.0**	**0**	**5**	**2**

*Tobacco company, corporate subsidiary, or parent.

	Tot. Fat (g)	Sat. Fat (g)	Chol. (mg)	Sod. (mg)	Cal.
HORSERADISH ***(cont'd)***					
Horseradish Sauce (1 tsp)					
Silver Spring (Silver Spring Gardens)	1.0	0.0	0	40	15
Miller Horseradish (1 tsp)					
Silver Spring (Silver Spring Gardens)	0.0	0.0	0	0	0
Prepared Horseradish (1 tsp)					
Kraft (Kraft General Foods)*	0.0	0.0	0	50	0
Silver Spring (Silver Spring Gardens)	0.0	0.0	0	10	0
HOT PEPPERS					
CHERRY PEPPERS					
Cherry Peppers (2 tbsp)					
Progresso (Pet)	2.0	0.0	0	30	20
Hot Cherry Peppers					
America's Choice (about 2 peppers)	0.0	0.0	0	480	10
Progresso (Pet) (1 pepper)	0.0	0.0	0	250	15
CHILI PEPPERS					
Hot chili peppers, canned (1 pepper)					
Most brands (USDA)	**0.1**	**0.0**	**0**	**(3)**	**18**
Hot chili peppers, raw (1 pepper)	0.1	0.0	0	3	18
Hot Yellow Chili Peppers (4 peppers)					
Del Monte	0.0	0.0	0	610	10
JALAPEÑO PEPPERS					
Green Jalapeño Wheels (1 oz)					
Chi-Chi's (Hormel)	0.0	0.0	0	110	10
Green Jalapeños, Whole (1 oz)					
Chi-Chi's (Hormel)	0.0	0.0	0	110	10
Jalapeño peppers, canned (¼ cup)					
Most brands (USDA)	**0.2**	**0.0**	**0**	**202**	**9**
Peeled Jalapeños (3 jalapeños)					
Old El Paso (Pet)	0.0	0.0	0	200	10
Pickled Jalapeño Nacho Slices (about 17 slices)					
Clemente Jacques (Van den Bergh Foods)	0.0	0.0	0	270	10

*Tobacco company, corporate subsidiary, or parent.

	Tot. Fat (g)	Sat. Fat (g)	Chol. (mg)	Sod. (mg)	Cal.
Pickled Jalapeño Peppers (about 2 peppers) Clemente Jacques (Van den Bergh Foods)	0.0	0.0	0	290	10
Pickled Jalapeño Slices (2 tbsp) Old El Paso (Pet)	0.0	0.0	0	400	15
Pickled Jalapeños (2 jalapeños) Old El Paso (Pet)	0.0	0.0	0	380	5
Red Jalapeño Wheels (1 oz) Chi-Chi's (Hormel)	0.0	0.0	0	110	10
Red Jalapeños, Whole (1 oz) Chi-Chi's (Hormel)	0.0	0.0	0	110	15
Whole Jalapeño Peppers (about 2 peppers) Clemente Jacques (Van den Bergh Foods)	0.0	0.0	0	270	10
OTHER HOT PEPPERS					
Tuscan Peppers (3 peppers) Progresso (Pet)	0.0	0.0	0	330	10
HOT SAUCES					
Jalapeño Sauce (1 tsp) Tabasco brand (McIlhenny Co)	0.0	0.0	0	70	0
Pepper Sauce (1 tsp) Tabasco brand (McIlhenny Co)	0.0	0.0	0	30	0
JAMS—*see* "SWEET TOPPINGS AND SAUCES," FRUIT SPREADS, page 376					
JELLIES—*see* "SWEET TOPPINGS AND SAUCES," FRUIT SPREADS, page 376					
KETCHUPS					
Ketchup (1 tbsp) **Most brands** (USDA)	**0.1**	**0.0**	**0**	**156**	**16**
Low-sodium ketchup (1 tbsp) **Most brands** (USDA)	**0.1**	**0.0**	**0**	**3**	**16**

	Tot. Fat (g)	Sat. Fat (g)	Chol. (mg)	Sod. (mg)	Cal.
KETCHUPS *(cont'd)*					
Spicy Ketchup (1 tbsp)					
McIlhenny Farms brand (McIlhenny Co)	0.0	0.0	0	130	25
Tomato Ketchup (1 tbsp)					
Del Monte	0.0	0.0	0	190	15
Weight Watchers (H.J. Heinz)	0.0	0.0	0	115	8
MARINADES					
DRY MARINADES					
Barbecue Marinade in Minutes (½ tsp)					
Adolph's (Van den Bergh Foods)	0.0	0.0	0	310	5
Cajun Marinade in Minutes (½ tsp)					
Adolph's (Van den Bergh Foods)	0.0	0.0	0	170	5
Chicken Marinade Mix (¾ tsp)					
Adolph's (Van den Bergh Foods)	0.0	0.0	0	290	5
Chicken Sodium Free Marinade Mix (¾ tsp)					
Adolph's (Van den Bergh Foods)	0.0	0.0	0	0	5
Garlic Dijon Marinade in Minutes (¾ tsp)					
Adolph's (Van den Bergh Foods)	0.0	0.0	0	210	10
Garlic Marinade in Minutes (½ tsp)					
Adolph's (Van den Bergh Foods)	0.0	0.0	0	460	0
Hot 'N Spicy Marinade in Minutes (¾ tsp)					
Adolph's (Van den Bergh Foods)	0.0	0.0	0	130	5
Italian Herb Marinade in Minutes (¼ tsp)					
Adolph's (Van den Bergh Foods)	0.0	0.0	0	270	0
Lemon Herb Marinade in Minutes for Seafood (½ tsp)					
Adolph's (Van den Bergh Foods)	0.0	0.0	0	170	10
Lemon Pepper Marinade in Minutes (½ tsp)					
Adolph's (Van den Bergh Foods)	0.0	0.0	0	180	10
Mandarin Marinade (1 tbsp)					
House of Tsang (Hormel)	0.0	0.0	0	680	25

	Tot. Fat (g)	Sat. Fat (g)	Chol. (mg)	Sod. (mg)	Cal.
Meat Marinade Mix (½ tsp)					
Adolph's (Van den Bergh Foods)	0.0	0.0	0	390	0
Meat Sodium Free Marinade Mix (½ tsp)					
Adolph's (Van den Bergh Foods)	0.0	0.0	0	0	5
Mesquite Marinade in Minutes (¾ tsp)					
Adolph's (Van den Bergh Foods)	0.0	0.0	0	230	10
Parmesan Herb Marinade in Minutes (¾ tsp)					
Adolph's (Van den Bergh Foods)	0.0	0.0	0	230	10
Scampi Marinade in Minutes for Seafood (½ tsp)					
Adolph's (Van den Bergh Foods)	0.0	0.0	0	240	10
Steak Sauce Marinade in Minutes (¼ tsp)					
Adolph's (Van den Bergh Foods)	0.0	0.0	0	350	0
Teriyaki Marinade in Minutes (1½ tsp)					
Adolph's (Van den Bergh Foods)	0.0	0.0	0	380	15
Liquid Marinades					
Hawaiian Marinade with Tropical Fruit Juices (1 tbsp)					
Lawry's (Lawry's Foods)	0.0	0.0	0	250	20
Hickory Grill Marinade in Minutes (1 tbsp)					
Adolph's (Van den Bergh Foods)	0.5	0.0	0	200	20
Lemon Garlic Marinade in Minutes (1 tbsp)					
Adolph's (Van den Bergh Foods)	2.5	0.0	0	80	20
Mesquite Marinade in Minutes (1 tbsp)					
Adolph's (Van den Bergh Foods)	2.5	0.0	0	270	45
Red Wine Marinade with Cabernet Sauvignon (1 tbsp)					
Lawry's (Lawry's Foods)	0.0	0.0	0	270	5
Teriyaki Marinade in Minutes (1 tbsp)					
Adolph's (Van den Bergh Foods)	0.0	0.0	0	740	20
Teriyaki Sauce and Marinade (1 tbsp)					
Ka-me (Shaffer, Clarke & Co) ...	0.0	0.0	0	480	10

	Tot. Fat (g)	Sat. Fat (g)	Chol. (mg)	Sod. (mg)	Cal.
MARMALADES—see "SWEET TOPPINGS AND SAUCES," FRUIT SPREADS, page 376					
MUSTARDS					
Chinese Mustards					
Chinese mustard (1 tsp)					
Most brands (USDA)	**0.2**	**0.0**	**0**	**63**	**4**
Dijon Mustards					
Country Dijon Mustard (1 tsp)					
Grey Poupon (Nabisco Foods)*	0.0	0.0	0	120	5
Dijon Mustard (1 tsp)					
Grey Poupon (Nabisco Foods)*	0.0	0.0	0	120	5
Silver Spring (Silver Spring Gardens)	0.0	0.0	0	100	0
Horseradish Mustards					
Horseradish Mustard (1 tsp)					
Most brands (USDA)	**0.2**	**0.0**	**0**	**63**	**4**
Kraft (Kraft General Foods)*	0.0	0.0	0	55	0
Pure Prepared Horseradish Style Mustard (1 tsp)					
America's Choice (A & P)	0.0	0.0	0	60	0
Hot Mustards					
Hot Mustard Sauce (Chinese style) (1 tsp)					
Ka-me (Shaffer, Clarke & Co)	0.0	0.0	0	80	0
Jalapeño Mustard (1 tsp)					
Silver Spring (Silver Spring Gardens)	0.0	0.0	0	85	0
Sweet 'N Hot Mustard (1 tsp)					
Silver Spring (Silver Spring Gardens)	0.0	0.0	0	45	5
Regular Mustards					
Pure Prepared All American Mustard (1 tsp)					
America's Choice (A & P)	0.0	0.0	0	60	0
Pure Prepared Mustard (1 tsp)					
Kraft (Kraft General Foods)*	0.0	0.0	0	60	0
Regular mustard (1 tsp)					
Most brands (USDA)	**0.2**	**0.0**	**0**	**63**	**4**

*Tobacco company, corporate subsidiary, or parent.

	Tot. Fat (g)	Sat. Fat (g)	Chol. (mg)	Sod. (mg)	Cal.
OTHER MUSTARDS					
Beer 'N Brat Mustard (1 tsp)					
Silver Spring (Silver Spring Gardens)	0.0	0.0	0	55	0
Dill Mustard (1 tsp)					
Silver Spring (Silver Spring Gardens)	0.0	0.0	0	60	0
Polish Mustard (1 tsp)					
Silver Spring (Silver Spring Gardens)	0.0	0.0	0	70	10
Pure Prepared Spicy Brown Mustard (1 tsp)					
America's Choice (A & P)	0.0	0.0	0	60	0
Spicy Brown Mustard (1 tsp)					
Grey Poupon (Nabisco Foods)*	0.0	0.0	0	60	5
OLIVES—*see* "FATS AND OILS," OLIVES, page 197					
PEPPERS—*see* HOT PEPPERS, page 92					
PICANTE SAUCES—*see* CHILI/PICANTE/SALSA/TACO SAUCES, page 87					
PICKLED VEGETABLES					
Pickled cocktail onions (1 onion)					
Most brands (USDA)	**0.0**	**0.0**	**0**	**5**	**12**
Tomato Halves (1 oz)					
Claussen (Claussen Pickle Co)*	0.0	0.0	0	320	5
PICKLES—*see also* RELISHES, page 101					
BREAD AND BUTTER PICKLES					
Bread & Butter Pickle (about 9 slices)					
Gedney State Fair (M.A. Gedney Co)	0.0	0.0	0	180	35
Bread and butter pickles (4 slices)					
Most brands (USDA)	**tr**	**0.0**	**0**	**202**	**22**

*Tobacco company, corporate subsidiary, or parent.

	Tot. Fat (g)	Sat. Fat (g)	Chol. (mg)	Sod. (mg)	Cal.
BREAD AND BUTTER PICKLES *(cont'd)*					
Bread'N Butter Chips (4 slices)					
Claussen (Claussen Pickle Co)*	0.0	0.0	0	170	20
Hot Bread & Butter Pickle (about 9 slices)					
Gedney State Fair (M.A. Gedney Co)	0.0	0.0	0	180	35
No Salt Added Bread & Butter Slices (about 5 slices)					
America's Choice (A & P)	0.0	0.0	0	10	30
Old Fashioned Bread & Butter Slices (about 3 slices)					
America's Choice (A & P)	0.0	0.0	0	170	30
Sweet Bread & Butter Slices (about 5 slices)					
America's Choice (A & P)	0.0	0.0	0	170	30
DILL PICKLES—*see also* KOSHER DILL PICKLES, page 99					
Dill Hamburger Chips (5 chips)					
Del Monte	0.0	0.0	0	310	5
Dill Pickle Slices (about ½ pickle)					
America's Choice (A & P)	0.0	0.0	0	390	0
Dill Pickles					
Most brands (1 lrg pickle) (USDA)	**0.1**	**0.0**	**0**	**833**	**12**
Del Monte (1 pickle)	0.0	0.0	0	590	5
Gedney State Fair (M.A. Gedney Co) (about 1 med pickle)	0.0	0.0	0	290	5
Dill pickles, low-sodium (1 lrg pickle)					
Most brands (USDA)	**0.1**	**0.0**	**0**	**12**	**12**
Dill Spears (about 1 spear)					
Gedney (M.A. Gedney Co)	0.0	0.0	0	290	5
Grandma's Baby Baby Dill Pickle (about 4 sml pickles)					
Gedney State Fair (M.A. Gedney Co)	0.0	0.0	0	290	5
Hamburger Dill Pickle Slices (about 7 slices)					
America's Choice (A & P)	0.0	0.0	0	390	0

*Tobacco company, corporate subsidiary, or parent.

	Tot. Fat (g)	Sat. Fat (g)	Chol. (mg)	Sod. (mg)	Cal.
Hamburger Dill Slices/Chips (10 slices)					
Claussen (Claussen Pickle Co)*	0.0	0.0	0	420	5
Midget Dill Pickle (about 1 med pickle)					
Gedney (M.A. Gedney Co)	0.0	0.0	0	290	5
Milwaukee Plain Dills (1 oz)					
Vlasic (Campbell Soup Co)	0.0	0.0	0	260	5
No Garlic Baby Dill Pickles (about 1 pickle)					
America's Choice (A & P)	0.0	0.0	0	220	0
No Garlic Dill Pickles (about ½ pickle)					
America's Choice (A & P)	0.0	0.0	0	220	0
No Garlic Dill Spears (about 1 spear)					
America's Choice (A & P)	0.0	0.0	0	220	0
Polish Dill Spears (about 1 spear)					
America's Choice (A & P)	0.0	0.0	0	220	0
Whole Dill Pickles					
America's Choice (A & P) (½ pickle)	0.0	0.0	0	390	0
Gedney (M.A. Gedney Co) (about ½ lrg pickle)	0.0	0.0	0	290	5
KOSHER DILL PICKLES—*see also* DILL PICKLES, page 98					
Kosher Baby Dill Pickles (about 1 pickle)					
America's Choice (A & P)	0.0	0.0	0	220	0
Kosher Dill Halves (1 oz)					
Claussen (Claussen Pickle Co)*	0.0	0.0	0	330	5
Kosher Dill Pickles (about ½ pickle)					
America's Choice (A & P)	0.0	0.0	0	220	0
Kosher Dill Slices (4 slices)					
Claussen (Claussen Pickle Co)*	0.0	0.0	0	320	5
Kosher Dill Spears					
America's Choice (A & P) (about 1 spear)	0.0	0.0	0	220	0
Claussen (Claussen Pickle Co)* (1 spear)	0.0	0.0	0	310	5
Kosher Dill Wholes (1 oz)					
Claussen (Claussen Pickle Co)*	0.0	0.0	0	330	5

*Tobacco company, corporate subsidiary, or parent.

	Tot. Fat (g)	Sat. Fat (g)	Chol. (mg)	Sod. (mg)	Cal.
KOSHER DILL PICKLES *(cont'd)*					
Kosher Midget Dill Pickle (about 1 med pickle)					
Gedney State Fair (M.A. Gedney Co)	0.0	0.0	0	290	5
Kosher Mini Dills (1 pickle)					
Claussen (Claussen Pickle Co)*	0.0	0.0	0	300	5
Old Fashioned Kosher Dill Pickle Spears (about 1 spear)					
America's Choice (A & P)	0.0	0.0	0	340	0
Old Fashioned Kosher Dill Pickles (about ½ pickle)					
America's Choice (A & P)	0.0	0.0	0	220	30
Tiny Kosher Dill Pickles (1 pickle)					
Del Monte	0.0	0.0	0	200	5
SOUR PICKLES					
New York Deli Style Half Sours (1 oz)					
Claussen (Claussen Pickle Co)*	0.0	0.0	0	260	5
Sour pickles (1 med)					
Most brands (USDA)	**0.0**	**0.0**	**0**	**423**	**4**
Sour pickles, low sodium (1 med)					
Most brands (USDA)	**0.0**	**0.0**	**0**	**6**	**4**
SWEET PICKLES					
Pantry Sweet Pickles (about 5 slices)					
Gedney (M.A. Gedney Co)	0.0	0.0	0	190	30
Sweet Cucumber Sticks (about 1¼ spears)					
America's Choice (A & P)	0.0	0.0	0	170	30
Sweet Gherkins					
Most brands (USDA) (1 med pickle)	**0.0**	**0.0**	**0**	**141**	**18**
America's Choice (A & P) (about 1½ pickles)	0.0	0.0	0	180	35
Gedney (M.A. Gedney Co) (about 2 pickles)	0.0	0.0	0	180	30
Sweet Midgets (about 2 pickles)					
America's Choice (A & P)	0.0	0.0	0	180	35
Sweet Mixed Pickles (about 3 pieces)					
America's Choice (A & P)	0.0	0.0	0	180	35

*Tobacco company, corporate subsidiary, or parent.

	Tot. Fat (g)	Sat. Fat (g)	Chol. (mg)	Sod. (mg)	Cal.
Sweet Pickles (1 oz)					
Vlasic (Campbell Soup Co)	0.0	0.0	0	170	40
America's Choice (A & P)	0.0	0.0	0	180	35
Sweet Salad Cubes (1 tbsp)					
America's Choice (A & P)	0.0	0.0	0	140	20
Whole Sweet Pickles (1 pickle)					
Del Monte	0.0	0.0	0	230	45
OTHER PICKLES					
Hot & Sweet Snackers (about 4 slices)					
Gedney (M.A. Gedney Co)	0.0	0.0	0	180	30
Hot 'N Sweet Sliced Pickles (about 5 slices)					
McIlhenny Farms brand (McIlhenny Co)	0.0	0.0	0	30	40
Watermelon rind pickles (1 piece)					
Most brands (USDA)	**0.1**	**0.0**	**0**	**214**	**44**
PIMIENTOS					
Pimientos (3/4 tsp)					
Osage (Cherokee)	0.0	0.0	0	0	0
PRESERVES—*see* "SWEET TOPPINGS AND SAUCES," FRUIT SPREADS, page 376					
RELISHES					
PICKLE RELISHES—*see also* OTHER RELISHES, BELOW					
Dill Pickle Relish (1 tbsp)					
Gedney (M.A. Gedney Co)	0.0	0.0	0	270	0
Hamburger Relish (1 tbsp)					
Del Monte	0.0	0.0	0	220	20
Hot Dog Relish					
Most brands (1 tbsp) (USDA)	**0.1**	**0.0**	**0**	**164**	**14**
Del Monte (1 tbsp)	0.0	0.0	0	140	15
Gedney (M.A. Gedney Co) (1 tbsp)	0.0	0.0	0	100	18
Silver Spring (Silver Spring Gardens) (1 tsp)	0.0	0.0	0	45	5

	Tot. Fat (g)	Sat. Fat (g)	Chol. (mg)	Sod. (mg)	Cal.
PICKLE RELISHES *(cont'd)*					
Sour pickle relish (1 tbsp)					
Most brands (USDA)	**0.0**	**0.0**	**0**	**192**	**3**
Sweet Pickle Relish (1 tbsp)					
Most brands (USDA)	**0.1**	**0.0**	**0**	**122**	**19**
America's Choice (A & P)	0.0	0.0	0	140	20
Claussen (Claussen Pickle Co)*	0.0	0.0	0	85	15
Del Monte	0.0	0.0	0	125	20
OTHER RELISHES					
Chow chow, sour (1 tbsp)					
Most brands (USDA)	**0.2**	**0.0**	**0**	**201**	**4**
Chow chow, sweet (1 tbsp)					
Most brands (USDA)	**0.1**	**0.0**	**0**	**81**	**18**
Chutney (1 tbsp)					
Most brands (USDA)	**0.1**	**0.0**	**0**	**9**	**21**
Corn Relish (1 tbsp)					
Most brands (USDA)	**0.5**	**0.0**	**0**	**135**	**20**
Green Giant (Grand Metropolitan PLC)	0.0	0.0	0	40	20
Cranberry-orange relish (½ cup)					
Most brands (USDA)	**0.1**	**0.0**	**0**	**44**	**246**
Jalapeño Relish (1 tbsp)					
Old El Paso (Pet)	0.0	0.0	0	110	5

SALSAS—*see* CHILI/PICANTE/SALSA/TACO SAUCES, page 87

SANDWICH SPREADS—*see* "SALAD DRESSINGS AND SANDWICH SPREADS," MAYONNAISE/MAYONNAISE-TYPE SALAD DRESSINGS, page 332

SOY SAUCES

	Tot. Fat (g)	Sat. Fat (g)	Chol. (mg)	Sod. (mg)	Cal.
SOY SAUCES					
Dark Soy Sauce (1 tbsp)					
House of Tsang (Hormel)	0.0	0.0	0	860	10
Dark Soy Sauce (Chinese) (1 tbsp)					
Ka-me (Shaffer, Clarke & Co)	0.0	0.0	0	1020	10

*Tobacco company, corporate subsidiary, or parent.

	Tot. Fat (g)	Sat. Fat (g)	Chol. (mg)	Sod. (mg)	Cal.
Ginger Flavored Soy Sauce (1 tbsp)					
House of Tsang (Hormel)	0.0	0.0	0	730	20
Mild Soy Sauce (1 tbsp)					
Ka-me (Shaffer, Clarke & Co) ...	0.0	0.0	0	490	5
Soy Sauce (1 tbsp)					
Chun King (Chun King Corp) ...	0.0	0.0	0	1050	5
Soy Sauce (Japanese) (1 tbsp)					
Ka-me (Shaffer, Clarke & Co) ...	0.0	0.0	0	520	5
LIGHT/LOW-SODIUM SOY SAUCES					
Light Soy Sauce (1 tbsp)					
House of Tsang (Hormel)	0.0	0.0	0	900	5
Light Soy Sauce (Chinese) (1 tbsp)					
Ka-me (Shaffer, Clarke & Co) ...	0.0	0.0	0	1170	5
Lite Soy Sauce (1 tbsp)					
Chun King (Chun King Corp) ...	0.0	0.0	0	630	5
Low Sodium Ginger Flavored Soy Sauce (1 tbsp)					
House of Tsang (Hormel)	0.0	0.0	0	280	10
Low Sodium Mushroom Flavored Soy Sauce (1 tbsp)					
House of Tsang (Hormel)	0.0	0.0	0	280	10
Low Sodium Soy Sauce (1 tbsp)					
House of Tsang (Hormel)	0.0	0.0	0	280	5
STEAK SAUCES					
Bold Steak Sauce (1 tbsp)					
A-1 (Nabisco Foods)*	0.0	0.0	0	190	20
100% Natural Steak Sauce Tenderizer (¼ tsp)					
Adolph's (Van den Bergh Foods)	0.0	0.0	0	310	0
Steak Sauce (1 tbsp)					
A-1 (Nabisco Foods)*	0.0	0.0	0	250	15
TACO SAUCES—*see* CHILI/PICANTE/SALSA/TACO SAUCES, page 87					
TOMATO PASTE					
Italian Tomato Paste (2 tbsp)					
Contadina (Nestlé Food Company)	1.0	0.0	0	320	40

*Tobacco company, corporate subsidiary, or parent.

	Tot. Fat (g)	Sat. Fat (g)	Chol. (mg)	Sod. (mg)	Cal.
TOMATO PASTE *(cont'd)*					
No-salt-added tomato paste (½ cup)					
Most brands (USDA)	**1.2**	**0.2**	**0**	**86**	**110**
Tomato paste (½ cup)					
Most brands (USDA)	**1.2**	**0.2**	**0**	**1035**	**110**
Tomato Paste Italian Style (2 oz)					
Hunt's (Hunt-Wesson)	<1.0	0.0	0	430	50
Tomato Paste with Garlic (2 oz)					
Hunt's (Hunt-Wesson)	<1.0	0.0	0	440	50
TOMATO PUREE					
Organic Tomato Puree (¼ cup)					
Muir Glen	0.0	0.0	0	20	20
Tomato puree (½ cup)					
Most brands (USDA)	**0.1**	**0.0**	**0**	**499**	**51**
VINEGARS					
Chinese Seasoned Vinegar (1 tbsp)					
Ka-me (Shaffer, Clarke & Co)	0.0	0.0	0	60	5
Garlic Flavored Vinegar (1 tbsp)					
Progresso (Pet)	0.0	0.0	0	0	0
Red Wine Vinegar (1 tbsp)					
Progresso (Pet)	0.0	0.0	0	0	0
Rice Wine Vinegar (Chinese) (1 tbsp)					
Ka-me (Shaffer, Clarke & Co)	0.0	0.0	0	0	5
Rice Wine Vinegar (Japanese) (1 tbsp)					
Ka-me (Shaffer, Clarke & Co)	0.0	0.0	0	0	0
Seasoned Rice Vinegar (Japanese) (1 tbsp)					
Ka-me (Shaffer, Clarke & Co)	0.0	0.0	0	180	10
Vinegar (1 tbsp)					
Most brands (USDA)	**0.0**	**0.0**	**0**	**0**	**2**
White Wine Vinegar (1 tbsp)					
Progresso (Pet)	0.0	0.0	0	0	0

CRACKERS

How do our crackers crumble? From saltines and cheese crackers to popcorn, rice, and other grain cakes, you can rest easy about munching on the crackers listed in this chapter. They're all low in fat, saturated fat, and cholesterol.

Like all the other entries in this book, the crackers entries that follow list sodium content. The AHA does not have criteria for sodium but recommends a total of no more than 3,000 mg a day.

If you find products that were introduced after this book went to press, use the generic listings and the following tables to help evaluate them.

AHA Criteria for Crackers*

	Tot. Fat (g)	Sat. Fat (g)	Chol. (mg)
Crackers not used as snacks, such as saltines and oyster crackers	3	<0.5	<2
Crackers usually used as snacks	3	1	<2

*Per serving.

Crackers You'll Want to Limit

Some crackers, like the examples below, are too high in fat, saturated fat, and/or cholesterol to meet AHA

Crackers

criteria. They aren't included in this book, and we recommend that you don't eat them often.

Compare the amounts of fat, saturated fat, cholesterol, sodium, and calories in these examples with the more healthful alternatives listed on the following pages.

Sample Crackers to Limit

	Tot. Fat (g)	Sat. Fat (g)	Chol. (mg)	Sod. (mg)	Cal.
Rye cracker sandwich with cheese filling (1 oz, or 4 sandwiches)	6.4*	1.6*	2*	296	136
Wheat cracker sandwich with peanut butter filling (1 oz, or 4 sandwiches)	7.6*	1.6*	0	228	140

Adapted from USDA Handbook No. 8 series.

*These values exceed AHA criteria for crackers.

	Tot. Fat (g)	Sat. Fat (g)	Chol. (mg)	Sod. (mg)	Cal.
BREADSTICKS, HARD—*see* "BREADS AND BREAD PRODUCTS," BREADSTICKS, page 54					
CRACKER CRUMBS—*see* "BREADS AND BREAD PRODUCTS," BREAD CRUMBS/ CRACKER CRUMBS, page 46					
CRACKERS					
CHEESE CRACKERS					
Cheese Crackers (38 crackers)					
Nabisco SnackWell's (Nabisco Foods)*	2.0	0.5	0	340	130
Cheese Rice Crunch Crackers (16 pieces)					
Ka-me (Shaffer, Clarke and Co)	1.5	0.0	0	180	120
Fat-Free Cheese Crackers (7 crackers)					
Health Valley (Health Valley Foods)	0.0	0.0	0	80	50
Fat-Free Healthy Pizza Crackers, Spicy Cheese Style (6 crackers)					
Health Valley (Health Valley Foods)	0.0	0.0	0	80	50
CRISPBREADS					
Crispy Thin All Natural Whole Grain Crispbread (3 pieces)					
Kavli (O.Kavli)	0.0	0.0	0	45	60
Dark Crispbread (3 pieces)					
Finn Crisp (Shaffer, Clarke & Co)	0.0	0.0	0	0	60
Dark Crispbread with Caraway (3 pieces)					
Finn Crisp (Shaffer, Clarke & Co)	0.0	0.0	0	0	60
Fat Free Crispini (½ cup)					
Burns & Ricker	0.0	0.0	0	400	110
5-Grain All Natural Crispbread (1 piece)					
Kavli (O.Kavli)	0.0	0.0	0	30	40
Flavorful Fiber Crisp Bread (2 slices)					
Ryvita (Shaffer, Clarke & Co)	0.5	0.0	0	20	50

*Tobacco company, corporate subsidiary, or parent.

	Tot. Fat (g)	Sat. Fat (g)	Chol. (mg)	Sod. (mg)	Cal.
CRISPBREADS *(cont'd)*					
Hearty Thick All Natural Whole Grain Crispbread (2 pieces) Kavli (O.Kavli)	0.5	0.0	0	55	70
Salt Free Stone Ground Wheat Crispini (5 pieces) Burns & Ricker	<1.0	<1.0	0	0	110
Seeds & Spice Crispini (5 pieces) Burns & Ricker	3.0	<1.0	0	120	110
Sesame Crispini (5 pieces) Burns & Ricker	3.0	<1.0	0	120	110
Sesame Garlic Crispini (5 pieces) Burns & Ricker	3.0	<1.0	0	120	110
Tasty Dark Rye Crisp Bread (2 slices) Ryvita (Shaffer, Clarke & Co)	0.5	0.0	0	35	60
Tasty Light Rye Crisp Bread (2 slices) Ryvita (Shaffer, Clarke & Co)	0.0	0.0	0	20	60
Toasted Sesame Rye Crisp Bread (2 slices) Ryvita (Shaffer, Clarke & Co)	1.5	0.0	0	35	70
GARLIC/ONION CRACKERS					
Fat Free Bite Size Onion Snack Crackers (10 crackers) Auburn Farms 7-Grainers (Auburn Farms)	0.0	0.0	0	105	60
Fat Free Garlic & Herb Crackers (22 crackers) Venus (Venus Wafers)	0.0	0.0	0	120	110
Fat-Free Onion Crackers (7 crackers) Health Valley (Health Valley Foods)	0.0	0.0	0	80	50
Onion Rice Crunch Crackers (16 pieces) Ka-me (Shaffer, Clarke & Co)	1.0	0.0	0	75	120
GRAHAM CRACKERS—*see* "DESSERTS," COOKIES, page 159					
HOT/SPICY CRACKERS					
Fat-Free Hot 3 Chilies Fire Crackers (6 crackers) Health Valley (Health Valley Foods)	0.0	0.0	0	80	50

	Tot. Fat (g)	Sat. Fat (g)	Chol. (mg)	Sod. (mg)	Cal.
Fat-Free Medium Jalapeño Fire Crackers (6 crackers) Health Valley (Health Valley Foods)	0.0	0.0	0	80	50
Fat-Free Mild Chili Fire Crackers (6 crackers) Health Valley (Health Valley Foods)	0.0	0.0	0	80	50
Fat Free Salsa & Hot Chipotle Spicy Snack Crackers (20 crackers) Auburn Farms 7-Grainers (Auburn Farms)	0.0	0.0	0	280	110
LAHVOSH					
Lahvosh Hearts (1 oz) Valley (Valley Bakery)	1.0	0.0	0	140	110
Lahvosh Rounds					
2″ (1 oz) Valley (Valley Bakery) . .	1.0	0.0	0	140	110
3″ (1 oz) Valley (Valley Bakery) . .	1.0	0.0	0	140	110
5″ (1.2 oz) Valley (Valley Bakery)	1.5	0.0	0	180	140
15″ (1.8 oz) Valley (Valley Bakery)	2.0	0.0	0	250	190
Lahvosh Sweetheart Crispies (1 oz) Valley (Valley Bakery)	2.5	1.0	0	130	120
Lahvosh Wheat Rounds					
3″ (1 oz) Valley (Valley Bakery) . .	1.0	0.0	0	140	110
5″ (1.2 oz) Valley (Valley Bakery)	1.5	0.0	0	180	130
15″ (1.8 oz) Valley (Valley Bakery)	2.0	0.0	0	250	190
OYSTER CRACKERS					
Oyster Crackers (14 g) Lance	2.0	0.5	0	135	60
Soup & Chili Crackers (80 pieces) Delicious (Delicious Cookie Co) .	3.0	1.0	0	250	120
Soup & Oyster Crackers					
Nabisco Premium (Nabisco Foods)* (23 crackers) .	1.5	0.0	0	230	60
Sunshine Krispy (Sunshine) (17 crackers)	1.5	0.0	0	200	60
PIZZA CRACKERS					
Fat-Free Healthy Pizza Crackers, Garlic & Herbs Style (6 crackers) Health Valley (Health Valley Foods)	0.0	0.0	0	80	50

*Tobacco company, corporate subsidiary, or parent.

	Tot. Fat (g)	Sat. Fat (g)	Chol. (mg)	Sod. (mg)	Cal.
PIZZA CRACKERS *(cont'd)*					
Fat-Free Healthy Pizza Crackers, Italiano Style (6 crackers)					
Health Valley (Health Valley Foods)	0.0	0.0	0	80	50
Fat Free 7-Grainers Spicy Pizza Snack Crackers (20 crackers)					
Auburn Farms	0.0	0.0	0	280	110
RICE CRACKERS					
Baked Brown Rice Snaps (5 crackers)					
Edward & Sons (Edward & Sons Trading Co)	<1.0	(0.0)	0	1	35
Plain Rice Crunch Crackers (16 pieces)					
Ka-me (Shaffer, Clarke & Co)	1.5	0.0	0	15	120
Seaweed Rice Crunch Crackers (16 pieces)					
Ka-me (Shaffer, Clarke & Co)	1.5	0.0	0	100	120
Sesame Rice Crunch Crackers (16 pieces)					
Ka-me (Shaffer, Clarke & Co)	1.5	0.0	0	85	120
Unsalted Rice Crunch Crackers (16 pieces)					
Ka-me (Shaffer, Clarke & Co)	0.5	0.0	0	0	120
SALTINES					
Cracked Pepper Saltines (5 crackers)					
Sunshine Krispy (Sunshine)	1.5	0.0	0	180	60
Fat Free Saltines (5 crackers)					
Keebler Zesta	0.0	0.0	0	90	50
Nabisco Premium (Nabisco Foods)*	0.0	0.0	0	130	50
Sunshine Krispy (Sunshine) .0.0	0.0	0	135	60	
Low Sodium Saltine Crackers (5 crackers)					
Nabisco Premium (Nabisco Foods)*	1.0	0.0	0	35	60
Multigrain Saltine Crackers (5 crackers)					
Nabisco Premium (Nabisco Foods)*	1.5	0.0	0	150	60

*Tobacco company, corporate subsidiary, or parent.

	Tot. Fat (g)	Sat. Fat (g)	Chol. (mg)	Sod. (mg)	Cal.
Original Saltine Crackers (5 crackers)					
Nabisco Premium (Nabisco Foods)*	1.5	0.0	0	180	60
Saltines (5 crackers)					
America's Choice (A & P)	0.0	0.0	0	135	60
Sunshine Krispy (Sunshine)	1.5	0.0	0	180	60
Unsalted Saltines (5 crackers)					
Sunshine Krispy (Sunshine)	1.5	0.0	0	120	60
Unsalted Tops Saltine Crackers (5 crackers)					
Nabisco Premium (Nabisco Foods)*	1.5	0.0	0	135	60
Whole Wheat Saltines (5 crackers)					
Sunshine Krispy (Sunshine)	1.5	0.0	0	130	60
VEGETABLE CRACKERS					
Fat Free Bite Size Veggie Snack Crackers (10 crackers)					
Auburn Farms 7-Grainers (Auburn Farms)	0.0	0.0	0	105	60
Fat Free Garden Vegetable Crackers (10 crackers)					
Venus (Venus Wafers)	0.0	0.0	0	150	110
Fat-Free No Salt Vegetable Crackers (5 crackers)					
Health Valley (Health Valley Foods)	0.0	0.0	0	15	50
Fat-Free Vegetable Crackers (7 crackers)					
Health Valley (Health Valley Foods)	0.0	0.0	0	80	50
WATER CRACKERS					
Bremner Wafers (13 crackers)					
Bremner (Bremner Biscuit)	3.0	0.5	0	200	130
Table Water Crackers, King Size (2 pieces)					
Carr's (Shaffer, Clarke & Co)	1.0	0.0	0	90	60
Table Water Crackers, Bite Size (5 pieces)					
Carr's (Shaffer, Clarke & Co)	1.5	0.0	0	100	70

*Tobacco company, corporate subsidiary, or parent.

	Tot. Fat (g)	Sat. Fat (g)	Chol. (mg)	Sod. (mg)	Cal.
WATER CRACKERS *(cont'd)*					
Table Water Crackers with Cracked Pepper (5 pieces)					
Carr's (Shaffer, Clarke & Co) . . .	1.5	0.0	0	100	70
Table Water Crackers with Sesame (5 pieces)					
Carr's (Shaffer, Clarke & Co) . . .	1.5	0.0	0	95	70
WHEAT CRACKERS					
Fat-Free Whole Wheat Crackers (7 crackers)					
Health Valley (Health Valley Foods)	0.0	0.0	0	80	50
Garden Vegetable Stoneground Wheat Crackers (12 crackers)					
Lifestream Natural Foods	2.0	0.0	0	210	120
Reduced Fat Triscuit Wafers (8 wafers)					
Nabisco (Nabisco Foods)*	3.0	0.5	0	180	130
Salt Free Stoned Wheat Crackers (10 crackers)					
Venus (Venus Wafers)	2.5	0.5	0	0	120
Sesame Seed Stoneground Wheat Crackers (12 crackers)					
Lifestream Natural Foods	2.5	0.0	0	170	130
Wheat & Onion Stoneground Wheat Crackers (12 crackers)					
Lifestream Natural Foods	2.0	0.0	0	160	120
Wheat Crackers					
Nabisco SnackWell's (Nabisco Foods)* (5 crackers) . .	0.0	0.0	0	170	60
Ry-Krisp (Ralston Foods) (2 crackers)	1.5	0.0	0	150	70
OTHER CRACKERS					
Classic Golden Crackers (6 crackers)					
Nabisco SnackWell's (Nabisco Foods)*	1.0	0.0	0	140	60
Cracked Pepper Crackers (7 crackers)					
Nabisco SnackWell's (Nabisco Foods)*	0.0	0.0	0	150	60

*Tobacco company, corporate subsidiary, or parent.

	Tot. Fat (g)	Sat. Fat (g)	Chol. (mg)	Sod. (mg)	Cal.
Crown Pilot (1 cracker) Nabisco (Nabisco Foods)*	1.5	0.0	0	85	70
Fat Free Bite Size Original Snack Crackers (10 crackers) Auburn Farms 7-Grainers (Auburn Farms)	0.0	0.0	0	110	60
Fat Free Bite Size Rye Snack Crackers (10 crackers) Auburn Farms 7-Grainers (Auburn Farms)	0.0	0.0	0	105	60
Fat Free Cracked Pepper Crackers (22 crackers) Venus (Venus Wafers)	0.0	0.0	0	120	110
Fat-Free Herb Crackers (7 crackers) Health Valley (Health Valley Foods)	0.0	0.0	0	80	50
Fat Free Multi-Grain Crackers (10 crackers) Venus (Venus Wafers)	0.0	0.0	0	170	110
Fat Free Pesto & Dill Spicy Snack Crackers (20 crackers) Auburn Farms 7-Grainers (Auburn Farms)	0.0	0.0	0	250	110
Fat Free Sun Dried Tomato & Basil Spicy Snack Crackers (20 crackers) Auburn Farms 7-Grainers (Auburn Farms)	0.0	0.0	0	250	110
Original Crackers (2 crackers) Ry-Krisp (Ralston Foods)	0.0	0.0	0	75	60
Original Sesame Crackers (5 crackers) Ak-mak (Ak-mak Bakeries)	2.3	0.5	0	214	116
Reduced Fat Wheat Toasteds (10 crackers) Keebler	3.0	1.0	0	300	120
Royal Lunch Milk Crackers (1 cracker) Nabisco (Nabisco Foods)*	2.0	0.0	0	65	50
Salt Free Bran Wafers (10 wafers) Venus (Venus Wafers)	2.0	0.5	0	0	120

*Tobacco company, corporate subsidiary, or parent.

	Tot. Fat (g)	Sat. Fat (g)	Chol. (mg)	Sod. (mg)	Cal.
OTHER CRACKERS *(cont'd)*					
Seasoned Crackers (2 crackers)					
Ry-Krisp (Ralston Foods)	1.5	0.0	0	90	60
Sesame Twins (4 crackers)					
Lance	2.0	0.5	0	125	70
Sour Dough Crackers (4 crackers)					
Lance	3.0	0.5	0	100	70
Teething Toast (1 toast)					
Nabisco Zwieback (Nabisco Foods)*	1.0	0.0	0	10	35
Uneeda Biscuit (2 crackers)					
Nabisco (Nabisco Foods)*	1.5	0.0	0	110	60
GRAIN CAKES—*see* POPCORN/RICE/OTHER GRAIN CAKES, below					
POPCORN/RICE/OTHER GRAIN CAKES					
POPCORN CAKES					
Butter-Flavor Popcorn Cakes					
Natural Butter Flavor Popped Corn Cakes (1 cake)					
Snack Lovers (TKI Foods)	0.0	0.0	0	55	50
Unsalted Butter Flavor Corn Cakes (1 cake)					
Mother's (Quaker Oats Company)	0.0	0.0	0	0	35
Caramel Popcorn Cakes					
Caramel Corn Mini Rice Cakes (5 mini cakes)					
Quaker (Quaker Oats Company)	0.0	0.0	0	25	50
Caramel Flavored Corn Cakes (1 cake)					
Quaker (Quaker Oats Company)	0.0	0.0	0	30	50
Natural Caramel Flavor Popped Corn Cakes (1 cake)					
Snack Lovers (TKI Foods)	0.0	0.0	0	10	60
Other Popcorn Cakes					
Mild White Cheddar Corn Cakes (1 cake)					
Quaker (Quaker Oats Company)	0.0	0.0	0	100	40

*Tobacco company, corporate subsidiary, or parent.

	Tot. Fat (g)	Sat. Fat (g)	Chol. (mg)	Sod. (mg)	Cal.
Nacho Corn Cakes (1 cake)					
Quaker (Quaker Oats Company)	0.0	0.0	0	80	40
Natural White Cheddar Flavor Popped Corn Cakes (1 cake)					
Snack Lovers (TKI Foods)	0.0	0.0	0	45	50
Unsalted Popped Corn Cakes (1 cake)					
Mother's (Quaker Oats Company)	0.0	0.0	0	0	35
RICE CAKES					
Apple Rice Cakes					
Apple Cinnamon Rice Cakes (1 cake)					
Quaker (Quaker Oats Company)	0.0	0.0	0	0	50
Apple Crisp Mini Rice Cakes (5 cakes)					
Pritikin (Quaker Oats Company) .	0.0	0.0	0	20	50
Apple Mini Rice Cakes (5 mini cakes)					
Mother's (Quaker Oats Company)	0.0	0.0	0	40	50
Butter-Flavor Rice Cakes					
Buttered Popcorn Mini Rice Cakes (6 cakes)					
Quaker (Quaker Oats Company)	0.0	0.0	0	120	50
Caramel Rice Cakes					
Caramel Mini Rice Cakes (5 mini cakes)					
Mother's (Quaker Oats Company)	0.0	0.0	0	40	50
Caramel Nut Flavor Mini Rice Cakes (5 cakes)					
Pritikin (Quaker Oats Company) .	0.0	0.0	0	45	50
Cheese-Flavor Rice Cakes					
White Cheddar Mini Rice Cakes (6 mini cakes)					
Quaker (Quaker Oats Company)	0.0	0.0	0	120	50
Cinnamon Rice Cakes					
Cinnamon Crunch Mini Rice Cakes (5 mini cakes)					
Quaker (Quaker Oats Company)	0.0	0.0	0	25	50
Cinnamon Crunch Rice Cake (1 cake)					
Quaker (Quaker Oats Company)	0.0	0.0	0	25	50
Cinnamon Mini Rice Cakes (5 mini cakes)					
Mother's (Quaker Oats Company)	0.0	0.0	0	40	50

	Tot. Fat (g)	Sat. Fat (g)	Chol. (mg)	Sod. (mg)	Cal.
RICE CAKES *(cont'd)*					
Plain Rice Cakes					
Plain Rice Cakes (1 cake)					
Pritikin (Quaker Oats Company) .	0.0	0.0	0	20	35
Plain Unsalted Mini Rice Cakes (7 mini cakes)					
Mother's (Quaker Oats Company)	0.0	0.0	0	0	60
Plain Unsalted Rice Cakes (1 cake)					
Pritikin (Quaker Oats Company) .	0.0	0.0	0	0	35
Toasted Original Unsalted Whole Brown Rice Cakes (2 cakes)					
Lifestream Natural Foods	0.5	0.0	0	5	110
Toasted Original Whole Brown Rice Cakes (2 cakes)					
Lifestream Natural Foods	0.5	0.0	0	30	110
Sesame Rice Cakes					
Sesame Low Sodium Rice Cakes (1 cake)					
Pritikin (Quaker Oats Company) .	0.0	0.0	0	20	35
Sesame Unsalted Rice Cakes (1 cake)					
Pritikin (Quaker Oats Company) .	0.0	0.0	0	0	35
Toasted Sesame Unsalted Whole Brown Rice Cakes (2 cakes)					
Lifestream Natural Foods	0.5	0.0	0	5	110
Toasted Sesame Whole Brown Rice Cakes (2 cakes)					
Lifestream Natural Foods	0.5	0.0	0	35	110
Other Rice Cakes					
Honey Nut Mini Rice Cakes (5 mini cakes)					
Quaker (Quaker Oats Company)	0.0	0.0	0	25	50
Lightly Salted Multigrain Rice Cakes (1 cake)					
Mother's (Quaker Oats Company)	0.0	0.0	0	30	35
Multigrain Rice Cakes (1 cake)					
Pritikin (Quaker Oats Company) .	0.0	0.0	0	20	35
Multigrain Unsalted Rice Cakes (1 cake)					
Pritikin (Quaker Oats Company) .	0.0	0.0	0	0	35

	Tot. Fat (g)	Sat. Fat (g)	Chol. (mg)	Sod. (mg)	Cal.
Toasted Multigrain Whole Brown Rice Cakes (2 cakes) Lifestream Natural Foods	0.5	0.0	0	25	110
OTHER GRAIN CAKES					
Unsalted Wheat Cakes (1 cake) Mother's (Quaker Oats Company)	0.0	0.0	0	0	35
Wheat Grain Cakes (1 cake) Quaker (Quaker Oats Company)	0.0	0.0	0	45	35

RICE CAKES—*see* POPCORN/RICE/OTHER GRAIN CAKES, page 114

Crackers

DAIRY PRODUCTS AND DAIRY SUBSTITUTES

At one time, "low-fat dairy products" was a contradiction in terms. Dairy products meant whole milk, which meant high fat. But not today!

Walking down your grocery aisles, you'll find skim and 1% milk, dozens of nonfat and low-fat cheeses and sour creams, and just about every flavor of nonfat yogurt imaginable. It's easier than ever to get the calcium you need without the fat and cholesterol you *don't.* As long as you stick with the skim, low-fat, or nonfat products listed in these tables, you can enjoy your favorite dairy products every day.

Like all the other entries in this book, the dairy products and dairy substitutes entries that follow list sodium content. The AHA does not have criteria for sodium but recommends a total of no more than 3,000 mg a day.

Generic Listings

By far, most of the foods in this book are brand name products. However, if a product is listed without a brand name, it means that most brands of that product contain about the same amount of fat, saturated fat, and cholesterol and that these amounts are within the criteria cited below.

If you find products that were introduced after this book went to press, use the generic listings and the following tables to help you evaluate them.

AHA Criteria for Dairy Products and Dairy Substitutes*

	Tot. Fat (g)	Sat. Fat (g)	Chol. (mg)
Buttermilk, cheese (except as listed below), milk, milk-based products, sour cream, and yogurt	3	2	20
Coffee creamers, liquid and powdered	3	<0.5	<2
Condensed or evaporated milk, undiluted, and whipped toppings	<0.5	<0.5	<2
Hard cheeses, grated, such as Parmesan and Romano	3	1	20

*Per serving.

Dairy Products and Dairy Substitutes You'll Want to Limit

Some dairy products and dairy substitutes, like the examples below, are too high in fat, saturated fat, and/or cholesterol to meet AHA criteria. They aren't included in this book, and we recommend that you don't eat them often.

Compare the amounts of fat, saturated fat, cholesterol, sodium, and calories in these examples with the more healthful alternatives listed on the following pages.

Sample Dairy Products and Dairy Substitutes to Limit

	Tot. Fat (g)	Sat. Fat (g)	Chol. (mg)	Sod. (mg)	Cal.
Coffee cream (1 tbsp)	2.9	1.8*	10*	6	29
Creamed cottage cheese (½ cup)	5.1*	3.2*	17	457	117
Cultured sour cream (1 oz, or about 2½ tbsp)	5.9*	3.7*	12	14	61
Evaporated whole milk (2 tbsp)	2.4*	1.5*	9*	33	42
Pimiento pasteurized process cheese (1 oz)	8.8*	5.6*	27*	405	106
Whole milk (1 cup)	8.2*	5.1*	33*	120	150

Adapted from USDA Handbook No. 8 series.

*These values exceed AHA criteria for dairy products.

	Tot. Fat (g)	Sat. Fat (g)	Chol. (mg)	Sod. (mg)	Cal.
BUTTERMILK—*see* MILKS/ BUTTERMILKS, page 129					
CHEESES					
AMERICAN CHEESES					
Chunk/Shredded/Sliced American Cheeses					
American Flavor Fat Free Non-Dairy Slices (1 slice)					
Heart Beat Foods Smart Beat (GFA Brands)	0.0	0.0	0	180	25
American Flavor Lactose Free Fat Free Non-Dairy Slices (1 slice)					
Heart Beat Foods Smart Beat (GFA Brands)	0.0	0.0	0	180	25
American Flavor Low Sodium Reduced Calorie Slices (1 slice)					
Heart Beat Foods Smart Beat (GFA Brands)	2.0	<1.0	0	90	35
Fat Free Pasteurized Process Skim Milk American Cheese Product Singles (⅔ oz)					
Alpine Lace (Alpine Lace Brands)	0.0	0.0	<5	280	25
Fat Free Pasteurized Skim Milk American Processed Cheese Product (1 oz)					
Alpine Lace (Alpine Lace Brands)	0.0	0.0	<5	280	45
Fat Free White Cheese Slices (0.75 oz)					
Weight Watchers (H.J. Heinz)	0.0	0.0	0	310	30
Fat Free Yellow Cheese Slices (0.75 oz)					
Weight Watchers (H.J. Heinz)	0.0	0.0	0	310	30
Grated American Cheese Food (1 tbsp)					
Kraft (Kraft General Foods)*	1.5	1.0	<5	135	25
Low Sodium White American Cheese Slices (0.75 oz)					
Weight Watchers (H.J. Heinz)	2.0	1.0	5	110	50
Low Sodium Yellow American Cheese Slices (0.75 oz)					
Weight Watchers (H.J. Heinz)	2.0	1.0	5	110	50

*Tobacco company, corporate subsidiary, or parent.

	Tot. Fat (g)	Sat. Fat (g)	Chol. (mg)	Sod. (mg)	Cal.
AMERICAN CHEESES *(cont'd)*					
Nonfat Pasteurized Process Cheese Slice Singles					
Kraft Free (Kraft General Foods)* (⅔ oz)	0.0	0.0	<5	290	30
Kraft Free (Kraft General Foods)* (¾ oz)	0.0	0.0	<5	320	30
Nonfat Pasteurized Process Cheese Slice Singles (White)					
Kraft Free (Kraft General Foods)* (⅔ oz)	0.0	0.0	<5	290	30
Kraft Free (Kraft General Foods)* (¾ oz)	0.0	0.0	<5	320	30
Pasteurized Process Cheese Product (1 oz)					
Velveeta Light (Kraft General Foods)*	3.0	2.0	10	420	60
Process Cheese Loaf (1″ slice)					
Healthy Choice (Beatrice Cheese)	0.0	0.0	<5	390	35
White American Singles (¾ oz)					
Healthy Choice (Beatrice Cheese)	0.0	0.0	<5	290	30
Yellow American Singles					
Healthy Choice (Beatrice Cheese) (⅔ oz)	0.0	0.0	<5	270	25
Healthy Choice (Beatrice Cheese) (¾ oz)	0.0	0.0	<5	290	30
Spreadable American Cheeses					
Light Pasteurized Process Cheese Product (2 tbsp)					
Kraft Cheez Whiz (Kraft General Foods)*	3.0	2.0	15	540	80
CHEDDAR CHEESES					
Chunk/Shredded/Sliced Cheddar Cheeses					
Cheddar Antioxidant Fortified Fat Free Cheese (1 oz)					
Healthy Farms (Lifeline Food)	0.0	0.0	<5	220	40
Cheddar Fat Free Cheese (1 oz)					
Lifetime (Lifeline Food)	0.0	0.0	<5	220	40

*Tobacco company, corporate subsidiary, or parent.

	Tot. Fat (g)	Sat. Fat (g)	Chol. (mg)	Sod. (mg)	Cal.
Cheddar Fat-Free Shredded Natural Non-Fat Cheese (¼ cup) Kraft Healthy Favorites (Kraft General Foods)*	0.0	0.0	<5	220	45
Fancy Shredded Cheddar Cheese (¼ cup) Healthy Choice (Beatrice Cheese)	0.0	0.0	<5	200	45
Fat Free Pasteurized Process Skim Milk Cheddar Cheese Product, Shredded (¼ cup) Alpine Lace (Alpine Lace Brands)	0.0	0.0	<5	280	45
Fat Free Pasteurized Process Skim Milk Cheese Product, Cheddar, Chunk (⅛ bar) Alpine Lace (Alpine Lace Brands)	0.0	0.0	<5	280	45
Fat Free Pasteurized Skim Milk Cheddar Processed Cheese Product, deli cut (1 oz) Alpine Lace (Alpine Lace Brands)	0.0	0.0	<5	280	45
Fat Free Sharp Cheddar Cheese Slices (0.75 oz) Weight Watchers (H.J. Heinz) . .	0.0	0.0	0	310	30
Mellow Cheddar Flavor Fat Free Non-Dairy Slices (1 slice) Heart Beat Foods Smart Beat (GFA Brands)	0.0	0.0	0	180	25
Salsa Cheddar Antioxidant Fortified Fat Free Cheese (1 oz) Healthy Farms (Lifeline Food) . . .	0.0	0.0	<5	220	40
Sharp Cheddar Antioxidant Fortified Fat Free Cheese (1 oz) Healthy Farms (Lifeline Food) . . .	0.0	0.0	<5	220	40
Sharp Cheddar Artificially Flavored Nonfat Pasteurized Process Cheese Slice Singles (¾ oz) Kraft Free (Kraft General Foods)*	0.0	0.0	<5	290	30
Sharp Cheddar Fat Free Cheese (1 oz) Lifetime (Lifeline Food)	0.0	0.0	<5	220	40

*Tobacco company, corporate subsidiary, or parent.

	Tot. Fat (g)	Sat. Fat (g)	Chol. (mg)	Sod. (mg)	Cal.
CHEDDAR CHEESES *(cont'd)*					
Sharp Cheddar Flavor Fat Free Non-Dairy Slices (1 slice)					
Heart Beat Foods Smart Beat (GFA Brands)	0.0	0.0	0	230	25
Shredded Cheddar Cheese (¼ cup)					
Healthy Choice (Beatrice Cheese)	0.0	0.0	<5	200	45
Imitation Cheddar Cheese					
Cheddar Cheese Alternative, shredded (1 oz)					
Formägg (Galaxy Foods)	3.0	0.0	0	190	60
COTTAGE CHEESES					
Dry Curd Cottage Cheeses					
Dry curd cottage cheese (½ cup)					
Most brands (USDA)	**0.3**	**0.2**	**5**	**10**	**62**
Dry Curd Cottage Cheese Less than ½% Milk Fat with Added Skim Milk (¼ cup)					
Breakstone's (Kraft General Foods)*	0.0	0.0	5	25	45
Regular Cottage Cheeses					
Lowfat Cottage Cheese (½ cup)					
Nancy's (Springfield Creamery)	1.0	0.5	5	460	80
Lowfat Cottage Cheese 1% Milkfat (½ cup)					
Kraft Light n' Lively (Kraft General Foods)*	1.5	1.0	15	380	80
Lowfat Large Curd Cottage Cheese 2% Milkfat (½ cup)					
Breakstone's (Kraft General Foods)*	2.5	1.5	15	380	90
Lowfat Small Curd Cottage Cheese 2% Milkfat (½ cup)					
Breakstone's (Kraft General Foods)*	2.5	1.5	15	380	90
Knudsen (Kraft General Foods)*	2.5	1.5	15	400	100
Sealtest (Kraft General Foods)*	2.5	1.5	15	380	90
No Fat Cottage Cheese (½ cup)					
Cabot (Cabot Creamery)	0.0	0.0	5	410	70

*Tobacco company, corporate subsidiary, or parent.

	Tot. Fat (g)	Sat. Fat (g)	Chol. (mg)	Sod. (mg)	Cal.
1% Fat Cottage Cheese (½ cup)					
Most brands (USDA)	**1.2**	**0.7**	**5**	**459**	**82**
Weight Watchers (H.J. Heinz) . .	1.0	0.5	5	460	90
Nonfat Cottage Cheese (½ cup)					
Crowley (Crowley Foods)	0.0	0.0	10	500	90
Knudsen Free (Kraft General Foods)*	0.0	0.0	10	370	80
Kraft Light n'Lively Free (Kraft General Foods)*	0.0	0.0	10	440	80
2% fat cottage cheese (½ cup)					
Most brands (USDA)	**2.2**	**1.4**	**9**	**459**	**101**
Regular Cottage Cheese with Fruit					
Lowfat Cottage Cheese & Peach 1.5% Milkfat (4 oz)					
Knudsen (Kraft General Foods)*	1.5	1.0	10	290	110
Lowfat Cottage Cheese & Pineapple 1.5% Milkfat (4 oz)					
Knudsen (Kraft General Foods)*	1.5	1.0	10	290	110
Lowfat Cottage Cheese & Strawberry 1.5% Milkfat (4 oz)					
Knudsen (Kraft General Foods)*	1.5	1.0	10	280	110
Lowfat Cottage Cheese & Tropical Fruit 1.5% Milkfat (4 oz)					
Knudsen (Kraft General Foods)*	2.0	1.5	10	300	120
Lowfat Cottage Cheese 1% Milkfat with Peach & Pineapple (½ cup)					
Kraft Light n' Lively (Kraft General Foods)*	1.0	1.0	10	350	120
Nonfat Cottage Cheese with Aspartame Sweetened Peach (½ cup)					
Crowley (Crowley Foods)	0.0	0.0	5	410	90
Nonfat Cottage Cheese with Aspartame Sweetened Pear (½ cup)					
Crowley (Crowley Foods)	0.0	0.0	5	410	90

*Tobacco company, corporate subsidiary, or parent.

	Tot. Fat (g)	Sat. Fat (g)	Chol. (mg)	Sod. (mg)	Cal.
COTTAGE CHEESES *(cont'd)*					
Nonfat Cottage Cheese with Aspartame Sweetened Pineapple (½ cup)					
Crowley (Crowley Foods)	0.0	0.0	5	440	90
Nonfat Cottage Cheese with Aspartame Sweetened Spiced Apple (½ cup)					
Crowley (Crowley Foods)	0.0	0.0	5	420	90
Regular Cottage Cheeses with Vegetables					
Lowfat Cottage Cheese 1% Milkfat with Garden Salad (½ cup)					
Kraft Light n' Lively (Kraft General Foods)*	1.5	1.0	15	410	90
CREAM CHEESES					
Flavored Cream Cheeses					
Fat Free Cream Cheese with Garden Vegetables (2 tbsp)					
Alpine Lace (Alpine Lace Brands)	0.0	0.0	<5	165	30
Fat Free Garlic & Herbs Cream Cheese (2 tbsp)					
Alpine Lace (Alpine Lace Brands)	0.0	0.0	<5	165	30
Fat Free Mexican Nacho Cream Cheese (2 tbsp)					
Alpine Lace (Alpine Lace Brands)	0.0	0.0	<5	165	30
Herbs & Garlic Cream Cheese (2 tbsp)					
Healthy Choice (Beatrice Cheese)	0.0	0.0	<5	200	25
Strawberry Cream Cheese (2 tbsp)					
Healthy Choice (Beatrice Cheese)	0.0	0.0	<5	200	35
Plain Cream Cheeses					
Cream Cheese (1 oz)					
Weight Watchers (H.J. Heinz)	2.0	1.0	10	40	35
Fat Free Cream Cheese (2 tbsp)					
Alpine Lace (Alpine Lace Brands)	0.0	0.0	<5	165	30
America's Choice (A & P)	0.0	0.0	<5	150	30
Fat Free Cream Cheese (Brick) (1 oz)					
Kraft Philadelphia Brand Free (Kraft General Foods)*	0.0	0.0	<5	135	25

*Tobacco company, corporate subsidiary, or parent.

	Tot. Fat (g)	Sat. Fat (g)	Chol. (mg)	Sod. (mg)	Cal.
Fat Free Cream Cheese (Soft) (2 tbsp)					
Kraft Philadelphia Brand Free (Kraft General Foods)*	0.0	0.0	<5	160	30
Plain Cream Cheese (2 tbsp)					
Healthy Choice (Beatrice Cheese)	0.0	0.0	<5	200	25
MONTEREY JACK CHEESES					
Chunk/Shredded/Sliced Monterey Jack Cheeses					
Monterey Jack Fat Free Cheese (1 oz)					
Lifetime (Lifeline Food)	0.0	0.0	<5	220	40
MOZZARELLA CHEESES					
Chunk/Shredded/Sliced Mozzarella Cheeses					
Fancy Shredded Mozzarella Cheese (¼ cup)					
Healthy Choice (Beatrice Cheese)	0.0	0.0	<5	200	45
Fat Free Pasteurized Process Skim Milk Cheese Product, Mozzarella, Chunk (⅛ bar)					
Alpine Lace (Alpine Lace Brands)	0.0	0.0	<5	280	45
Fat Free Pasteurized Process Skim Milk Shredded Mozzarella Cheese Product (¼ cup)					
Alpine Lace (Alpine Lace Brands)	0.0	0.0	<5	280	45
Fat Free Pasteurized Skim Milk Mozzarella Processed Cheese Product, deli cut (1 oz)					
Alpine Lace (Alpine Lace Brands)	0.0	0.0	<5	280	45
Mozzarella Cheese Ball (1″ cube)					
Healthy Choice (Beatrice Cheese)	0.0	0.0	<5	200	45
Mozzarella Fat-Free Shredded Natural Non-Fat Cheese (¼ cup)					
Kraft Healthy Favorites (Kraft General Foods)*	0.0	0.0	<5	280	50
Shredded Mozzarella Cheese (¼ cup)					
Healthy Choice (Beatrice Cheese)	0.0	0.0	<5	200	45
Imitation Mozzarella Cheeses					
Mozzarella Cheese Alternative, shredded (1 oz)					
Formägg (Galaxy Foods)	3.0	0.0	0	140	60

*Tobacco company, corporate subsidiary, or parent.

	Tot. Fat (g)	Sat. Fat (g)	Chol. (mg)	Sod. (mg)	Cal.
PARMESAN/ROMANO CHEESES					
Fat Free Grated Parmesan Italian Topping (1 tbsp)					
Weight Watchers (H.J. Heinz) . .	0.0	0.0	5	45	15
Grated House Italian (⅓ Less Fat) (2 tsp)					
Kraft (Kraft General Foods)*	1.0	0.5	<5	115	25
Grated Italian Blend (2 tsp)					
Kraft (Kraft General Foods)*	1.5	1.0	<5	95	25
Grated Parmesan Cheese Alternative (2 tsp)					
Formägg (Galaxy Foods)	0.5	0.0	0	80	15
100% Grated Parmesan Cheese (2 tsp)					
DiGiorno (Kraft General Foods)*	1.5	1.0	5	85	20
Kraft (Kraft General Foods)*	1.5	1.0	5	90	25
100% Grated Romano Cheese (2 tsp)					
DiGiorno (Kraft General Foods)*	1.5	1.0	5	90	20
100% Shredded Parmesan Cheese (2 tsp)					
DiGiorno (Kraft General Foods)*	1.5	1.0	<5	75	20
Kraft (Kraft General Foods)*	1.5	1.0	<5	75	20
100% Shredded Romano Cheese (2 tsp)					
DiGiorno (Kraft General Foods)*	1.5	1.0	5	70	20
Parmesan Cheese (2 tsp)					
DiGiorno (Kraft General Foods)*	1.0	1.0	5	55	20
Romano Cheese (2 tsp)					
DiGiorno (Kraft General Foods)*	1.5	1.0	5	75	20
RICOTTA CHEESES					
Fat Free Ricotta (¼ cup)					
Miceli's (Miceli Dairy Products) . .	0.0	0.0	15	65	50
ROMANO CHEESES—*see* PARMESAN/ ROMANO CHEESES, page 127					
STRING CHEESES					
Mozzarella String Cheese (1 stick)					
Healthy Choice (Beatrice Cheese)	0.0	0.0	<5	200	45
Pizza String Cheese (1 stick)					
Healthy Choice (Beatrice Cheese)	0.0	0.0	<5	200	45

*Tobacco company, corporate subsidiary, or parent.

	Tot. Fat (g)	Sat. Fat (g)	Chol. (mg)	Sod. (mg)	Cal.
SWISS CHEESES					
Chunk/Shredded/Sliced Swiss Cheeses					
Fat Free Swiss Cheese Slices (0.75 oz)					
Weight Watchers (H.J. Heinz)	0.0	0.0	0	280	30
Swiss Antioxidant Fortified Fat Free Cheese (1 oz)					
Healthy Farms (Lifeline Food)	0.0	0.0	<5	220	40
Swiss Artificially Flavored Nonfat Pasteurized Process Cheese Slice Singles (¾ oz)					
Kraft Free (Kraft General Foods)*	0.0	0.0	<5	290	30
Swiss Fat Free Cheese (1 oz)					
Lifetime (Lifeline Food)	0.0	0.0	<5	220	40
OTHER CHEESES					
Fancy Shredded Pizza Cheese (¼ cup)					
Healthy Choice (Beatrice Cheese)	0.0	0.0	<5	200	45
Garden Vegetable Fat Free Cheese (1 oz)					
Lifetime (Lifeline Food)	0.0	0.0	<5	220	40
Mild Mexican Fat Free Cheese (1 oz)					
Lifetime (Lifeline Food)	0.0	0.0	<5	220	40
Shredded Mexican Cheese (¼ cup)					
Healthy Choice (Beatrice Cheese)	0.0	0.0	<5	200	45
Swiss Knight Light (1 oz)					
Swiss Knight (Gerber Cheese Co)	2.5	1.0	10	270	45
COFFEE CREAMERS					
Coffee Creamer (1 tsp)					
N-Rich (Hunt-Wesson)	<1.0	0.3	0	0	10
Dairy Creamer Instant Nonfat Milk (1 pkt)					
Weight Watchers (H.J. Heinz)	0.0	0.0	(0)	15	10

FROZEN DAIRY DESSERTS—*see* "FROZEN DESSERTS," ICE CREAMS/ICE MILKS, page 214

*Tobacco company, corporate subsidiary, or parent.

	Tot. Fat (g)	Sat. Fat (g)	Chol. (mg)	Sod. (mg)	Cal.
MILKS/BUTTERMILKS					
BUTTERMILKS					
Buttermilk, cultured (1 cup)					
Most brands (USDA)	**2.2**	**1.3**	**9**	**257**	**99**
Cultured Buttermilk Blend (4 tbsp dry)					
Saco (Saco Foods)	1.0	0.0	4	166	80
CHOCOLATE MILKS					
Fat Free Cholesterol Free No Sugar Added Chocolate Milk (1 cup)					
Golden Jersey (U.S. Dairy)	0.0	0.0	0	155	110
DRY MILKS					
Mix'n Drink Pure Skim Milk (⅓ cup)					
Saco (Saco Foods)	0.0	0.0	<5	125	80
Nonfat Dry Milk					
Most brands (USDA) (¼ cup)	**<1.0**	**0.0**	**0**	**161**	**109**
Carnation (Nestlé Food Company) (⅓ cup)	0.0	0.0	<5	125	80
Sanalac (Hunt-Wesson) (8 oz liquid)	<1.0	0.0	4	125	80
EVAPORATED MILKS					
Evaporated Skim Milk (2 tbsp)					
Most brands (USDA)	**0.1**	**0.0**	**1**	**37**	**25**
Pet	0.0	0.0	<5	35	25
Lowfat Evaporated Milk (2 tbsp)					
Carnation (Nestlé Food Company)	0.5	0.0	5	35	25
Skimmed Evaporated Milk (2 tbsp)					
Carnation (Nestlé Food Company)	0.0	0.0	0	40	25
REGULAR MILKS					
Fat Free Cholesterol Free Milk (1 cup)					
Golden Jersey (U.S. Dairy)	0.0	0.0	0	120	100
Fat Free Skim Milk with Solids Added (1 cup)					
Borden	0.0	0.0	10	125	90
Nonfat milk (1 cup)					
Most brands (USDA)	**0.4**	**0.3**	**4**	**126**	**86**
½% fat milk (1 cup)					
Most brands (USDA)	**1.0**	**1.0**	**7**	**125**	**94**
½% Plus Lowfat Milk (1 cup)					
Robinson (Robinson Dairy)	1.0	0.5	10	125	90
1% fat milk (1 cup)					
Most brands (USDA)	**2.6**	**1.6**	**10**	**123**	**102**

	Tot. Fat (g)	Sat. Fat (g)	Chol. (mg)	Sod. (mg)	Cal.
Organic Nonfat Milk (1 cup)					
Horizon (Natural Horizons)	0.0	0.0	4	130	90
Skim milk, nonfat (1 cup)					
Most brands (USDA)	**0.4**	**0.3**	**4**	**126**	**86**
MILK SUBSTITUTES					
EdenBlend (8 fl oz)					
EdenBlend (Eden Foods)	3.0	0.5	0	85	120
EdenRice (8 fl oz)					
EdenRice (Eden Foods)	3.0	0.0	0	85	110
Extra Vanilla (8 fl oz)					
Edensoy (Eden Foods)	3.0	0.0	0	90	140
Fat Free Chocolate Vegelicious Ready-to-Serve Beverage (8 oz)					
A&A Amazing Foods	0.0	0.0	0	200	140
Fat-Free Soy Moo (1 cup)					
Health Valley (Health Valley Foods)	0.0	0.0	0	60	110
Fat Free Vegelicious Ready-to-Serve Beverage (8 oz)					
A&A Amazing Foods	0.0	0.0	0	100	90
Vanilla (8 fl oz)					
Edensoy (Eden Foods)	3.0	0.0	0	90	150
Vegelicious Beverage Mix, made with water (8 oz)					
A&A Amazing Foods	2.5	0.0	0	115	90
SOUR CREAMS					
Fat Free Sour Cream (2 tbsp)					
Breakstone's Free (Kraft General Foods)*	0.0	0.0	<5	25	35
Knudsen Free (Kraft General Foods)*	0.0	0.0	0	25	35
Sealtest Free (Kraft General Foods)*	0.0	0.0	<5	25	35
Light Sour Cream					
Knudsen Light (Kraft General Foods)* (2 tbsp)	2.5	2.0	10	20	40
Sealtest Light (Kraft General Foods)* (2 tbsp)	2.5	2.0	10	20	40
Weight Watchers (H.J. Heinz) (1 oz)	2.0	1.0	5	40	35

*Tobacco company, corporate subsidiary, or parent.

	Tot. Fat (g)	Sat. Fat (g)	Chol. (mg)	Sod. (mg)	Cal.
SOUR CREAMS *(cont'd)*					
No Fat Sour Cream (2 tbsp)					
Land O'Lakes (Land O'Lakes Foods)	0.0	0.0	<5	45	30
Nonfat Sour Cream (2 tbsp)					
Crowley (Crowley Foods)	0.0	0.0	0	45	20
Real Dairy No Fat Sour Cream (2 tbsp)					
Naturally Yours (International Delight)	0.0	0.0	0	25	20
WHIPPED TOPPINGS					
Whipped Topping Mix, made with skim milk (2 tbsp)					
Dream Whip (Kraft General Foods)*	0.5	0.5	0	10	18
YOGURT DRINKS					
Blueberry Nonfat Yogurt Drink (1 cup)					
Nancy's (Springfield Creamery)	0.0	0.0	5	150	180
Boysenberry Nonfat Yogurt Drink (1 cup)					
Nancy's (Springfield Creamery)	0.0	0.0	5	140	180
Cherry Nonfat Yogurt Drink (1 cup)					
Nancy's (Springfield Creamery)	0.0	0.0	5	140	190
Raspberry Nonfat Yogurt Drink (1 cup)					
Nancy's (Springfield Creamery)	0.0	0.0	5	140	180
Strawberry Nonfat Yogurt Drink (1 cup)					
Nancy's (Springfield Creamery)	0.0	0.0	5	140	170
YOGURTS					
FRUIT YOGURTS					
Apple Yogurts					
Apple Cinnamon Fruit on the Bottom Lowfat Yogurt (227 g)					
Dannon (The Dannon Company)	3.0	1.5	15	140	240
99% Fat Free Spiced Apple Yogurt (6 oz)					
Yoplait Original (General Mills)	1.5	1.0	10	105	170

*Tobacco company, corporate subsidiary, or parent.

	Tot. Fat (g)	Sat. Fat (g)	Chol. (mg)	Sod. (mg)	Cal.
Banana Yogurts					
Banana Cream Pie Nonfat Yogurt with Aspartame (227 g) Dannon (The Dannon Company)	0.0	0.0	<5	125	100
Blueberry Yogurts					
Berry Blue Kidpack Lowfat Yogurt 1% Milkfat (4.4 oz) Kraft Light n' Lively (Kraft General Foods)*	1.0	0.5	10	65	150
Blueberries 'n Creme Nonfat Yogurt (1 cup) Weight Watchers Ultimate 90 (H.J. Heinz)	0.0	0.0	5	140	90
Blueberry 50 Calories Nonfat Yogurt with Aspartame Sweetener (4.4 oz) Kraft Light n' Lively Free (Kraft General Foods)*	0.0	0.0	<5	60	50
Blueberry Fruit on the Bottom Lowfat Yogurt (227 g) Dannon (The Dannon Company)	3.0	1.5	15	140	240
Blueberry Lowfat Yogurt (1 cup) Nancy's (Springfield Creamery) .	2.5	2.0	15	150	180
Blueberry Lowfat Yogurt Multipack 1% Milkfat (4.4 oz) Kraft Light n' Lively (Kraft General Foods)*	1.0	0.5	10	65	140
Blueberry Lowfat Yogurt 1% Milkfat (8 oz) Breyers (Kraft General Foods)* .	2.5	1.5	15	110	250
Blueberry Nonfat Swiss Aspartame Yogurt (1 container) Crowley (Crowley Foods)	0.0	0.0	<5	130	100
Blueberry Nonfat Yogurt (6 oz) Kraft Light n' Lively Free (Kraft General Foods)*	0.0	0.0	5	105	190
Blueberry Nonfat Yogurt with Aspartame (227 g) Dannon Light (The Dannon Company)	0.0	0.0	<5	140	100

*Tobacco company, corporate subsidiary, or parent.

	Tot. Fat (g)	Sat. Fat (g)	Chol. (mg)	Sod. (mg)	Cal.
FRUIT YOGURTS *(cont'd)*					
Blueberry Nonfat Yogurt with Aspartame Sweetener (6 oz)					
Knudsen Cal 70 (Kraft General Foods)*	0.0	0.0	5	80	70
Blueberry 70 Calories Nonfat Yogurt with Aspartame Sweetener (6 oz)					
Kraft Light n' Lively Free (Kraft General Foods)*	0.0	0.0	<5	80	70
Blueberry Yogurt (6 oz)					
Yoplait Light (General Mills)	0.0	0.0	<5	85	90
Fat Free Blueberry Yogurt					
Dannon Blended (The Dannon Company) (170 g)	0.0	0.0	<5	105	160
Yoplait Fruit on the Bottom (General Mills) (6 oz)	0.0	0.0	<5	105	160
Fat Free Swiss Style Blueberry Yogurt (1 container)					
Borden	0.0	0.0	5	105	100
Viva (Borden)	0.0	0.0	5	105	100
Lite 85 Nonfat Blueberry Yogurt (6 oz)					
Wells' Blue Bunny (Wells' Dairy)	0.0	0.0	<5	130	80
99% Fat Free Blueberry Yogurt (6 oz)					
Yoplait Original (General Mills)	1.5	1.0	10	105	170
No Fat Blueberry Yogurt (1 cup)					
Cabot (Cabot Creamery)	0.0	0.0	5	115	130
Organic Blueberry Yogurt (¾ cup)					
Horizon (Natural Horizons)	0.0	0.0	5	115	130
Boysenberry Yogurts					
Boysenberry Fruit on the Bottom Lowfat Yogurt (227 g)					
Dannon (The Dannon Company)	3.0	1.5	15	150	240
99% Fat Free Boysenberry Yogurt (6 oz)					
Yoplait Original (General Mills)	1.5	1.0	10	105	170
Cherry Yogurts					
Black Cherry Lowfat Yogurt 1% Milkfat (8 oz)					
Breyers (Kraft General Foods)*	2.5	1.5	15	110	260

*Tobacco company, corporate subsidiary, or parent.

	Tot. Fat (g)	Sat. Fat (g)	Chol. (mg)	Sod. (mg)	Cal.
Black Cherry Nonfat Swiss Aspartame Yogurt (1 container) Crowley (Crowley Foods)	0.0	0.0	<5	130	100
Black Cherry Nonfat Yogurt with Aspartame Sweetener (6 oz) Knudsen Cal 70 (Kraft General Foods)*	0.0	0.0	5	85	70
Black Cherry 70 Calories Nonfat Yogurt with Aspartame Sweetener (6 oz) Kraft Light n' Lively Free (Kraft General Foods)*	0.0	0.0	<5	85	70
Cherry Cheesecake with Graham Crunch (7 oz) Yoplait Crunch 'n Yogurt Light (General Mills)	1.0	0.0	<5	115	130
Cherry Fruit on the Bottom Lowfat Yogurt (227 g) Dannon (The Dannon Company)	3.0	1.5	15	135	240
Cherry Jubilee Nonfat Yogurt (1 cup) Weight Watchers Ultimate 90 (H.J. Heinz)	0.0	0.0	5	140	90
Cherry Kidpack Lowfat Yogurt 1% Milkfat (4.4 oz) Kraft Light n' Lively (Kraft General Foods)*	1.0	0.5	10	65	140
Cherry Vanilla Nonfat Swiss Aspartame Yogurt (1 container) Crowley (Crowley Foods)	0.0	0.0	<5	130	100
Cherry Vanilla Nonfat Yogurt with Aspartame (227 g) Dannon Light (The Dannon Company)	0.0	0.0	<5	140	100
Cherry Yogurt (6 oz) Yoplait Light (General Mills)	0.0	0.0	<5	85	90
Fat Free Cherry Yogurt (6 oz) Yoplait Fruit on the Bottom (General Mills)	0.0	0.0	<5	105	160
Light Cherry Vanilla Yogurt (6 oz) Yoplait Custard Style (General Mills)	0.0	0.0	0	85	90

*Tobacco company, corporate subsidiary, or parent.

	Tot. Fat (g)	Sat. Fat (g)	Chol. (mg)	Sod. (mg)	Cal.
Fruit Yogurts *(cont'd)*					
Lite 85 Nonfat Black Cherry Yogurt (6 oz) Wells' Blue Bunny (Wells' Dairy) .	0.0	0.0	<5	130	80
Lite 85 Nonfat Cherry Vanilla Yogurt (6 oz) Wells' Blue Bunny (Wells' Dairy) .	0.0	0.0	<5	130	80
99% Fat Free Cherry Yogurt (6 oz) Yoplait Original (General Mills) . .	1.5	1.0	10	105	170
No Fat Black Cherry Yogurt (1 cup) Cabot (Cabot Creamery)	0.0	0.0	5	115	130
Organic Cherry Yogurt (¾ cup) Horizon (Natural Horizons)	0.0	0.0	5	115	130
Lemon Yogurts					
Creamy Lemon Lowfat Yogurt 1.5% Milkfat (8 oz) Breyers (Kraft General Foods)* .	3.0	2.0	20	140	220
Fat Free Lemon Chiffon Yogurt (170 g) Dannon Blended (The Dannon Company)	0.0	0.0	<5	110	150
Lemon Chiffon Nonfat Yogurt (1 cup) Weight Watchers Ultimate 90 (H.J. Heinz)	0.0	0.0	5	140	90
Lemon Chiffon Nonfat Yogurt with Aspartame (227 g) Dannon Light (The Dannon Company)	0.0	0.0	<5	140	100
Lemon Chiffon with Blueberry Crunchies Nonfat Yogurt (227 g) Dannon Light 'N Crunchy (The Dannon Company)	0.0	0.0	<5	150	140
Lemon Flavored Nonfat Yogurt (6 oz) Kraft Light n' Lively Free (Kraft General Foods)*	0.0	0.0	5	105	170
Lemon Lowfat Yogurt (227 g) Dannon (The Dannon Company)	3.0	2.0	15	160	210
Lemon Nonfat Swiss Aspartame Yogurt (1 container) Crowley (Crowley Foods)	0.0	0.0	<5	130	100

*Tobacco company, corporate subsidiary, or parent.

	Tot. Fat (g)	Sat. Fat (g)	Chol. (mg)	Sod. (mg)	Cal.
Lemon Nonfat Yogurt (6 oz)					
Knudsen Free (Kraft General Foods)*	0.0	0.0	5	105	160
Lemon Nonfat Yogurt with Aspartame Sweetener (6 oz)					
Knudsen Cal 70 (Kraft General Foods)*	0.0	0.0	5	100	70
Lemon 70 Calories Nonfat Yogurt with Aspartame Sweetener (6 oz)					
Kraft Light n' Lively Free (Kraft General Foods)*	0.0	0.0	<5	120	70
Lite 85 Nonfat Lemon Yogurt (6 oz)					
Wells' Blue Bunny (Wells' Dairy)	0.0	0.0	<5	160	80
99% Fat Free Lemon Yogurt (6 oz)					
Yoplait Original (General Mills)	1.5	1.0	10	105	170
No Fat Lemon Yogurt (1 cup)					
Cabot (Cabot Creamery)	0.0	0.0	5	115	130
Mixed Berry Yogurts					
Fat Free Swiss Style Mixed Berry Yogurt (1 container)					
Borden	0.0	0.0	5	105	100
Viva (Borden)	0.0	0.0	5	105	100
Lite 85 Nonfat Mixed Berry Yogurt (6 oz)					
Wells' Blue Bunny (Wells' Dairy)	0.0	0.0	<5	140	80
Mixed Berries Fruit on the Bottom Lowfat Yogurt (227 g)					
Dannon (The Dannon Company)	3.0	1.5	15	150	240
Mixed Berry Lowfat Yogurt (6 oz)					
Yoplait Breakfast (General Mills)	2.0	1.0	10	125	200
Mixed Berry Lowfat Yogurt 1% Milkfat (8 oz)					
Breyers (Kraft General Foods)*	2.5	1.5	15	110	250
Mixed Berry Nonfat Swiss Aspartame Yogurt (1 container)					
Crowley (Crowley Foods)	0.0	0.0	<5	130	100
Mixed Berry Nonfat Yogurt (6 oz)					
Knudsen Free (Kraft General Foods)*	0.0	0.0	5	105	170
Kraft Light n' Lively Free (Kraft General Foods)*	0.0	0.0	5	105	170

*Tobacco company, corporate subsidiary, or parent.

	Tot. Fat (g)	Sat. Fat (g)	Chol. (mg)	Sod. (mg)	Cal.
Fruit Yogurts *(cont'd)*					
99% Fat Free Mixed Berry Yogurt (6 oz)					
Yoplait Original (General Mills) . .	1.5	1.0	10	105	170
No Fat Very Berry Yogurt (1 cup)					
Cabot (Cabot Creamery)	0.0	0.0	5	115	130
Wild Berry Kidpack Lowfat Yogurt 1% Milkfat (4.4 oz)					
Kraft Light n' Lively (Kraft General Foods)*	1.0	0.5	10	65	140
Mixed Fruit Yogurts—*see also* Strawberry-Banana Yogurts, page 146					
Banana Berry Kidpack Lowfat Yogurt 1% Milkfat (4.4 oz)					
Kraft Light n' Lively (Kraft General Foods)*	1.0	1.0	10	65	130
Cranberry Raspberry Nonfat Yogurt (1 cup)					
Weight Watchers Ultimate 90 (H.J. Heinz)	0.0	0.0	5	140	90
Cran/Raspberry Lowfat Yogurt (227 g)					
Dannon (The Dannon Company)	3.0	2.0	15	150	200
99% Fat Free Strawberry-Rhubarb Yogurt (6 oz)					
Yoplait Original (General Mills) . .	1.5	1.0	10	105	170
Nonfat Yogurt & Fruit Cup (9.5 oz)					
Nancy's (Springfield Creamery) .	0.0	0.0	5	180	175
Papaya-Pineapple Nonfat Yogurt (170 g)					
Dannon Tropifruta (The Dannon Company)	0.0	0.0	5	105	150
Tropical Fruit Lowfat Yogurt (6 oz)					
Yoplait Breakfast (General Mills) .	2.5	1.0	10	125	210
Tropical Fruit Nonfat Yogurt with Aspartame (227 g)					
Dannon Light (The Dannon Company)	0.0	0.0	<5	140	100

*Tobacco company, corporate subsidiary, or parent.

	Tot. Fat (g)	Sat. Fat (g)	Chol. (mg)	Sod. (mg)	Cal.
Tropical Punch Kidpack Lowfat Yogurt 1% Milkfat (4.4 oz) Kraft Light n' Lively (Kraft General Foods)*	1.0	0.5	10	65	140
Orange Yogurts					
Lite 85 Nonfat Orange Yogurt (6 oz) Wells' Blue Bunny (Wells' Dairy)	0.0	0.0	<5	130	80
99% Fat Free Orange Yogurt (6 oz) Yoplait Original (General Mills)	1.5	1.0	10	105	170
Orange Fruit on the Bottom Lowfat Yogurt (227 g) Dannon (The Dannon Company)	3.0	1.5	15	135	240
Outrageous Orange Kidpack Lowfat Yogurt 1% Milkfat (4.4 oz) Kraft Light n' Lively (Kraft General Foods)*	1.0	0.5	10	65	150
Peach Yogurts					
Fat Free Peach Yogurt (170 g) Dannon Blended (The Dannon Company)	0.0	0.0	<5	100	150
Fat Free Peach Yogurt (6 oz) Yoplait Fruit on the Bottom (General Mills)	0.0	0.0	<5	105	160
Fat Free Swiss Style Peach Yogurt (1 container)					
Borden	0.0	0.0	5	105	100
Viva (Borden)	0.0	0.0	5	105	100
Light Peach Yogurt (6 oz) Yoplait Custard Style (General Mills)	0.0	0.0	0	85	90
Lite 85 Nonfat Peach Yogurt (6 oz) Wells' Blue Bunny (Wells' Dairy)	0.0	0.0	<5	130	80
99% Fat Free Peach Yogurt (6 oz) Yoplait Original (General Mills)	1.5	1.0	10	105	170
No Fat Peach Yogurt (1 cup) Cabot (Cabot Creamery)	0.0	0.0	5	115	130
Organic Peach Yogurt (¾ cup) Horizon (Natural Horizons)	0.0	0.0	5	110	130

*Tobacco company, corporate subsidiary, or parent.

	Tot. Fat (g)	Sat. Fat (g)	Chol. (mg)	Sod. (mg)	Cal.
FRUIT YOGURTS *(cont'd)*					
Peach 50 Calories Nonfat Yogurt with Aspartame Sweetener (4.4 oz)					
Kraft Light n' Lively Free (Kraft General Foods)*	0.0	0.0	<5	60	50
Peach Fruit on the Bottom Lowfat Yogurt (227 g)					
Dannon (The Dannon Company)	3.0	1.5	15	140	240
Peach Lowfat Yogurt (1 cup)					
Nancy's (Springfield Creamery)	2.5	2.0	15	150	170
Peach Lowfat Yogurt Multipack 1% Milkfat (4.4 oz)					
Kraft Light n' Lively (Kraft General Foods)*	1.0	0.5	10	65	140
Peach Lowfat Yogurt 1% Milkfat (8 oz)					
Breyers (Kraft General Foods)*	2.5	1.5	15	110	250
Peach Nonfat Swiss Aspartame Yogurt (1 container)					
Crowley (Crowley Foods)	0.0	0.0	<5	130	100
Peach Nonfat Yogurt					
Knudsen Free (Kraft General Foods)* (6 oz)	0.0	0.0	5	105	170
Kraft Light n' Lively Free (Kraft General Foods)* (6 oz)	0.0	0.0	5	105	170
Weight Watchers Ultimate 90 (H.J. Heinz) (1 cup)	0.0	0.0	5	140	90
Peach Nonfat Yogurt with Aspartame (227 g)					
Dannon Light (The Dannon Company)	0.0	0.0	<5	140	100
Peach Nonfat Yogurt with Aspartame Sweetener (6 oz)					
Knudsen Cal 70 (Kraft General Foods)*	0.0	0.0	5	80	70
Peach 70 Calories Nonfat Yogurt with Aspartame Sweetener (6 oz)					
Kraft Light n' Lively Free (Kraft General Foods)*	0.0	0.0	<5	80	70
Peach Yogurt (6 oz)					
Yoplait Light (General Mills)	0.0	0.0	<5	85	90

*Tobacco company, corporate subsidiary, or parent.

	Tot. Fat (g)	Sat. Fat (g)	Chol. (mg)	Sod. (mg)	Cal.
Peach Yogurt with Granola (7 oz) Yoplait Crunch 'n Yogurt (General Mills)	1.5	0.0	<5	115	220
Piña Colada Yogurts					
Lite 85 Nonfat Piña Colada Yogurt (6 oz) Wells' Blue Bunny (Wells' Dairy)	0.0	0.0	<5	130	80
99% Fat Free Piña Colada Yogurt (6 oz) Yoplait Original (General Mills)	1.5	1.0	10	105	170
Piña Colada Nonfat Yogurt (170 g) Dannon Tropifruta (The Dannon Company)	0.0	0.0	5	105	150
Pineapple Yogurts—*see also* Piña Colada Yogurts, *above*					
Lite 85 Nonfat Pineapple Yogurt (6 oz) Wells' Blue Bunny (Wells' Dairy)	0.0	0.0	<5	130	80
99% Fat Free Pineapple Yogurt (6 oz) Yoplait Original (General Mills)	1.5	1.0	10	105	170
Pineapple Lowfat Yogurt Multipack 1% Milkfat (4.4 oz) Kraft Light n' Lively (Kraft General Foods)*	1.0	0.5	5	60	140
Pineapple Lowfat Yogurt 1% Milkfat (8 oz) Breyers (Kraft General Foods)*	2.5	1.5	15	110	250
Pineapple Nonfat Yogurt with Aspartame Sweetener (6 oz) Knudsen Cal 70 (Kraft General Foods)*	0.0	0.0	5	80	70
Raspberry Yogurts					
All Natural Nonfat Raspberry Yogurt (1 cup) Crowley (Crowley Foods)	0.0	0.0	5	220	230
Fat Free Raspberry Yogurt Dannon Blended (The Dannon Company) (170 g)	0.0	0.0	<5	100	160
Yoplait Fruit on the Bottom (General Mills) (6 oz)	0.0	0.0	<5	105	160

*Tobacco company, corporate subsidiary, or parent.

	Tot. Fat (g)	Sat. Fat (g)	Chol. (mg)	Sod. (mg)	Cal.
FRUIT YOGURTS *(cont'd)*					
Fat Free Swiss Style Raspberry Yogurt (1 container)					
Borden	0.0	0.0	5	105	100
Viva (Borden)	0.0	0.0	5	105	100
Lite 85 Nonfat Raspberry Yogurt (6 oz)					
Wells' Blue Bunny (Wells' Dairy)	0.0	0.0	<5	130	80
99% Fat Free Raspberry Yogurt (6 oz)					
Yoplait Original (General Mills)	1.5	1.0	10	105	170
No Fat Raspberry Yogurt (1 cup)					
Cabot (Cabot Creamery)	0.0	0.0	5	115	130
Organic Raspberry Yogurt (¾ cup)					
Horizon (Natural Horizons)	0.0	0.0	5	115	120
Raspberries 'n Creme Nonfat Yogurt (1 cup)					
Weight Watchers Ultimate 90 (H.J. Heinz)	0.0	0.0	5	140	90
Raspberry Fruit on the Bottom Lowfat Yogurt (227 g)					
Dannon (The Dannon Company)	3.0	1.5	15	150	240
Raspberry Lowfat Yogurt (1 cup)					
Nancy's (Springfield Creamery)	2.5	2.0	15	150	180
Raspberry Nonfat Swiss Aspartame Yogurt (1 container)					
Crowley (Crowley Foods)	0.0	0.0	<5	130	100
Raspberry Nonfat Yogurt with Aspartame (227 g)					
Dannon Light (The Dannon Company)	0.0	0.0	<5	150	100
Raspberry with Granola Crunchies Nonfat Yogurt (227 g)					
Dannon Light 'N Crunchy (The Dannon Company)	0.0	0.0	<5	135	150
Raspberry Yogurt (6 oz)					
Yoplait Light (General Mills)	0.0	0.0	<5	85	90
Raspberry Yogurt with Granola (7 oz)					
Yoplait Crunch 'n Yogurt (General Mills)	1.0	0.0	<5	115	130

	Tot. Fat (g)	Sat. Fat (g)	Chol. (mg)	Sod. (mg)	Cal.
Red Raspberry 50 Calories Nonfat Yogurt with Aspartame Sweetener (4.4 oz)					
Kraft Light n' Lively Free (Kraft General Foods)*	0.0	0.0	<5	60	50
Red Raspberry Lowfat Yogurt Multipack 1% Milkfat (4.4 oz)					
Kraft Light n' Lively (Kraft General Foods)*	1.0	1.0	10	65	130
Red Raspberry Lowfat Yogurt 1% Milkfat (8 oz)					
Breyers (Kraft General Foods)*	2.5	1.5	15	110	250
Red Raspberry Nonfat Yogurt (6 oz)					
Kraft Light n' Lively Free (Kraft General Foods)*	0.0	0.0	5	105	180
Red Raspberry Nonfat Yogurt (6 oz)					
Knudsen Free (Kraft General Foods)*	0.0	0.0	5	105	160
Red Raspberry Nonfat Yogurt with Aspartame Sweetener (6 oz)					
Knudsen Cal 70 (Kraft General Foods)*	0.0	0.0	5	75	70
Red Raspberry 70 Calories Nonfat Yogurt with Aspartame Sweetener (6 oz)					
Kraft Light n' Lively Free (Kraft General Foods)*	0.0	0.0	<5	80	70
Strawberry Yogurts—*see also* Strawberry-Banana Yogurts, page 146					
All Natural Nonfat Strawberry Yogurt (1 cup)					
Crowley (Crowley Foods)	0.0	0.0	5	220	220
Fat Free Strawberry Yogurt					
Dannon Blended (The Dannon Company) (170 g)	0.0	0.0	<5	105	150
Yoplait Fruit on the Bottom (General Mills) (6 oz)	0.0	0.0	<5	105	160
Fat Free Swiss Style Strawberry Yogurt (1 container)					
Borden	0.0	0.0	5	105	100
Viva (Borden)	0.0	0.0	5	105	100

*Tobacco company, corporate subsidiary, or parent.

	Tot. Fat (g)	Sat. Fat (g)	Chol. (mg)	Sod. (mg)	Cal.
FRUIT YOGURTS *(cont'd)*					
Light Strawberry Yogurt (6 oz)					
Yoplait Custard Style (General Mills)	0.0	0.0	0	85	90
Lite 85 Nonfat Strawberry Yogurt (6 oz)					
Wells' Blue Bunny (Wells' Dairy)	0.0	0.0	<5	130	80
99% Fat Free Strawberry Yogurt (6 oz)					
Yoplait Original (General Mills)	1.5	1.0	10	105	170
No Fat Strawberry Yogurt (1 cup)					
Cabot (Cabot Creamery)	0.0	0.0	5	115	130
Organic Strawberry Yogurt (¾ cup)					
Horizon (Natural Horizons)	0.0	0.0	5	105	120
Strawberry 50 Calories Nonfat Yogurt with Aspartame Sweetener (4.4 oz)					
Kraft Light n' Lively Free (Kraft General Foods)*	0.0	0.0	<5	60	50
Strawberry Fruit Basket Nonfat Yogurt with Aspartame Sweetener (6 oz)					
Knudsen Cal 70 (Kraft General Foods)*	0.0	0.0	5	90	70
Strawberry Fruit Cup 50 Calories Nonfat Yogurt with Aspartame Sweetener (4.4 oz)					
Kraft Light n' Lively Free (Kraft General Foods)*	0.0	0.0	<5	60	50
Strawberry Fruit Cup Lowfat Yogurt Multipack 1% Milkfat (4.4 oz)					
Kraft Light n' Lively (Kraft General Foods)*	1.0	0.5	10	60	140
Strawberry Fruit Cup Nonfat Yogurt (6 oz)					
Kraft Light n' Lively Free (Kraft General Foods)*	0.0	0.0	5	105	170
Strawberry Fruit Cup Nonfat Yogurt with Aspartame (227 g)					
Dannon Light (The Dannon Company)	0.0	0.0	<5	140	100

*Tobacco company, corporate subsidiary, or parent.

	Tot. Fat (g)	Sat. Fat (g)	Chol. (mg)	Sod. (mg)	Cal.
Strawberry Fruit Cup 70 Calories Nonfat Yogurt with Aspartame Sweetener (6 oz)					
Kraft Light n' Lively Free (Kraft General Foods)*	0.0	0.0	<5	80	70
Strawberry Fruit on the Bottom Lowfat Yogurt (227 g)					
Dannon (The Dannon Company)	3.0	1.5	15	135	240
Strawberry Lowfat Yogurt (1 cup)					
Nancy's (Springfield Creamery)	2.5	2.0	15	150	170
Strawberry Lowfat Yogurt Multipack 1% Milkfat (4.4 oz)					
Kraft Light n' Lively (Kraft General Foods)*	1.0	1.0	10	65	140
Strawberry Lowfat Yogurt 1% Milkfat (8 oz)					
Breyers (Kraft General Foods)*	2.5	1.5	15	110	250
Strawberry Nonfat Swiss Aspartame Yogurt (1 container)					
Crowley (Crowley Foods)	0.0	0.0	<5	130	100
Strawberry Nonfat Yogurt					
Dannon Tropifruta (The Dannon Company) (170 g)	0.0	0.0	5	105	150
Knudsen Free (Kraft General Foods)* (6 oz)	0.0	0.0	5	105	160
Kraft Light n' Lively Free (Kraft General Foods)* (6 oz)	0.0	0.0	5	105	180
Weight Watchers Ultimate 90 (H.J. Heinz) (1 cup)	0.0	0.0	5	140	90
Strawberry Nonfat Yogurt with Aspartame (227 g)					
Dannon Light (The Dannon Company)	0.0	0.0	<5	140	100
Strawberry Nonfat Yogurt with Aspartame Sweetener (6 oz)					
Knudsen Cal 70 (Kraft General Foods)*	0.0	0.0	5	85	70
Strawberry 70 Calories Nonfat Yogurt with Aspartame Sweetener (6 oz)					
Kraft Light n' Lively Free (Kraft General Foods)*	0.0	0.0	<5	85	70

*Tobacco company, corporate subsidiary, or parent.

	Tot. Fat (g)	Sat. Fat (g)	Chol. (mg)	Sod. (mg)	Cal.
FRUIT YOGURTS *(cont'd)*					
Strawberry Yogurt (6 oz)					
Yoplait Light (General Mills)	0.0	0.0	<5	85	90
Strawberry Yogurt with Cereal Nuggets (7 oz)					
Yoplait Crunch 'n Yogurt (General Mills)	0.5	0.0	<5	160	200
Strawberry Yogurt with Granola (7 oz)					
Yoplait Crunch 'n Yogurt (General Mills)	1.5	0.0	<5	115	220
Yoplait Crunch 'n Yogurt Light (General Mills)	1.0	0.0	<5	115	130
Wild Strawberry Kidpack Lowfat Yogurt (4.4 oz)					
Kraft Light n' Lively (Kraft General Foods)*	1.0	0.5	10	65	140
Strawberry-Banana Yogurts—*see also* Strawberry Yogurts, page 143					
All Natural Nonfat Strawberry Banana Yogurt (1 cup)					
Crowley (Crowley Foods)	0.0	0.0	5	220	230
Fat Free Strawberry/Banana (6 oz)					
Yoplait Fruit on the Bottom (General Mills)	0.0	0.0	<5	105	160
Fat Free Strawberry/Banana Yogurt (170 g)					
Dannon Blended (The Dannon Company)	0.0	0.0	<5	105	150
Fat Free Swiss Style Strawberry/Banana Yogurt (1 container)					
Borden	0.0	0.0	5	105	100
Viva (Borden)	0.0	0.0	5	105	100
Lite 85 Nonfat Strawberry Banana Yogurt (6 oz)					
Wells' Blue Bunny (Wells' Dairy)	0.0	0.0	<5	130	80
Lowfat Strawberry/Banana Yogurt (6 oz)					
Yoplait Breakfast (General Mills)	2.0	1.0	10	115	200
99% Fat Free Strawberry/Banana Yogurt (6 oz)					
Yoplait Original (General Mills)	1.5	1.0	10	105	170

*Tobacco company, corporate subsidiary, or parent.

	Tot. Fat (g)	Sat. Fat (g)	Chol. (mg)	Sod. (mg)	Cal.
No Fat Strawberry Banana Yogurt (1 cup)					
Cabot (Cabot Creamery)	0.0	0.0	10	120	130
Strawberry Banana 50 Calories Nonfat Yogurt with Aspartame Sweetener (4.4 oz)					
Kraft Light n' Lively Free (Kraft General Foods)*	0.0	0.0	<5	60	50
Strawberry/Banana Fruit on the Bottom Lowfat Yogurt (227 g)					
Dannon (The Dannon Company)	3.0	1.5	15	140	230
Strawberry Banana Lowfat Yogurt 1% Milkfat (8 oz)					
Breyers (Kraft General Foods)*	2.5	1.5	15	115	250
Strawberry Banana Lowfat Yogurt Multipack 1% Milkfat (4.4 oz)					
Kraft Light n' Lively (Kraft General Foods)*	1.0	0.5	10	60	140
Strawberry Banana Nonfat Swiss Aspartame Yogurt (1 container)					
Crowley (Crowley Foods)	0.0	0.0	<5	130	100
Strawberry-Banana Nonfat Yogurt (170 g)					
Dannon Tropifruta (The Dannon Company)	0.0	0.0	5	105	150
Strawberry/Banana Nonfat Yogurt with Aspartame (227 g)					
Dannon Light (The Dannon Company)	0.0	0.0	<5	140	100
Strawberry Banana Nonfat Yogurt with Aspartame Sweetener (6 oz)					
Knudsen Cal 70 (Kraft General Foods)*	0.0	0.0	5	85	70
Strawberry Banana 70 Calories Nonfat Yogurt with Aspartame Sweetener (6 oz)					
Kraft Light n' Lively Free (Kraft General Foods)*	0.0	0.0	<5	85	70
Strawberry/Banana (6 oz)					
Yoplait Light (General Mills)	0.0	0.0	<5	85	90

*Tobacco company, corporate subsidiary, or parent.

	Tot. Fat (g)	Sat. Fat (g)	Chol. (mg)	Sod. (mg)	Cal.
FRUIT YOGURTS *(cont'd)*					
Strawberry/Banana Nonfat Yogurt (1 cup) Weight Watchers Ultimate 90 (H.J. Heinz)	0.0	0.0	5	140	90
Other Fruit Yogurts					
Grape Kidpack Lowfat Yogurt 1% Milkfat (4.4 oz) Kraft Light n' Lively (Kraft General Foods)*	1.0	1.0	10	65	130
Guava Nonfat Yogurt (170 g) Dannon Tropifruta (The Dannon Company)	0.0	0.0	5	105	150
Mango Nonfat Yogurt (170 g) Dannon Tropifruta (The Dannon Company)	0.0	0.0	5	105	150
Multi-Pack Yogurt, all flavors (4 oz) Yoplait Light (General Mills)	0.0	0.0	0	55	60
99% Fat Free Yogurt Multi-Pack (4 oz) Yoplait Original (General Mills)	1.0	0.5	5	70	110
Pear Fruit on the Bottom Lowfat Yogurt (227 g) Dannon (The Dannon Company)	3.0	1.5	15	135	240
Plum Fruit on the Bottom Lowfat Yogurt (227 g) Dannon (The Dannon Company)	3.0	1.5	15	160	240
NONFRUIT YOGURTS					
Cappuccino/Coffee Yogurts					
Cappuccino Nonfat Swiss Aspartame Yogurt (1 container) Crowley (Crowley Foods)	0.0	0.0	<5	130	100
Cappuccino Nonfat Yogurt (1 cup) Weight Watchers Ultimate 90 (H.J. Heinz)	0.0	0.0	5	140	90
Cappuccino Nonfat Yogurt with Aspartame (227 g) Dannon Light (The Dannon Company)	0.0	0.0	<5	140	100

*Tobacco company, corporate subsidiary, or parent.

	Tot. Fat (g)	Sat. Fat (g)	Chol. (mg)	Sod. (mg)	Cal.
Cappuccino with Chocolate Crunchies 99% Fat Free Yogurt (227 g) Dannon Light 'N Crunchy (The Dannon Company)	1.0	0.0	5	160	150
Cappuccino with Chocolate Nuggets (7 oz) Yoplait Crunch 'n Yogurt Light (General Mills)	1.5	0.0	<5	150	130
Coffee Lowfat Yogurt (227 g) Dannon (The Dannon Company)	3.0	2.0	15	160	210
Coffee Lowfat Yogurt 1.5% Milkfat (8 oz) Breyers (Kraft General Foods)* .	3.0	2.0	20	135	250
Organic Cappuccino Yogurt (¾ cup) Horizon (Natural Horizons)	0.0	0.0	5	125	110
Chocolate Yogurts					
Chocolate Nonfat Swiss Aspartame Yogurt (1 container) Crowley (Crowley Foods)	0.0	0.0	<5	130	100
Coffee Yogurts—*see* Cappuccino/ Coffee Yogurts, page 148					
Plain Yogurts					
All Natural Nonfat Plain Yogurt (1 cup) Crowley (Crowley Foods)	0.0	0.0	5	220	140
Lite 85 Nonfat Plain Yogurt (1 cup) Wells' Blue Bunny (Wells' Dairy) .	0.0	0.0	<5	170	110
No Fat Yogurt (1 cup) Cabot (Cabot Creamery)	0.0	0.0	5	135	100
Nonfat Plain Yogurt (6 oz) Yoplait Original (General Mills) ..	0.0	0.0	5	140	100
Nonfat Yogurt (1 cup) Nancy's (Springfield Creamery) .	0.0	0.0	5	180	120
Organic Plain Yogurt (¾ cup) Horizon (Natural Horizons)	0.0	0.0	5	115	80
Plain Lowfat Yogurt 1.5% Milkfat (8 oz) Breyers (Kraft General Foods)* .	3.0	2.0	20	150	130

*Tobacco company, corporate subsidiary, or parent.

	Tot. Fat (g)	Sat. Fat (g)	Chol. (mg)	Sod. (mg)	Cal.
NONFRUIT YOGURTS *(cont'd)*					
Plain Nonfat Yogurt					
Dannon (The Dannon Company) (227 g)	0.0	0.0	5	150	110
Weight Watchers Ultimate 90 (H.J. Heinz) (1 cup)	0.0	0.0	5	150	90
Yoplait (General Mills) (1 cup)	0.0	0.0	10	190	140
Unflavored Yogurts—*see* Plain Yogurts, *above*					
Vanilla Yogurts					
All Natural Nonfat Vanilla Yogurt (1 cup)					
Crowley (Crowley Foods)	0.0	0.0	5	220	220
Fat Free French Vanilla Yogurt (170 g)					
Dannon Blended (The Dannon Company)	0.0	0.0	<5	100	150
Light Vanilla Yogurt (6 oz)					
Yoplait Custard Style (General Mills)	0.0	0.0	0	85	90
Lite 85 Nonfat Vanilla Yogurt (6 oz)					
Wells' Blue Bunny (Wells' Dairy)	0.0	0.0	<5	130	80
99% Fat Free Vanilla Yogurt (6 oz)					
Yoplait Original (General Mills)	2.0	1.0	10	140	170
No Fat French Vanilla Yogurt (1 cup)					
Cabot (Cabot Creamery)	0.0	0.0	10	115	130
Organic Vanilla Yogurt (¾ cup)					
Horizon (Natural Horizons)	0.0	0.0	5	125	120
Vanilla Lowfat Yogurt					
Dannon (The Dannon Company (227 g)	3.0	2.0	15	160	210
Nancy's (Springfield Creamery) (1 cup)	3.0	2.0	15	160	140
Vanilla Lowfat Yogurt 1.5% Milkfat (8 oz)					
Breyers (Kraft General Foods)*	3.0	2.0	20	135	220
Vanilla Nonfat Swiss Aspartame Yogurt (1 container)					
Crowley (Crowley Foods)	0.0	0.0	<5	130	100

*Tobacco company, corporate subsidiary, or parent.

	Tot. Fat (g)	Sat. Fat (g)	Chol. (mg)	Sod. (mg)	Cal.
Vanilla Nonfat Yogurt					
Knudsen Free (Kraft General Foods)* (6 oz)	0.0	0.0	5	100	170
Kraft Light n' Lively Free (Kraft General Foods)* (6 oz)	0.0	0.0	5	105	160
Weight Watchers Ultimate 90 (H.J. Heinz) (1 cup)	0.0	0.0	5	140	90
Yoplait (General Mills) (1 cup)	0.0	0.0	10	160	210
Vanilla Nonfat Yogurt with Aspartame (227 g)					
Dannon Light (The Dannon Company)	0.0	0.0	<5	140	100
Vanilla Nonfat Yogurt with Aspartame Sweetener (6 oz)					
Knudsen Cal 70 (Kraft General Foods)*	0.0	0.0	5	80	70
Vanilla with Blueberry Crunchies Nonfat Yogurt (227 g)					
Dannon Light 'N Crunchy (The Dannon Company)	0.0	0.0	<5	150	140
Vanilla with Chocolate Crunchies 99% Fat Free Yogurt (227 g)					
Dannon Light 'N Crunchy (The Dannon Company)	1.0	0.0	5	160	150
Vanilla Yogurt with Chocolate Flavor Crunchies (7 oz)					
Yoplait Crunch 'n Yogurt (General Mills)	1.5	0.5	<5	180	220
Vanilla Yogurt with Granola (7 oz)					
Yoplait Crunch 'n Yogurt (General Mills)	1.5	0.0	<5	120	220
Other Nonfruit Yogurts					
Creme Caramel Nonfat Yogurt with Aspartame (227 g)					
Dannon Light (The Dannon Company)	0.0	0.0	<5	125	100
Lowfat Maple Yogurt (1 cup)					
Nancy's (Springfield Creamery)	3.0	2.0	15	160	180

*Tobacco company, corporate subsidiary, or parent.

DESSERTS

Have an eternal "sweet tooth"? Thanks to the overwhelming demand for low-fat goodies, you can now go to your supermarket and find desserts that are low in fat, saturated fat, and cholesterol but high in taste.

From brownies and cakes to cookies and pies, the desserts on the following pages will satisfy your sweet tooth but be good to your heart. Just make sure that you prepare them according to package directions or with skim milk. And even if the package directions don't say so, always prepare mixes by substituting skim milk or 1% milk for whole milk and using egg whites or egg substitute instead of whole eggs.

Unfortunately, there's a downside to many low-fat desserts: They have almost the same number of calories as the high-fat versions. Proceed with caution!

Like all the other entries in this book, the desserts entries that follow list sodium content. The AHA does not have criteria for sodium but recommends a total of no more than 3,000 mg a day.

Generic Listings

By far, most of the foods in this book are brand name products. However, if a product is listed without a brand name, it means that most brands of that product contain about the same amount of fat, saturated fat, and cholesterol and that these amounts are within the criteria cited below.

If you find products that were introduced after this book went to press, use the generic listings and the following tables to help you evaluate them.

AHA Criteria for Desserts*

	Tot. Fat (g)	Sat. Fat (g)	Chol. (mg)
Brownies, cakes and cupcakes, cookies, graham crackers, pies, and quick-type sweet breads, such as muffins	3	1	<2
Custards, gelatins, mousses, and puddings, prepared	3	1	20
Frostings	<0.5	<0.5	<2

*Per serving.

Desserts You'll Want to Limit

Some desserts, like the examples below, are too high in fat, saturated fat, and/or cholesterol to meet AHA criteria. They aren't included in this book, and we recommend that you don't eat them often.

Compare the amounts of fat, saturated fat, cholesterol, sodium, and calories in these examples with the more healthful alternatives listed on the following pages.

Sample Desserts to Limit

	Tot. Fat (g)	Sat. Fat (g)	Chol. (mg)	Sod. (mg)	Cal.
Brownie from mix, made with oil and egg (about 2″ × 2½″)	7.9*	1.6*	11*	100	167
Cheesecake, made from no-bake mix with whole milk; graham cracker crust made with butter (about ⅙ of 8″-diam cheesecake)	15.9*	8.8*	(39)*	475	341
Cherry fried pie (about 5″ × 3¾″)	20.7*	3.1*	(13)*	479	404
Coconut cream pie, made from no-bake mix with whole milk; crust made with butter (⅙ of 9″-diam pie)	22.0*	12.8*	(148)*	412	345
Creme-filled sponge snack cake (2.8 oz, or about 2 cakes)	9.2*	2.2*	13*	291	291
Fudge cake, made from mix with egg, without frosting (1⁄10 of 9″ cake)	9.3*	2.1*	43*	455	244
Glazed cake doughnut (about 3⅜″ diam)	12.6*	2.9*	17*	221	235
Peanut butter cookie (1 oz, or about 2 cookies)	6.7*	1.5*	(0)	118	135
Pecan shortbread cookie (1 oz, or about 2 cookies)	9.2*	2.0*	9*	80	154

Adapted from USDA Handbook No. 8 series.

*These values exceed AHA criteria for desserts.

	Tot. Fat (g)	Sat. Fat (g)	Chol. (mg)	Sod. (mg)	Cal.
BLONDIES—*see* BROWNIES, below					
BROWNIES					
Cream Cheese Fudgy Brownie (1 brownie)					
Formägg (Galaxy Foods)	3.0	0.0	0	30	130
Fat Free Apple Spice Blondie (1 bar)					
Greenfield Healthy Foods	0.0	0.0	0	65	120
Fat Free Brownie (1 bar)					
Greenfield Healthy Foods	0.0	0.0	0	65	120
Fat Free Butterscotch Brownies (1 brownie)					
Auburn Farms Jammers (Auburn Farms)	0.0	0.0	0	65	100
Fat Free Cappuccino Fudge Brownies (1 brownie)					
Auburn Farms Jammers (Auburn Farms)	0.0	0.0	0	90	100
Fat-Free Caramel Brownie (1 bar)					
Health Valley (Health Valley Foods)	0.0	0.0	0	30	110
Fat-Free Cherry Brownie (1 bar)					
Health Valley (Health Valley Foods)	0.0	0.0	0	30	110
Fat Free Chocolate Chip Blondie (1 bar)					
Greenfield Healthy Foods	0.0	0.0	0	65	120
Fat Free Chocolate Fudge Brownies (1 brownie)					
Auburn Farms Jammers (Auburn Farms)	0.0	0.0	0	95	90
Fat-Free Fudge Brownie (1 bar)					
Health Valley (Health Valley Foods)	0.0	0.0	0	30	110
Fat-Free Raspberry Brownie (1 bar)					
Health Valley (Health Valley Foods)	0.0	0.0	0	30	110
Fat Free Raspberry Fudge Brownies (1 brownie)					
Auburn Farms Jammers (Auburn Farms)	0.0	0.0	0	95	90

	Tot. Fat (g)	Sat. Fat (g)	Chol. (mg)	Sod. (mg)	Cal.
BROWNIES *(cont'd)*					
Fat-Free Strawberry Brownie (1 bar)					
Health Valley (Health Valley Foods)	0.0	0.0	0	30	110
Fudge Brownies (1/10 strip)					
Entenmann's (Kraft General Foods)*	0.0	0.0	0	140	110
Mint Frosted Brownie (1 brownie)					
Weight Watchers (H.J. Heinz)	2.0	0.0	5	130	100
Swiss Mocha Fudge Brownie (1 brownie)					
Weight Watchers (H.J. Heinz)	2.0	0.0	5	140	90
CAKES/CUPCAKES—*see also* SNACK CAKES, page 184					
CAKE MIXES					
Angel Food Cake Mixes					
Angel Food Cake Mix, made with water (1/10 of cake)					
Pillsbury Moist Supreme (Grand Metropolitan PLC)	0.0	0.0	0	330	140
Pillsbury Plus (Grand Metropolitan PLC)	0.0	0.0	0	360	150
Chocolate Swirl Angel Food Cake Mix (1/12 of pkg)					
Betty Crocker (General Mills)	0.0	0.0	0	280	150
Confetti Angel Food Cake Mix (1/12 of pkg)					
Betty Crocker (General Mills)	0.0	0.0	0	300	150
Lemon Custard Angel Food Cake Mix (1/12 of pkg)					
Betty Crocker (General Mills)	0.0	0.0	0	290	140
One Step Angel Food Cake Mix (1/12 of pkg)					
Betty Crocker (General Mills)	0.0	0.0	0	280	140
Traditional Angel Food Cake Mix (1/12 of pkg)					
Betty Crocker (General Mills)	0.0	0.0	0	160	130
Banana Cake Mixes					
Banana Cake Mix (1/6 of cake)					
Sweet'N Low (Bernard Foods)	3.0	1.0	0	30	150

*Tobacco company, corporate subsidiary, or parent.

	Tot. Fat (g)	Sat. Fat (g)	Chol. (mg)	Sod. (mg)	Cal.
Chocolate/Devil's Food Cake Mixes					
Chocolate Cake Mix (1/6 of cake)					
Sweet'N Low (Bernard Foods) .	3.0	1.0	0	30	150
Lemon Cake Mixes					
Lemon Cake Mix (1/6 of cake)					
Sweet'N Low (Bernard Foods) .	3.0	1.0	0	30	150
White Cake Mixes					
White Cake Mix (1/6 of cake)					
Sweet'N Low (Bernard Foods) .	3.0	1.0	0	30	150
Yellow Cake Mixes					
Yellow Cake Mix (1/6 of cake)					
Sweet'N Low (Bernard Foods) .	3.0	1.0	0	30	150
PREPARED CAKES/CUPCAKES					
Angel Food Cakes/Cupcakes, Prepared					
Angel food cake, plain or flavored (1/2 of a 10"-diam cake)					
Most brands (USDA)	**0.1**	**0.0**	**0**	**255**	**129**
Chocolate/Devil's Food Cakes/ Cupcakes, Prepared					
Chocolate Crunch Cake (1/8 cake)					
Entenmann's (Kraft General Foods)*	0.0	0.0	0	170	130
Chocolate Cup Cakes Light (1 cake)					
Hostess (Continental Baking Co)	1.5	0.0	0	170	120
Chocolate Loaf (1/8 loaf)					
Entenmann's (Kraft General Foods)*	0.0	0.0	0	250	130
Fudge Iced Chocolate Cake (1/6 cake)					
Entenmann's (Kraft General Foods)*	0.0	0.0	0	270	210
Mocha Iced Chocolate Cake (1/6 cake)					
Entenmann's (Kraft General Foods)*	0.0	0.0	0	270	200
Fruit Cakes/Cupcakes, Prepared					
Apple Spice Crumb Cake (1/8 cake)					
Entenmann's (Kraft General Foods)*	0.0	0.0	0	140	130

*Tobacco company, corporate subsidiary, or parent.

	Tot. Fat (g)	Sat. Fat (g)	Chol. (mg)	Sod. (mg)	Cal.
PREPARED CAKES/CUPCAKES *(cont'd)*					
Banana Crunch Cake (1/8 cake)					
Entenmann's (Kraft General Foods)*	0.0	0.0	0	150	140
Banana Loaf (1/8 loaf)					
Entenmann's (Kraft General Foods)*	0.0	0.0	0	190	150
Blueberry Crunch Cake (1/8 cake)					
Entenmann's (Kraft General Foods)*	0.0	0.0	0	200	140
Raisin Loaf (1/8 loaf)					
Entenmann's (Kraft General Foods)*	0.0	0.0	0	150	140
Other Cakes/Cupcakes, Prepared					
Carrot Cake (1/8 cake)					
Entenmann's (Kraft General Foods)*	0.0	0.0	0	230	170
Fudge Iced Golden Cake (1/6 cake)					
Entenmann's (Kraft General Foods)*	0.0	0.0	0	200	220
Golden Chocolatey Chip Loaf (1/8 loaf)					
Entenmann's (Kraft General Foods)*	0.0	0.0	0	220	130
Golden French Crumb Cake (1/8 cake)					
Entenmann's (Kraft General Foods)*	0.0	0.0	0	150	140
Golden Loaf (1/8 loaf)					
Entenmann's (Kraft General Foods)*	0.0	0.0	0	160	120
Louisiana Crunch Cake (1/6 cake)					
Entenmann's (Kraft General Foods)*	0.0	0.0	0	220	220
Marble Loaf (1/8 loaf)					
Entenmann's (Kraft General Foods)*	0.0	0.0	0	190	130

CANDIES—*see* "SWEETS," page 385

*Tobacco company, corporate subsidiary, or parent.

	Tot. Fat (g)	Sat. Fat (g)	Chol. (mg)	Sod. (mg)	Cal.
COFFEE CAKES—*see* "BREADS AND BREAD PRODUCTS," COFFEE CAKES/DANISHES/ SWEET ROLLS, page 57					
COOKIES					
CHOCOLATE CHIP COOKIES					
Fat-Free Double Chocolate Healthy Chip Cookies (3 cookies) Health Valley (Health Valley Foods)	0.0	0.0	0	20	100
Fat-Free Old Fashioned Healthy Chips Cookies (3 cookies) Health Valley (Health Valley Foods)	0.0	0.0	0	20	100
Fat-Free Original Healthy Chip Cookies (3 cookies) Health Valley (Health Valley Foods)	0.0	0.0	0	20	100
Oatmeal Chocolatey Chip Cookies (2 cookies) Entenmann's (Kraft General Foods)*	0.0	0.0	0	110	80
CHOCOLATE/DEVIL'S FOOD COOKIES—*see also* SANDWICH COOKIES, page 167					
Chewy Chocolate Cookies (2 cookies) Auburn Farms Jammers (Auburn Farms)	0.0	0.0	0	80	80
Chocolate Brownie Cookies (2 cookies) Entenmann's (Kraft General Foods)*	0.0	0.0	0	90	80
Chocolate Cheese Cake Chocolate Chip Cookies (1 cookie) Formägg (Galaxy Foods)	3.0	0.0	0	50	110
Chocolate Mint Cookies (2 cookies) Auburn Farms Jammers (Auburn Farms)	0.0	0.0	0	95	90

*Tobacco company, corporate subsidiary, or parent.

	Tot. Fat (g)	Sat. Fat (g)	Chol. (mg)	Sod. (mg)	Cal.
CHOCOLATE/DEVIL'S FOOD COOKIES *(cont'd)*					
Cream Cheese Fudgy Brownie Cookies (1 cookie) Formägg (Galaxy Foods)	2.0	0.0	0	30	100
Devil's Food Cookie Cakes (1 cookie) Nabisco SnackWell's (Nabisco Foods)*	0.0	0.0	0	25	50
Devil's Food Cookies (2 cookies) Auburn Farms Jammers (Auburn Farms)	0.0	0.0	0	80	80
Double Fudge Cookie Cakes (1 cookie) Nabisco SnackWell's (Nabisco Foods)*	0.0	0.0	0	70	50
Fat-Free Chocolate Cookies with Caramel Centers (2 cookies) Health Valley (Health Valley Foods)	0.0	0.0	0	20	70
Fat-Free Chocolate Cookies with Cherry Centers (2 cookies) Health Valley (Health Valley Foods)	0.0	0.0	0	20	70
Fat-Free Chocolate Cookies with Fudge Centers (2 cookies) Health Valley (Health Valley Foods)	0.0	0.0	0	20	70
Fat-Free Chocolate Cookies with Mint Fudge Centers (2 cookies) Health Valley (Health Valley Foods)	0.0	0.0	0	20	70
Fat-Free Chocolate Cookies with Raspberry Centers (2 cookies) Health Valley (Health Valley Foods)	0.0	0.0	0	20	70
Fat-Free Chocolate Cookies with Strawberry Centers (2 cookies) Health Valley (Health Valley Foods)	0.0	0.0	0	20	70

*Tobacco company, corporate subsidiary, or parent.

	Tot. Fat (g)	Sat. Fat (g)	Chol. (mg)	Sod. (mg)	Cal.
Fat Free Devils Food Cookies (1 cookie) Keebler	0.0	0.0	0	80	70
Fruit Cookies					
Apple Cookies					
Apple Filled Oatmeal Cookies (1 cookie) Archway	3.0	0.5	<5	105	110
Apple Raisin Bar (1 oz) Weight Watchers (H.J. Heinz)	3.0	1.0	0	115	100
Apple Snack Bars (1 bar) Sun Belt Fruit Boosters (McKee Baking)	2.0	0.0	0	60	130
Apple Spice Cookies (2 cookies) Auburn Farms Jammers (Auburn Farms)	0.0	0.0	0	90	80
Fat-Free Apple Bakes (1 bar) Health Valley (Health Valley Foods)	0.0	0.0	0	30	70
Fat Free Apple Bars (6 bars) Lance	0.0	0.0	0	75	140
Fat-Free Apple-Cinnamon Mini Fruit Center Cookies (2 cookies) Health Valley (Health Valley Foods)	0.0	0.0	0	25	70
Fat-Free Apple Fruit Center Cookies (1 cookie) Health Valley (Health Valley Foods)	0.0	0.0	0	20	70
Fat Free Apple Newtons (2 cookies) Nabisco (Nabisco Foods)*	0.0	0.0	0	60	100
Fat-Free Apple-Raisin Jumbo Cookies (1 cookie) Health Valley (Health Valley Foods)	0.0	0.0	0	35	80
Fat-Free Apple Spice Cookies (3 cookies) Health Valley (Health Valley Foods)	0.0	0.0	0	50	100

*Tobacco company, corporate subsidiary, or parent.

	Tot. Fat (g)	Sat. Fat (g)	Chol. (mg)	Sod. (mg)	Cal.
FRUIT COOKIES *(cont'd)*					
Fruit Filled Apple Cookies (0.7 oz) Weight Watchers (H.J. Heinz)	0.0	0.0	0	40	70
Golden Fruit Apple Biscuits (1 cookie) Sunshine	1.5	0.0	0	55	80
Apricot Cookies					
Fat-Free Apricot Delight Cookies (3 cookies) Health Valley (Health Valley Foods)	0.0	0.0	0	50	100
Fat-Free Apricot Fruit Center Cookies (1 cookie) Health Valley (Health Valley Foods)	0.0	0.0	0	20	70
Blueberry Cookies					
Blueberry Apple Bakes (1 bar) Health Valley (Health Valley Foods)	0.0	0.0	0	25	110
Blueberry Snack Bars (1 bar) Sun Belt Fruit Boosters (McKee Baking)	2.0	0.0	0	60	130
Cranberry Cookies					
Cream Cheese Oatmeal Cranberry Cookies (1 cookie) Formägg (Galaxy Foods)	2.0	0.0	0	80	100
Fat Free Cranberry Bars (6 bars) Lance	0.0	0.0	0	45	140
Fat Free Cranberry Newtons (2 cookies) Nabisco (Nabisco Foods)*	0.0	0.0	0	95	100
Golden Fruit Cranberry Biscuits (1 cookie) Sunshine	1.0	0.0	0	55	70
Date Cookies					
Fat-Free Date Bakes (1 bar) Health Valley (Health Valley Foods)	0.0	0.0	0	30	70

*Tobacco company, corporate subsidiary, or parent.

	Tot. Fat (g)	Sat. Fat (g)	Chol. (mg)	Sod. (mg)	Cal.
Fat-Free Date Delight Cookies (3 cookies)					
Health Valley (Health Valley Foods)	0.0	0.0	0	50	100
Fat-Free Date Fruit Center Cookies (1 cookie)					
Health Valley (Health Valley Foods)	0.0	0.0	0	20	70
Fig Cookies					
Fat Free Fig Cake (½ of 2⅛-oz cake)					
Lance	0.0	0.0	0	85	100
Fat Free Fig Newtons (2 cookies)					
Nabisco (Nabisco Foods)*	0.0	0.0	0	115	100
Fig Bar					
Keebler (1 bar)	1.5	0.5	0	70	60
Lance (½ of 2-oz bar)	2.0	0.5	0	85	100
Fig Bars					
America's Choice (A & P) (2 bars)	3.0	0.0	0	55	120
Sunshine (2 cookies)	2.5	0.5	0	60	110
Fig Cake (½ of 2⅛-oz cake)					
Lance	2.0	0.5	0	70	110
Fig Newtons (2 cookies)					
Nabisco (Nabisco Foods)*	2.5	1.0	0	120	110
Fruit Filled Fig Cookies (0.7 oz)					
Weight Watchers Smart Snackers (H.J. Heinz)	0.0	0.0	0	50	70
Raisin Cookies					
Fat-Free Raisin Apple Center Cookies (1 cookie)					
Health Valley (Health Valley Foods)	0.0	0.0	0	20	70
Fat-Free Raisin Bakes (1 bar)					
Health Valley (Health Valley Foods)	0.0	0.0	0	30	70
Fat-Free Raisin-Raisin Jumbo Cookies (1 cookie)					
Health Valley (Health Valley Foods)	0.0	0.0	0	35	80

*Tobacco company, corporate subsidiary, or parent.

	Tot. Fat (g)	Sat. Fat (g)	Chol. (mg)	Sod. (mg)	Cal.
Fruit Cookies *(cont'd)*					
Golden Fruit Raisin Biscuits (1 cookie)					
Sunshine	1.5	0.0	0	40	80
Raspberry Cookies					
Fat-Free Raspberry Fruit Center Cookies (1 cookie)					
Health Valley (Health Valley Foods)	0.0	0.0	0	20	70
Fat-Free Raspberry Jumbo Cookies (1 cookie)					
Health Valley (Health Valley Foods)	0.0	0.0	0	35	80
Fat Free Raspberry Newtons (2 cookies)					
Nabisco (Nabisco Foods)*	0.0	0.0	0	115	100
Fruit Filled Raspberry Cookies (0.7 oz)					
Weight Watchers Smart Snackers (H.J. Heinz)	0.0	0.0	0	45	70
Raspberry Bakes (1 bar)					
Health Valley (Health Valley Foods)	0.0	0.0	0	25	110
Strawberry Cookies					
Fat-Free Strawberry Mini Fruit Center Cookies (2 cookies)					
Health Valley (Health Valley Foods)	0.0	0.0	0	25	70
Fat Free Strawberry Newtons (2 cookies)					
Nabisco (Nabisco Foods)*	0.0	0.0	0	115	100
Strawberry Bakes (1 bar)					
Health Valley (Health Valley Foods)	0.0	0.0	0	25	110
Strawberry Snack Bars (1 bar)					
Sun Belt Fruit Boosters (McKee Baking)	2.0	0.0	0	60	130
Other Fruit Cookies					
Fat-Free Hawaiian Fruit Cookies (3 cookies)					
Health Valley (Health Valley Foods)	0.0	0.0	0	50	100

*Tobacco company, corporate subsidiary, or parent.

	Tot. Fat (g)	Sat. Fat (g)	Chol. (mg)	Sod. (mg)	Cal.
Fat-Free Orange-Pineapple Mini Fruit Center Cookies (2 cookies) Health Valley (Health Valley Foods)	0.0	0.0	0	25	70
Fat-Free Peach-Apricot Mini Fruit Center Cookies (2 cookies) Health Valley (Health Valley Foods)	0.0	0.0	0	25	70
Fat-Free Raspberry-Apple Mini Fruit Center Cookies (2 cookies) Health Valley (Health Valley Foods)	0.0	0.0	0	25	70
Fat-Free Tropical Fruit Center Cookies (1 cookie) Health Valley (Health Valley Foods)	0.0	0.0	0	20	70
GINGER SNAPS					
Ginger Snaps (4 cookies) Delicious (Delicious Cookie Co)	3.0	0.5	<2	170	130
Old Fashion Ginger Snaps (4 cookies) Nabisco (Nabisco Foods)*	2.5	0.5	0	170	120
GRAHAM CRACKERS					
Cinnamon Graham Cookies (2 cookies) Auburn Farms Jammers (Auburn Farms)	0.0	0.0	0	85	90
Cinnamon Graham Snacks (20 pieces) Nabisco SnackWell's (Nabisco Foods)*	0.0	0.0	0	90	110
Cinnamon Grahams (10 crackers) Nabisco Honey Maid (Nabisco Foods)*	3.0	0.5	0	210	140
Fat-Free Amaranth Graham Crackers (8 crackers) Health Valley (Health Valley Foods)	0.0	0.0	0	30	100
Fat-Free Oat Bran Graham Crackers (8 crackers) Health Valley (Health Valley Foods)	0.0	0.0	0	30	100

*Tobacco company, corporate subsidiary, or parent.

	Tot. Fat (g)	Sat. Fat (g)	Chol. (mg)	Sod. (mg)	Cal.
GRAHAM CRACKERS *(cont'd)*					
Grahams (8 crackers)					
Nabisco (Nabisco Foods)*	3.0	0.5	0	180	120
Honey Grahams (8 crackers)					
Nabisco (Nabisco Foods)*	3.0	0.5	0	180	120
Low Fat Cinnamon Crisp (8 crackers)					
Keebler	1.5	0.5	0	190	110
Low Fat Honey Graham Cracker (9 crackers)					
Keebler	1.5	0.5	0	210	120
Original Graham Selects Old Fashioned Graham Crackers (8 crackers)					
Keebler	3.0	1.0	0	135	130
MOLASSES COOKIES					
Molasses Cookies (2 cookies)					
Auburn Farms Jammers (Auburn Farms)	0.0	0.0	0	40	80
Old Fashioned Molasses (1 cookie)					
Archway	3.0	1.0	5	150	120
OATMEAL/OATMEAL AND RAISIN COOKIES					
Oatmeal Cookies					
Oatmeal Date Lites Cookies (1 cookie)					
Natural Lady Foods	1.0	0.0	0	80	80
Oatmeal and Raisin Cookies					
Cream Cheese Oatmeal Raisin Cookies (1 cookie)					
Formägg (Galaxy Foods)	2.0	0.0	0	80	100
Fat-Free Raisin Oatmeal Cookies (3 cookies)					
Health Valley (Health Valley Foods)	0.0	0.0	0	50	100
Oatmeal Raisin Cookies					
Auburn Farms Jammers (Auburn Farms) (2 cookies)	0.5	0.0	0	70	80
Entenmann's (Kraft General Foods)* (2 cookies)	0.0	0.0	0	120	80
Weight Watchers Smart Snackers (H.J. Heinz) (0.7 oz)	2.0	0.0	0	90	120

*Tobacco company, corporate subsidiary, or parent.

	Tot. Fat (g)	Sat. Fat (g)	Chol. (mg)	Sod. (mg)	Cal.
Oatmeal Raisin Cookies (2 cookies)					
Nabisco SnackWell's (Nabisco Foods)*	2.5	0.0	0	135	110
SANDWICH COOKIES					
Chocolate Sandwich Cookies with Chocolate Creme (2 cookies)					
Nabisco SnackWell's (Nabisco Foods)*	2.5	0.5	0	190	100
Creme Sandwich Cookies (2 cookies)					
Nabisco SnackWell's (Nabisco Foods)*	2.5	0.5	0	95	110
Reduced Fat Chocolate Sandwich Cookies with Fudge Creme (2 cookies)					
Keebler Elfin Delights	2.5	0.5	0	100	110
Reduced Fat Chocolate Sandwich Cookies with Vanilla Creme (2 cookies)					
Keebler Elfin Delights	2.5	0.5	0	120	110
Reduced Fat Creme Sandwich Cookie (2 cookies)					
Keebler Elfin Delights	2.5	0.5	0	90	110
Vanilla Sandwich Cookies (1.06 oz)					
Weight Watchers Smart Snackers (H.J. Heinz)	3.0	1.0	0	80	140
VANILLA COOKIES—*see also* SANDWICH COOKIES, above					
Vanilla Wafer (8 cookies)					
Delicious (Delicious Cookie Co)	1.5	1.0	<2	90	110
OTHER COOKIES					
Choconut (3 cookies)					
Almondina (YZ Enterprises)	1.1	0.0	0	10	80
Cinnamon Lites Cookies (1 cookie)					
Natural Lady Foods	1.0	0.0	0	65	90
Cookie Jar Hermits (1 cookie)					
Archway	3.0	0.5	<5	160	110
Fortune Cookies (1 cookie)					
La Choy (Hunt-Wesson)	<1.0	0.0	0	1	15
P'Nutty Crisp Cookies (2 cookies)					
Auburn Farms Jammers (Auburn Farms)	0.5	0.0	0	90	90

*Tobacco company, corporate subsidiary, or parent.

	Tot. Fat (g)	Sat. Fat (g)	Chol. (mg)	Sod. (mg)	Cal.
OTHER COOKIES *(cont'd)*					
Pfeffernusse (2 cookies)					
Archway	1.0	0.0	0	100	140
CREAM PIE FILLINGS—*see* PUDDINGS, page 175					
CUPCAKES—*see* CAKES/ CUPCAKES, page 156					
CUSTARDS—*see* PUDDINGS, page 175					
DANISHES—*see* "BREADS AND BREAD PRODUCTS," COFFEE CAKES/DANISHES/SWEET ROLLS, page 57					
FROZEN YOGURTS—*see* "FROZEN DESSERTS," FROZEN YOGURTS, page 204					
FRUIT GLAZES/PIE FILLINGS					
Apples, sweetened, sliced (½ cup)					
Most brands (USDA)	**0.5**	**0.1**	**0**	**3**	**68**
Creamy Glaze for Bananas (2 tbsp)					
Marie's (Campbell Soup Co)	0.0	0.0	0	30	40
Glaze for Blueberries (2 tbsp)					
Marie's (Campbell Soup Co)	0.0	0.0	10	30	40
Glaze for Peaches (2 tbsp)					
Marie's (Campbell Soup Co)	0.0	0.0	10	50	40
Glaze for Strawberries (2 tbsp)					
Marie's (Campbell Soup Co)	0.0	0.0	0	30	40
Pumpkin Pie Mix (½ cup)					
Most brands (USDA)	**0.2**	**0.1**	**0**	**280**	**141**
Libby's (Nestlé Food Company)	0.0	0.0	0	150	100

	Tot. Fat (g)	Sat. Fat (g)	Chol. (mg)	Sod. (mg)	Cal.
GELATIN					
SUGAR-FREE GELATIN MIXES					
Berry Blue Sugar Free Low Calorie Gelatin, made with water (½ cup)					
Jell-O (Kraft General Foods)* . . .	0.0	0.0	0	60	10
Cherry Sugar Free Low Calorie Gelatin, made with water (½ cup)					
Jell-O (Kraft General Foods)* . . .	0.0	0.0	0	70	10
Gelatin sweetened with aspartame, all flavors, made with water (½ cup)					
Most brands (USDA)	**0.0**	**0.0**	**0**	**(4)**	**8**
Gelatin sweetened with saccharin, all flavors, made with water (½ cup)					
Most brands (USDA)	**0.0**	**0.0**	**0**	**(2)**	**8**
Grape Sugar Free Low Calorie Gelatin, made with water (½ cup)					
Jell-O (Kraft General Foods)* . . .	0.0	0.0	0	50	10
Hawaiian Pineapple Sugar Free Low Calorie Gelatin, made with water (½ cup)					
Jell-O (Kraft General Foods)* . . .	0.0	0.0	0	50	10
Lemon Sugar Free Low Calorie Gelatin, made with water (½ cup)					
Jell-O (Kraft General Foods)* . . .	0.0	0.0	0	55	10
Lime Sugar Free Low Calorie Gelatin, made with water (½ cup)					
Jell-O (Kraft General Foods)* . . .	0.0	0.0	0	60	10
Mixed Fruit Sugar Free Low Calorie Gelatin, made with water (½ cup)					
Jell-O (Kraft General Foods)* . . .	0.0	0.0	0	50	10

*Tobacco company, corporate subsidiary, or parent.

	Tot. Fat (g)	Sat. Fat (g)	Chol. (mg)	Sod. (mg)	Cal.
SUGAR-FREE GELATIN MIXES *(cont'd)*					
Orange Sugar Free Low Calorie Gelatin, made with water (½ cup)					
Jell-O (Kraft General Foods)* . . .	0.0	0.0	0	65	10
Raspberry Sugar Free Low Calorie Gelatin, made with water (½ cup)					
Jell-O (Kraft General Foods)* . . .	0.0	0.0	0	55	10
Strawberry Banana Sugar Free Low Calorie Gelatin, made with water (½ cup)					
Jell-O (Kraft General Foods)* . . .	0.0	0.0	0	50	10
Strawberry Low Calorie Gelatin, made with water (½ cup)					
D-Zerta (Kraft General Foods)* .	0.0	0.0	0	5	10
Strawberry Sugar Free Low Calorie Gelatin, made with water (½ cup)					
Jell-O (Kraft General Foods)* . . .	0.0	0.0	0	55	10
Triple Berry Sugar Free Low Calorie Gelatin, made with water (½ cup)					
Jell-O (Kraft General Foods)* . . .	0.0	0.0	0	50	10
Watermelon Sugar Free Low Calorie Gelatin, made with water (½ cup)					
Jell-O (Kraft General Foods)* . . .	0.0	0.0	0	55	10
SUGAR-FREE GELATIN SNACKS					
Cherry Sugar Free Low Calorie Gelatin Snacks (1 snack)					
Jell-O (Kraft General Foods)* . . .	0.0	0.0	0	50	10
Orange Sugar Free Low Calorie Gelatin Snacks (1 snack)					
Jell-O (Kraft General Foods)* . . .	0.0	0.0	0	50	10
Raspberry Sugar Free Low Calorie Gelatin Snacks (1 snack)					
Jell-O (Kraft General Foods)* . . .	0.0	0.0	0	50	10
Strawberry Sugar Free Low Calorie Gelatin Snacks (1 snack)					
Jell-O (Kraft General Foods)* . . .	0.0	0.0	0	50	10

*Tobacco company, corporate subsidiary, or parent.

	Tot. Fat (g)	Sat. Fat (g)	Chol. (mg)	Sod. (mg)	Cal.
Sugar-Sweetened Gelatin Mixes					
Apricot Gelatin, made with water (½ cup)					
Jell-O (Kraft General Foods)* . . .	0.0	0.0	0	50	80
Berry Blue Gelatin, made with water (½ cup)					
Jell-O (Kraft General Foods)* . . .	0.0	0.0	0	50	80
Black Cherry Gelatin, made with water (½ cup)					
Jell-O (Kraft General Foods)* . . .	0.0	0.0	0	50	80
Black Raspberry Gelatin, made with water (½ cup)					
Jell-O (Kraft General Foods)* . . .	0.0	0.0	0	35	80
Blackberry Gelatin, made with water (½ cup)					
Jell-O (Kraft General Foods)* . . .	0.0	0.0	0	50	80
Cherry Gelatin, made with water (½ cup)					
Jell-O (Kraft General Foods)* . . .	0.0	0.0	0	70	80
Cranberry Gelatin, made with water (½ cup)					
Jell-O (Kraft General Foods)* . . .	0.0	0.0	0	70	80
Gelatin sweetened with sugar, all flavors, made with water (½ cup)					
Most brands (USDA)	**0.0**	**0.0**	**0**	**(61)**	**71**
Grape Gelatin, made with water (½ cup)					
Jell-O (Kraft General Foods)* . . .	0.0	0.0	0	45	80
Lemon Gelatin, made with water (½ cup)					
Jell-O (Kraft General Foods)* . . .	0.0	0.0	0	75	80
Lime Gelatin, made with water (½ cup)					
Jell-O (Kraft General Foods)* . . .	0.0	0.0	0	60	80
Mango Gelatin, made with water (½ cup)					
Jell-O (Kraft General Foods)* . . .	0.0	0.0	0	45	80
Mixed Fruit Gelatin, made with water (½ cup)					
Jell-O (Kraft General Foods)* . . .	0.0	0.0	0	50	80

*Tobacco company, corporate subsidiary, or parent.

	Tot. Fat (g)	Sat. Fat (g)	Chol. (mg)	Sod. (mg)	Cal.
Sugar-Sweetened Gelatin Mixes *(cont'd)*					
Orange Gelatin, made with water (½ cup)					
Jell-O (Kraft General Foods)* . . .	0.0	0.0	0	50	80
Orange Pineapple Gelatin, made with water (½ cup)					
Jell-O (Kraft General Foods)* . . .	0.0	0.0	0	65	80
Peach Gelatin, made with water (½ cup)					
Jell-O (Kraft General Foods)* . . .	0.0	0.0	0	50	80
Pineapple Gelatin, made with water (½ cup)					
Jell-O (Kraft General Foods)* . . .	0.0	0.0	0	45	80
Raspberry Gelatin, made with water (½ cup)					
Jell-O (Kraft General Foods)* . . .	0.0	0.0	0	50	80
Strawberry Banana Gelatin, made with water (½ cup)					
Jell-O (Kraft General Foods)* . . .	0.0	0.0	0	50	80
Strawberry Gelatin, made with water (½ cup)					
Jell-O (Kraft General Foods)* . . .	0.0	0.0	0	50	80
Tropical Punch Gelatin, made with water (½ cup)					
Jell-O (Kraft General Foods)* . . .	0.0	0.0	0	45	80
Watermelon Gelatin, made with water (½ cup)					
Jell-O (Kraft General Foods)* . . .	0.0	0.0	0	50	80
Wild Strawberry Gelatin, made with water (½ cup)					
Jell-O (Kraft General Foods)* . . .	0.0	0.0	0	75	80
Sugar-Sweetened Gelatin Snacks					
Berry Blue Gelooze (1 bottle)					
Betty Crocker (General Mills) . . .	0.0	0.0	0	65	130
Berry Blue Gelatin Snacks (1 snack)					
Jell-O (Kraft General Foods)* . . .	0.0	0.0	0	45	80
Blue Berry Gel Cup (1 can)					
Del Monte	0.0	0.0	0	80	90

*Tobacco company, corporate subsidiary, or parent.

	Tot. Fat (g)	Sat. Fat (g)	Chol. (mg)	Sod. (mg)	Cal.
Blue Raspberry Gel snacks (1 snack) Kraft Handi-Snacks (Kraft General Foods)*	0.0	0.0	0	40	80
Cherry Gelooze (1 bottle) Betty Crocker (General Mills)	0.0	0.0	0	65	130
Cherry Gel Cup (1 can) Del Monte	0.0	0.0	0	80	90
Cherry Gel Snacks (1 snack) Kraft Handi-Snacks (Kraft General Foods)*	0.0	0.0	0	40	80
Cherry Gelatin Snacks (1 snack) Jell-O (Kraft General Foods)*	0.0	0.0	0	45	80
Grape Gel Cup (1 can) Del Monte	0.0	0.0	0	80	90
Grape Gelatin Snacks (1 snack) Jell-O (Kraft General Foods)*	0.0	0.0	0	45	80
Orange Gel Cup (1 can) Del Monte	0.0	0.0	0	80	90
Orange Gel Snacks (1 snack) Kraft Handi-Snacks (Kraft General Foods)*	0.0	0.0	0	40	80
Orange Gelatin Snacks (1 snack) Jell-O (Kraft General Foods)*	0.0	0.0	0	45	80
Orange Gelooze (1 bottle) Betty Crocker (General Mills)	0.0	0.0	0	65	130
Raspberry Gel Cup (1 can) Del Monte	0.0	0.0	0	80	90
Raspberry Gelatin Snacks (1 snack) Jell-O (Kraft General Foods)*	0.0	0.0	0	45	80
Strawberry-Banana Gelatin Snacks (1 snack) Jell-O (Kraft General Foods)*	0.0	0.0	0	45	80
Strawberry Gelooze (1 bottle) Betty Crocker (General Mills)	0.0	0.0	0	65	130
Strawberry Gel Cup (1 can) Del Monte	0.0	0.0	0	80	90
Strawberry Gel Snacks (1 snack) Kraft Handi-Snacks (Kraft General Foods)*	0.0	0.0	0	45	80

*Tobacco company, corporate subsidiary, or parent.

	Tot. Fat (g)	Sat. Fat (g)	Chol. (mg)	Sod. (mg)	Cal.
SUGAR-SWEETENED GELATIN SNACKS *(cont'd)*					
Strawberry Gelatin Snacks (1 snack)					
Jell-O (Kraft General Foods)* . . .	0.0	0.0	0	45	80
GRAHAM CRACKERS—*see* COOKIES, GRAHAM CRACKERS, page 165					
ICE CREAMS—*see* "FROZEN DESSERTS," ICE CREAMS/ ICE MILKS, page 214					
ICE MILKS—*see* "FROZEN DESSERTS," ICE CREAMS/ ICE MILKS, page 214					
MOUSSES—*see* PUDDINGS, page 175					
MUFFINS					
MUFFIN MIXES					
Blueberry Muffin Mixes					
Blueberry Muffin Mix, made with water and egg white (1 muffin)					
Pillsbury Lovin' Lites (Grand Metropolitan PLC)	1.0	0.0	0	160	100
PREPARED MUFFINS					
Apple Muffins					
Fat-Free Apple Spice Muffin (1 muffin)					
Health Valley (Health Valley Foods)	0.0	0.0	0	55	170
Banana Muffins					
Fat-Free Banana Muffin (1 muffin)					
Health Valley (Health Valley Foods)	0.0	0.0	0	55	170
Blueberry Muffins					
Blueberry Muffins (1 muffin)					
Entenmann's (Kraft General Foods)*	0.0	0.0	0	220	120

 *Tobacco company, corporate subsidiary, or parent.

	Tot. Fat (g)	Sat. Fat (g)	Chol. (mg)	Sod. (mg)	Cal.
PIE FILLINGS—*see* FRUIT GLAZES/PIE FILLINGS, page 168; PUDDINGS, below					
PIES					
Apple Beehive Pie (⅕ pie)					
Entenmann's (Kraft General Foods)*	0.0	0.0	0	330	270
Cherry Beehive Pie (⅕ pie)					
Entenmann's (Kraft General Foods)*	0.0	0.0	0	310	270
PUDDING SNACKS—*see* PUDDINGS, below					
PUDDINGS (INCLUDES CREAM PIE FILLINGS, CUSTARDS, AND MOUSSES)					
BANANA PUDDINGS					
Instant Banana Puddings					
Banana Cream Instant Pudding & Pie Filling, made with skim milk (½ cup)					
Jell-O (Kraft General Foods)*	0.2	0.2	2	413	133
Banana Fat Free Sugar Free Instant Reduced Calorie Pudding & Pie Filling, made with skim milk (½ cup)					
Jell-O (Kraft General Foods)*	0.0	0.0	0	410	70
Instant Banana Cream Pudding & Pie Filling, made with skim milk (½ cup)					
Royal (Nabisco Foods)*	0.2	0.2	2	463	133
Sugar Free Instant Banana Cream Pudding & Pie Filling, made with skim milk (½ cup)					
Royal (Nabisco Foods)*	0.2	0.2	2	473	83
Regular Banana Puddings					
Banana Cream Cook & Serve Pudding & Pie Filling, made with skim milk (½ cup)					
Jell-O (Kraft General Foods)*	0.2	0.2	2	243	123

*Tobacco company, corporate subsidiary, or parent.

	Tot. Fat (g)	Sat. Fat (g)	Chol. (mg)	Sod. (mg)	Cal.
BANANA PUDDINGS *(cont'd)*					
Banana Cream Pudding & Pie Filling, made with skim milk (½ cup)					
Royal (Nabisco Foods)*	0.2	0.2	2	173	123
BUTTERSCOTCH PUDDINGS					
Instant Butterscotch Puddings					
Butterscotch Fat Free Sugar Free Instant Reduced Calorie Pudding & Pie Filling, made with skim milk (½ cup)					
Jell-O (Kraft General Foods)*	0.0	0.0	0	400	70
Butterscotch Instant Pudding & Pie Filling, made with skim milk (½ cup)					
Jell-O (Kraft General Foods)*	0.2	0.2	2	453	133
Instant Butterscotch Pudding & Pie Filling, made with skim milk (½ cup)					
Royal (Nabisco Foods)*	0.2	0.2	2	443	133
Sugar Free Instant Butterscotch Pudding & Pie Filling, made with skim milk (½ cup)					
Royal (Nabisco Foods)*	0.2	0.2	2	473	83
Ready-to-Eat Butterscotch Puddings					
Butterscotch Pudding Snacks (4 oz)					
Ultra Slim-Fast (Slim-Fast Foods)	<1.0	(0.0)	0	230	100
Regular Butterscotch Puddings					
Butterscotch Cook & Serve Pudding & Pie Filling, made with skim milk (½ cup)					
Jell-O (Kraft General Foods)*	0.2	0.2	2	193	133
Butterscotch Pudding & Pie Filling, made with skim milk (½ cup)					
Royal (Nabisco Foods)*	0.2	0.2	2	243	133
Butterscotch Pudding, made with skim milk (½ cup)					
My•T•Fine (Nabisco Foods)*	0.2	0.2	2	253	133

*Tobacco company, corporate subsidiary, or parent.

	Tot. Fat (g)	Sat. Fat (g)	Chol. (mg)	Sod. (mg)	Cal.
CHEESECAKE PUDDINGS					
Cheesecake Mousse Mix, made with skim milk (½ cup) Sans Sucre de Paris (Bernard Foods)	1.5	0.5	5	105	73
Chocolate Cheesecake Mousse Mix, made with skim milk (½ cup) Sans Sucre de Paris (Bernard Foods)	1.5	0.5	5	105	75
CHOCOLATE PUDDINGS					
Instant Chocolate Puddings					
Chocolate Fat Free Sugar Free Instant Reduced Calorie Pudding & Pie Filling, made with skim milk (½ cup) Jell-O (Kraft General Foods)*	0.0	0.0	0	390	80
Chocolate Fudge Fat Free Sugar Free Instant Reduced Calorie Pudding & Pie Filling, made with skim milk (½ cup) Jell-O (Kraft General Foods)*	0.0	0.0	0	390	80
Chocolate Fudge Instant Pudding & Pie Filling, made with skim milk (½ cup) Jell-O (Kraft General Foods)*	0.2	0.2	2	443	143
Chocolate Instant Pudding & Pie Filling, made with skim milk (½ cup) Jell-O (Kraft General Foods)*	0.2	0.2	2	473	143
Chocolate Instant Pudding, made with skim milk (½ cup) Weight Watchers (H.J. Heinz)	1.0	0.0	5	420	90
Chocolate Mousse Mix, made with skim milk (½ cup) Sans Sucre de Paris (Bernard Foods)	3.0	1.0	0	45	76
Chocolate Reduced Calorie Pudding, made with skim milk (½ cup) D-Zerta (Kraft General Foods)*	0.0	0.0	0	65	60

*Tobacco company, corporate subsidiary, or parent.

	Tot. Fat (g)	Sat. Fat (g)	Chol. (mg)	Sod. (mg)	Cal.
CHOCOLATE PUDDINGS *(cont'd)*					
Instant Chocolate Almond Pudding & Pie Filling, made with skim milk (½ cup)					
Royal (Nabisco Foods)*	1.2	0.2	2	493	143
Instant Chocolate Pudding & Pie Filling, made with skim milk (½ cup)					
Royal (Nabisco Foods)*	0.2	0.2	2	453	143
Instant Dark 'n Sweet Chocolate Pudding & Pie Filling, made with skim milk (½ cup)					
Royal (Nabisco Foods)*	0.2	0.2	2	513	143
Milk Chocolate Instant Pudding & Pie Filling, made with skim milk (½ cup)					
Jell-O (Kraft General Foods)* . . .	1.2	0.2	2	463	143
Sugar Free Instant Chocolate Pudding & Pie Filling, made with skim milk (½ cup)					
Royal (Nabisco Foods)*	0.2	0.2	2	493	88
White Chocolate Almond Mousse, made with skim milk (½ cup)					
Weight Watchers (H.J. Heinz) . .	3.0	1.0	(2)	105	70
Ready-to-Eat Chocolate Puddings					
Chocolate Fat Free Pudding Snacks (1 snack)					
Jell-O Free (Kraft General Foods)*	0.0	0.0	0	190	100
Chocolate Pudding Snacks (4 oz)					
Ultra Slim-Fast (Slim-Fast Foods)	<1.0	0.0	0	240	100
Chocolate-Vanilla Swirl Fat Free Pudding Snacks (1 snack)					
Jell-O Free (Kraft General Foods)*	0.0	0.0	0	210	100
Fat Free Chocolate Pudding (4 oz)					
Hershey's (Hershey Food Co) . .	0.0	0.0	0	180	100

*Tobacco company, corporate subsidiary, or parent.

	Tot. Fat (g)	Sat. Fat (g)	Chol. (mg)	Sod. (mg)	Cal.
Fat Free Chocolate Pudding Cup (1 cup)					
Del Monte	0.0	0.0	0	170	100
Fat Free Kiss Pudding (4 oz)					
Hershey's (Hershey Food Co)	0.0	0.0	0	170	100
Fat Free Special Dark Pudding (4 oz)					
Hershey's (Hershey Food Co)	0.0	0.0	0	170	100
Light Chocolate Fudge Pudding (4 oz)					
Swiss Miss (Hunt-Wesson)	1.0	0.3	0	120	100
Light Chocolate Pudding					
Del Monte (1 container)	1.0	0.0	0	140	100
Hunt's Snack Pack (Hunt-Wesson) (4 oz)	2.0	0.3	1	120	100
Swiss Miss (Hunt-Wesson) (4 oz)	1.0	0.3	0	120	100
Regular Chocolate Puddings					
Chocolate Almond Pudding, made with skim milk (½ cup)					
My·T·Fine (Nabisco Foods)*	1.2	0.2	2	198	133
Chocolate Cook & Serve Pudding & Pie Filling, made with skim milk (½ cup)					
Jell-O (Kraft General Foods)*	0.2	0.2	2	173	133
Chocolate Fudge Cook & Serve Pudding & Pie Filling, made with skim milk (½ cup)					
Jell-O (Kraft General Foods)*	0.2	0.2	2	178	133
Chocolate Fudge Pudding, made with skim milk (½ cup)					
My·T·Fine (Nabisco Foods)*	0.2	0.2	2	203	133
Chocolate Pudding & Pie Filling, made with skim milk (½ cup)					
Royal (Nabisco Foods)*	0.2	0.2	2	143	133
Chocolate Pudding, made with skim milk (½ cup)					
My·T·Fine (Nabisco Foods)*	0.2	0.2	2	203	133

*Tobacco company, corporate subsidiary, or parent.

	Tot. Fat (g)	Sat. Fat (g)	Chol. (mg)	Sod. (mg)	Cal.
CHOCOLATE PUDDINGS *(cont'd)*					
Chocolate Sugar Free Reduced Calorie Cook & Serve Pudding & Pie Filling, made with skim milk (½ cup) Jell-O (Kraft General Foods)* . . .	0.2	0.2	2	173	73
Dark 'n Sweet Chocolate Pudding & Pie Filling, made with skim milk (½ cup) (Nabisco Foods)*	0.2	0.2	2	163	133
Milk Chocolate Cook & Serve Pudding & Pie Filling, made with skim milk (½ cup) Jell-O (Kraft General Foods)* . . .	0.2	0.2	2	178	133
CUSTARD PUDDINGS					
Regular Custard Puddings					
Custard Dessert Mix, made with skim milk (½ cup) Jell-O Americana (Kraft General Foods)*	0.2	0.2	2	193	123
Flan Caramel Custard, made with skim milk (½ cup) Royal (Nabisco Foods)*	0.2	0.2	2	88	123
Flan Cook & Serve Pudding & Pie Filling, made with skim milk (½ cup) Jell-O (Kraft General Foods)* . . .	0.2	0.2	2	68	123
LEMON PUDDINGS					
Instant Lemon Puddings					
Instant Lemon Pudding & Pie Filling, made with skim milk (½ cup) Royal (Nabisco Foods)*	0.2	0.2	2	393	133
Lemon Instant Pudding & Pie Filling, made with skim milk (½ cup) Jell-O (Kraft General Foods)* . . .	0.2	0.2	2	363	133
Lemon Mousse Mix, made with skim milk (½ cup) Sans Sucre de Paris (Bernard Foods)	3.0	1.0	<5	50	70

*Tobacco company, corporate subsidiary, or parent.

	Tot. Fat (g)	Sat. Fat (g)	Chol. (mg)	Sod. (mg)	Cal.
Regular Lemon Puddings					
Lemon Flavored Pudding & Pie Filling, made with skim milk (1/6 of filling)					
My•T•Fine (Nabisco Foods)* . . .	0.2	0.2	2	178	93
Lemon Pie Filling, made with skim milk (1/6 of filling)					
Royal (Nabisco Foods)*	0.2	0.2	2	183	93
PISTACHIO PUDDINGS					
Instant Pistachio Puddings					
Instant Pistachio Pudding & Pie Filling, made with skim milk (1/2 cup)					
Royal (Nabisco Foods)*	0.7	0.2	2	413	133
Pistachio Fat Free Sugar Free Instant Reduced Calorie Pudding & Pie Filling, made with skim milk (1/2 cup)					
Jell-O (Kraft General Foods)* . . .	0.0	0.0	0	380	70
Pistachio Instant Pudding & Pie Filling, made with skim milk (1/2 cup)					
Jell-O (Kraft General Foods)* . . .	0.7	0.2	2	413	143
Sugar Free Instant Pistachio Pudding & Pie Filling, made with skim milk (1/2 cup)					
Royal (Nabisco Foods)*	0.7	0.2	2	473	83
STRAWBERRY PUDDINGS					
Strawberry Mousse Mix, made with skim milk (1/2 cup)					
Sans Sucre de Paris (Bernard Foods)	2.0	1.0	0	45	70
TAPIOCA PUDDINGS					
Ready-to-Eat Tapioca Puddings					
Fat Free Tapioca Pudding (4 oz)					
Hershey's (Hershey Food Co) . .	0.0	0.0	0	190	90
Light Tapioca Pudding (4 oz)					
Hunt's Snack Pack (Hunt-Wesson)	2.0	0.4	1	105	100

*Tobacco company, corporate subsidiary, or parent.

	Tot. Fat (g)	Sat. Fat (g)	Chol. (mg)	Sod. (mg)	Cal.
TAPIOCA PUDDINGS *(cont'd)*					
Regular Tapioca Puddings					
Tapioca Pudding Mix, made with skim milk (½ cup)					
Jell-O Americana (Kraft General Foods)*	0.2	0.2	2	168	123
Vanilla Tapioca Pudding, made with skim milk (½ cup)					
My•T•Fine (Nabisco Foods)*	0.2	0.2	2	223	123
Royal (Nabisco Foods)*	0.2	0.2	2	123	123
VANILLA PUDDINGS					
Instant Vanilla Puddings					
French Vanilla Instant Pudding & Pie Filling, made with skim milk (½ cup)					
Jell-O (Kraft General Foods)*	0.2	0.2	2	413	133
Instant Vanilla Pudding & Pie Filling, made with skim milk (½ cup)					
Royal (Nabisco Foods)*	0.2	0.2	2	383	133
Sugar Free Instant Vanilla Pudding & Pie Filling, made with skim milk (½ cup)					
Royal (Nabisco Foods)*	0.2	0.2	2	473	83
Vanilla Fat Free Sugar Free Instant Reduced Calorie Pudding & Pie Filling, made with skim milk (½ cup)					
Jell-O (Kraft General Foods)*	0.0	0.0	0	400	70
Vanilla Instant Pudding & Pie Filling, made with skim milk (½ cup)					
Jell-O (Kraft General Foods)*	0.2	0.2	2	413	133
Vanilla Instant Pudding, made with skim milk (½ cup)					
Weight Watchers (H.J. Heinz)	0.0	0.0	5	510	90
Ready-to-Eat Vanilla Puddings					
Fat Free Vanilla Pudding (4 oz)					
Hershey's (Hershey Food Co)	0.0	0.0	0	230	100
Fat Free Vanilla Pudding Cup (1 cup)					
Del Monte	0.0	0.0	0	160	100

*Tobacco company, corporate subsidiary, or parent.

	Tot. Fat (g)	Sat. Fat (g)	Chol. (mg)	Sod. (mg)	Cal.
Light Vanilla Pudding					
Del Monte (1 container)	1.0	0.0	0	190	90
Swiss Miss (Hunt-Wesson) (4 oz)	1.0	0.3	0	105	100
Vanilla-Chocolate Swirl Fat Free Pudding Snacks (1 snack)					
Jell-O Free (Kraft General Foods)*	0.0	0.0	0	220	100
Vanilla Fat Free Pudding Snacks (1 snack)					
Jell-O Free (Kraft General Foods)*	0.0	0.0	0	240	100
Regular Vanilla Puddings					
Vanilla Cook & Serve Pudding & Pie Filling, made with skim milk (½ cup)					
Jell-O (Kraft General Foods)*	0.2	0.2	2	198	123
Vanilla Pudding & Pie Filling, made with skim milk (½ cup)					
Royal (Nabisco Foods)*	0.2	0.2	2	223	123
Vanilla Pudding, made with skim milk (⅙ of pudding)					
My•T•Fine (Nabisco Foods)*	0.2	0.2	2	178	123
Vanilla Sugar Free Reduced Calorie Cook & Serve Pudding & Pie Filling, made with skim milk (½ cup)					
Jell-O (Kraft General Foods)*	0.2	0.2	2	178	63
OTHER PUDDINGS					
Butter Pecan Instant Pudding & Pie Filling, made with skim milk (½ cup)					
Jell-O (Kraft General Foods)*	0.7	0.7	2	413	143
Key Lime Pie Filling, made with skim milk (⅙ of filling)					
Royal (Nabisco Foods)*	0.2	0.2	2	183	93
Light Vanilla/Chocolate Parfait (4 oz)					
Swiss Miss (Hunt-Wesson)	1.0	0.3	0	110	100

*Tobacco company, corporate subsidiary, or parent.

	Tot. Fat (g)	Sat. Fat (g)	Chol. (mg)	Sod. (mg)	Cal.
OTHER PUDDINGS *(cont'd)*					
Rice Pudding Mix, made with skim milk (½ cup)					
Jell-O Americana (Kraft General Foods)*	0.2	0.2	2	163	143
SHERBETS—*see* "FROZEN DESSERTS," ICES/SHERBETS/SORBETS, page 223					
SORBETS—*see* "FROZEN DESSERTS," ICES/SHERBETS/SORBETS, page 223					
SNACK CAKES—*see also* CAKES/CUPCAKES, page 156					
Twinkie Lights (1 cake)					
Hostess (Continental Baking Co)	1.5	0.0	0	200	120
SWEET ROLLS—*see* "BREADS AND BREAD PRODUCTS," COFFEE CAKES/DANISHES/SWEET ROLLS, page 57					
TOASTER PASTRIES					
Apple-Cinnamon Fat Free Toaster Pastries (1 pastry)					
Auburn Farms Toast 'N Jammers (Auburn Farms)	0.0	0.0	0	200	180
Blueberry Fat Free Toaster Pastries (1 pastry)					
Auburn Farms Toast 'N Jammers (Auburn Farms)	0.0	0.0	0	200	180
Raspberry Fat Free Toaster Pastries (1 pastry)					
Auburn Farms Toast 'N Jammers (Auburn Farms)	0.0	0.0	0	200	180
Strawberry Fat Free Toaster Pastries (1 pastry)					
Auburn Farms Toast 'N Jammers (Auburn Farms)	0.0	0.0	0	200	180

*Tobacco company, corporate subsidiary, or parent.

EGG SUBSTITUTES

If you love eggs but not the cholesterol that comes with them, try egg substitutes. They're tasty and fluffy, and they cook just like the real thing. Best of all, they contain little if any total fat and no saturated fat or cholesterol. You'll find that the sodium contents vary slightly. The AHA does not have criteria for sodium but recommends a total of no more than 3,000 mg a day.

If you find products that were introduced after this book went to press, use the following tables to help you evaluate them.

AHA Criteria for Egg Substitutes*

	Tot. Fat (g)	Sat. Fat (g)	Chol. (mg)
All egg substitutes	3	1	<2

*Per serving.

You'll Want to Limit Whole Eggs

As you can see in the table below, whole eggs are high in cholesterol. We recommend that you eat no more than 3 or 4 egg yolks each week.

Compare the amounts of fat, saturated fat, cholesterol, sodium, and calories in this example with the more healthful alternatives listed on the following pages.

Whole Egg to Limit

	Tot. Fat (g)	Sat. Fat (g)	Chol. (mg)	Sod. (mg)	Cal.
Chicken egg, fried (1 large)	6.9*	1.7*	211*	162	91

Adapted from USDA Handbook No. 8 series.
*These values exceed AHA criteria for egg substitutes.

	Tot. Fat (g)	Sat. Fat (g)	Chol. (mg)	Sod. (mg)	Cal.
Better 'n Eggs, frozen (¼ cup) Morningstar Farms (Worthington Foods)	0.0	0.0	0	90	30
Better 'n Eggs, refrigerated (¼ cup) Morningstar Farms (Worthington Foods)	0.0	0.0	0	100	20
Cholesterol Free Egg Product (¼ cup) Healthy Choice (ConAgra)	0.0	0.0	0	95	25
Egg Beaters, frozen (¼ cup) Fleischmann's (Nabisco Foods)*	0.0	0.0	0	100	30
Egg Beaters, refrigerated (¼ cup) Fleischmann's (Nabisco Foods)*	0.0	0.0	0	100	30
Egg white, raw (1) **Most brands** (USDA)	**0.0**	**0.0**	**0**	**50**	**16**
99% Egg Product (¼ cup) America's Choice (A & P)	0.0	0.0	0	80	30
No Cholesterol Real Egg Product (¼ cup) Second Nature (International Delight)	2.0	0.0	0	110	60
No Fat Real Egg Product (¼ cup) Second Nature (International Delight)	0.0	0.0	0	115	40
Scramblers, frozen (¼ cup) Morningstar Farms (Worthington Foods)	0.0	0.0	0	95	35

*Tobacco company, corporate subsidiary, or parent.

FATS AND OILS

The two simple rules about fats and oils are:

1. Choose unsaturated oils and margarines.
2. Avoid highly saturated oils and fats.

We've made this easy with the charts on the following pages. You'll find cooking sprays and oils, butter substitutes, nut butters, and margarines that will help you cook to your heart's content. They're all low in saturated fat.

Like all the other entries in this book, the fats and oils entries that follow list sodium content. The AHA does not have criteria for sodium but recommends a total of no more than 3,000 mg a day.

The Butter/Margarine Controversy (Trans Fatty Acids)

Recently, certain studies found that stick margarines contain a kind of fat called trans fatty acids. This fat seems to raise blood cholesterol. After these studies were published, consumers began to worry about using margarine. Some wondered whether butter would be a better choice.

Although more studies are needed, we do know one thing: Butter is rich in both saturated fat and cholesterol. It will definitely help raise your blood cholesterol. In comparison, most margarine is made from vegetable oil and contains no cholesterol. We also know that the more liquid the margarine, the fewer trans fatty acids it contains. Therefore, if you choose a soft tub or liquid margarine rather than the stick form, you'll steer clear of a lot of the trans fatty acids. Our advice is to look for a margarine with liquid vegetable oil listed as the first ingredient. It should contain no more than 2 grams of saturated fat per tablespoon.

The bottom line: Margarine is still better than butter for your heart. And soft tub or liquid margarines are better for you than stick margarines are.

Generic Listings

By far, most of the foods in this book are brand name products. However, if a product is listed without a brand name, it means that most brands of that product contain about the same amount of fat, saturated fat, and cholesterol and that these amounts are within the criteria cited below.

If you find products that were introduced after this book went to press, use the generic listings and the following tables to help you evaluate them.

AHA Criteria for Fats and Oils*

	Tot. Fat (g)	Sat. Fat (g)	Chol. (mg)
Avocados, butter substitutes, cooking sprays, margarine, nut butters, nuts, oils, olives, and seeds	**	2	<2

*Per serving.

**No criterion; these foods are naturally high in fat but low in saturated fat.

Fats and Oils You'll Want to Limit

Some fats and oils, like the examples below, are too high in fat, saturated fat, and/or cholesterol to meet AHA criteria. They aren't included in this book, and we recommend that you don't eat them often.

Compare the amounts of fat, saturated fat, cholesterol, sodium, and calories in these examples with the more healthful alternatives listed on the following pages.

Sample Fats and Oils to Limit

	Tot. Fat (g)	Sat. Fat (g)	Chol. (mg)	Sod. (mg)	Cal.
Butter (3 pats, or 1 tbsp)	12.2	7.5*	33*	123	108
Cashew nuts, salted (1 oz)	13.2	2.6*	0	486	163
Cottonseed oil (1 tbsp)	13.6	8.9*	(0)	(0)	120
Oil-roasted macadamia nuts, salted (1 oz)	21.7	3.3*	0	74	204
Peanut oil (1 tbsp)	13.5	2.3*	(0)	0	119
Shortening, made from hydrogenated soybean and hydrogenated cottonseed oil (1 tbsp)	12.8	3.2*	(0)	(0)	113
Stick margarine, made from hydrogenated soybean oil, corn oil, and hydrogenated cottonseed oil (1 tbsp)	11.4	2.7*	(0)	133	101
Sweetened flaked coconut, canned (½ oz)	4.5	4.0*	0	3	63

Adapted from USDA Handbook No. 8 series.

*These values exceed AHA criteria for fats and oils.

	Tot. Fat (g)	Sat. Fat (g)	Chol. (mg)	Sod. (mg)	Cal.
ALMOND BUTTERS—*see* NUT BUTTERS, page 195					
AVOCADOS					
California avocado (2 tbsp puree)					
Most brands (USDA)	**4.6**	**0.7**	**0**	**3**	**48**
BUTTER SUBSTITUTES					
Butter Buds (1 tsp)					
Butter Buds (Cumberland Packing)	0.0	0.0	0	75	5
Butter Buds Sprinkles (1 tsp)					
Butter Buds (Cumberland Packing)	0.0	0.0	0	120	5
Natural Butter Flavor Sprinkles (1 tsp)					
Molly McButter (Alberto-Culver)	0.0	0.0	0	180	5
COOKING SPRAYS					
Buttery Spray (1-second spray)					
Weight Watchers (H.J. Heinz)	0.0	0.0	0	0	0
Cooking Spray (1-second spray)					
Weight Watchers (H.J. Heinz)	0.0	0.0	0	0	0
Lite Cooking Spray (0.27 g)					
Wesson (Hunt-Wesson)	<1.0	0.0	0	0	0
No Stick Cooking Spray (0.2 g)					
Mazola (Best Foods)	0.0	0.0	0	0	0
MARGARINES AND MARGARINE SPREADS					
DIET/LIGHT MARGARINES AND MARGARINE SPREADS					
Soft Tub/Diet/Light Margarines and Margarine Spreads					
Canola Choice (1 tbsp)					
Fleischmann's (Nabisco Foods)*	8.0	1.0	0	90	70
Canola Spread (1 tbsp)					
Sunrise (Dean Foods)	7.0	1.0	0	95	70
Diet Reduced Calorie Margarine (1 tbsp)					
Mazola (Best Foods)	6.0	1.0	0	130	50

*Tobacco company, corporate subsidiary, or parent.

	Tot. Fat (g)	Sat. Fat (g)	Chol. (mg)	Sod. (mg)	Cal.
DIET/LIGHT MARGARINES AND MARGARINE SPREADS *(cont'd)*					
Extra Light Spread (1 tbsp)					
Mazola (Best Foods)	6.0	1.0	0	100	50
Weight Watchers (H.J. Heinz)	4.0	1.0	0	75	45
Extra Light Unsalted Spread (1 tbsp)					
Weight Watchers (H.J. Heinz)	4.0	1.0	0	0	45
53% Vegetable Oil Spread (⅓ less fat) (1 tbsp)					
Kraft Parkay (Kraft General Foods)*	7.0	1.5	0	120	70
Light 40% Vegetable Oil Spread (1 tbsp)					
Kraft Parkay (Kraft General Foods)*	6.0	1.0	0	120	50
Lower Fat Margarine (1 tbsp)					
Fleischmann's (Nabisco Foods)*	4.5	0.0	0	55	40
Nucanola 52% Spread (1 tbsp)					
Nucoa (GFA Brands)	7.0	<1.0	0	90	70
Soft Diet Margarine (1 tbsp)					
Kraft Parkay (Kraft General Foods)*	6.0	1.0	0	110	50
Spread with Sweet Cream (1 tbsp)					
Land O'Lakes (Land O'Lakes Foods)	8.0	2.0	0	70	80
Super Light Margarine (1 tbsp)					
Nucoa Smart Beat (GFA Brands)	2.0	0.0	0	105	20
Unsalted Light Margarine (1 tbsp)					
Nucoa Smart Beat (GFA Brands)	3.0	0.0	0	0	25
Stick Diet/Light Margarines and Margarine Spreads					
Canola Choice (1 tbsp)					
Fleischmann's (Nabisco Foods)*	8.0	1.0	0	90	70
50% Vegetable Oil Spread (1 tbsp)					
Kraft Parkay (Kraft General Foods)*	7.0	1.5	0	110	60

*Tobacco company, corporate subsidiary, or parent.

	Tot. Fat (g)	Sat. Fat (g)	Chol. (mg)	Sod. (mg)	Cal.
47% Vegetable Oil and Dairy Spread (1 tbsp)					
Kraft Touch of Butter (Kraft General Foods)*	7.0	1.5	0	110	60
Light Spread (1 tbsp)					
Weight Watchers (H.J. Heinz)	7.0	1.0	0	130	60
Light Taste (1 tbsp)					
Blue Bonnet (Nabisco Foods)*	8.0	1.5	0	105	70
Fleischmann's (Nabisco Foods)*	8.0	1.5	0	90	70
Lower Fat Margarine (1 tbsp)					
Fleischmann's (Nabisco Foods)*	6.0	1.0	0	60	50
REGULAR MARGARINES AND MARGARINE SPREADS					
Soft Tub/Regular Margarines and Margarine Spreads					
Chiffon Soft Margarine (1 tbsp)					
Kraft (Kraft General Foods)*	11.0	2.0	0	105	100
Country Morning Blend (1 tbsp)					
Land O'Lakes (Land O'Lakes Foods)	11.0	2.0	0	80	100
Pure Vegetable Oil Spread (1 tbsp)					
Blue Bonnet (Nabisco Foods)*	10.0	1.5	0	80	80
70% Vegetable Oil and Dairy Spread (1 tbsp)					
Kraft Touch of Butter (Kraft General Foods)*	10.0	2.0	0	110	90
70% Vegetable Oil Spread (1 tbsp)					
Kraft Parkay (Kraft General Foods)*	10.0	2.0	0	110	90
Soft Margarine (1 tbsp)					
Kraft Parkay (Kraft General Foods)*	11.0	2.0	0	105	100
Stick Regular Margarines and Margarine Spreads					
Canola Margarine (1 tbsp)					
Sunrise (Dean Foods)	11.0	1.0	0	95	100
Margarine (1 tbsp)					
Mazola (Best Foods)	11.0	2.0	0	100	100

*Tobacco company, corporate subsidiary, or parent.

	Tot. Fat (g)	Sat. Fat (g)	Chol. (mg)	Sod. (mg)	Cal.
REGULAR MARGARINES AND MARGARINE SPREADS *(cont'd)*					
Move Over Butter (1 tbsp)					
Move Over Butter (Nabisco Foods)*	10.0	2.0	0	100	90
Pure Vegetable Oil Spread (1 tbsp)					
Blue Bonnet (Nabisco Foods)*	10.0	2.0	0	110	80
Spread with Sweet Cream Salted (1 tbsp)					
Land O'Lakes (Land O'Lakes Foods)	10.0	2.0	0	95	90
Spread with Sweet Cream Unsalted (1 tbsp)					
Land O'Lakes (Land O'Lakes Foods)	10.0	2.0	0	0	90
Sweet Unsalted Margarine (1 tbsp)					
Fleischmann's (Nabisco Foods)*	11.0	2.0	0	0	100
Unsalted Margarine (1 tbsp)					
Mazola (Best Foods)	11.0	2.0	0	0	100
Squeeze Regular Margarines and Margarine Spreads					
64% Vegetable Oil and Dairy Spread (1 tbsp)					
Kraft Touch of Butter (Kraft General Foods)*	9.0	1.5	0	115	80
Squeeze 64% Vegetable Oil Spread (1 tbsp)					
Kraft Parkay (Kraft General Foods)*	9.0	1.5	0	120	80
WHIPPED MARGARINES AND MARGARINE SPREADS					
Chiffon Whipped Margarine (1 tbsp)					
Kraft (Kraft General Foods)*	7.0	1.5	0	70	70
Whipped Margarine (1 tbsp)					
Kraft Parkay (Kraft General Foods)*	7.0	1.5	0	70	70

*Tobacco company, corporate subsidiary, or parent.

	Tot. Fat (g)	Sat. Fat (g)	Chol. (mg)	Sod. (mg)	Cal.
NUT BUTTERS					
Almond butter, salted (2 tbsp)					
Most brands (USDA)	18.9	1.8	0	144	202
Almond butter, unsalted (2 tbsp)					
Most brands (USDA)	18.9	1.8	0	4	202
NUTS					
Almonds, dry-roasted, salted (about 24 nuts)					
Most brands (USDA)	15.5	1.5	0	234	176
Almonds, honey-roasted (about 28 nuts)					
Most brands (USDA)	15.0	1.4	0	39	178
Chestnuts, roasted (30 g, or about 4 nuts)					
Most brands (USDA)	0.3	0.1	0	1	68
Filberts, dry-roasted, salted (30 g, or about 3½ tbsp)					
Most brands (USDA)	19.8	1.5	0	234	199
Filberts, dry-roasted, unsalted (30 g, or about 3½ tbsp)					
Most brands (USDA)	19.8	1.5	0	1	199
Hazelnuts, dry-roasted, salted (30 g)					
Most brands (USDA)	19.8	1.5	0	234	199
Hazelnuts, dry-roasted, unsalted (30 g)					
Most brands (USDA)	19.8	1.5	0	1	199
Pecans, dry-roasted, salted (about 33 nuts)					
Most brands (USDA)	19.4	1.6	0	234	198
Pecans, dry-roasted, unsalted (about 33 nuts)					
Most brands (USDA)	19.4	1.6	0	0	198
Pistachios, dry-roasted, salted (about 50 nuts)					
Most brands (USDA)	15.8	2.0	0	234	182

	Tot. Fat (g)	Sat. Fat (g)	Chol. (mg)	Sod. (mg)	Cal.
NUTS ***(cont'd)***					
Pistachios, dry-roasted, unsalted (about 50 nuts)					
Most brands (USDA)	**15.8**	**2.0**	**0**	**2**	**182**
Walnuts (15 halves)					
Most brands (USDA)	**17.0**	**1.1**	**0**	**0**	**182**
OILS					
CANOLA OILS					
Canola Oil (1 tbsp)					
Most brands (USDA)	**13.6**	**0.8**	**0**	**0**	**120**
Crisco Puritan (Procter & Gamble)	14.0	1.0	0	0	120
Nucoa Smart Beat (GFA Brands)	14.0	1.0	0	0	120
Wesson (Hunt-Wesson)	14.0	1.0	0	0	120
Pure Canola Oil (1 tbsp)					
America's Choice (A & P)	14.0	1.0	0	0	130
CORN OILS					
Corn Oil (1 tbsp)					
Most brands (USDA)	**13.6**	**1.7**	**0**	**0**	**120**
Mazola (Best Foods)	14.0	2.0	0	0	120
Wesson (Hunt-Wesson)	14.0	1.9	0	0	120
MIXED OILS					
Canola and Corn Oil Blend (1 tbsp)					
Crisco (Procter & Gamble)	14.0	1.5	0	0	120
OLIVE OILS					
Extra Mild Olive Oil (1 tbsp)					
Progresso (Pet)	14.0	2.0	0	0	120
Extra Virgin Olive Oil (1 tbsp)					
Progresso (Pet)	14.0	2.0	0	0	120
Olive Oil (1 tbsp)					
Most brands (USDA)	**13.5**	**1.8**	**0**	**0**	**119**
Wesson (Hunt-Wesson)	14.0	2.0	0	0	120
Olive Oil (Riviera Blend) (1 tbsp)					
Progresso (Pet)	14.0	2.0	0	0	120
SAFFLOWER OILS					
Safflower oil (1 tbsp)					
Most brands (USDA)	**13.6**	**1.2**	**0**	**0**	**120**

	Tot. Fat (g)	Sat. Fat (g)	Chol. (mg)	Sod. (mg)	Cal.
SESAME OILS					
Sesame Oil (1 tbsp)					
Most brands (USDA)	**13.6**	**1.9**	**0**	**0**	**120**
Ka-me (Shaffer, Clarke & Co)	14.0	2.0	0	0	130
SOYBEAN OILS					
Soybean oil (1 tbsp)					
Most brands (USDA)	**13.6**	**2.0**	**0**	**0**	**120**
SUNFLOWER OILS					
Sunflower Oil (1 tbsp)					
Most brands (USDA)	**13.6**	**1.4**	**0**	**0**	**120**
Wesson (Hunt-Wesson)	14.0	1.7	0	0	120
OTHER OILS					
Gourmet Popping and Topping Oils (1 tbsp)					
Orville Redenbacher's (Hunt-Wesson)	14.0	2.0	0	0	120
Hot Chili Oil (1 tbsp)					
Ka-me (Shaffer, Clarke & Co)	14.0	2.0	0	0	130
Vegetable Oil (1 tbsp)					
Wesson (Hunt-Wesson)	14.0	2.0	0	0	120
OLIVES					
BLACK/RIPE OLIVES					
Oil Cured Olives (6 olives)					
Progresso (Pet)	6.0	0.5	0	330	80
Olive Salad (2 tbsp)					
Progresso (Pet)	2.5	0.0	0	360	25
Ripe olives (2 extra large)					
Most brands (USDA)	**1.6**	**0.2**	**0**	**96**	**15**
Ripe Pitted Colossal Olives (2 olives)					
America's Choice (A & P)	2.0	0.0	0	110	20
Ripe Pitted Extra Large Olives (3 olives)					
America's Choice (A & P)	2.5	0.0	0	110	25
Ripe Pitted Jumbo Olives (3 olives)					
America's Choice (A & P)	2.0	0.0	0	135	25
Ripe Pitted Large Olives (4 olives)					
America's Choice (A & P)	2.5	0.0	0	115	25

	Tot. Fat (g)	Sat. Fat (g)	Chol. (mg)	Sod. (mg)	Cal.
BLACK/RIPE OLIVES *(cont'd)*					
Ripe Pitted Medium Olives (5 olives)					
America's Choice (A & P)	2.5	0.0	0	115	25
Ripe Pitted Small Olives (6 olives)					
America's Choice (A & P)	2.5	0.0	0	115	25
Ripe Pitted Super Colossal Olives (1 olive)					
America's Choice (A & P)	1.0	0.0	0	75	15
GREEN OLIVES					
Green olives (5 sml)					
Most brands (USDA)	**1.8**	**0.2**	**0**	**343**	**17**
SEEDS					
Sunflower seed kernels, salted (30 g, or about 3½ tbsp)					
Most brands (USDA)	**17.0**	**1.8**	**0**	**184**	**186**
Sunflower seed kernels, unsalted (30 g, or about 3½ tbsp)					
Most brands (USDA)	**17.0**	**1.8**	**0**	**1**	**186**

FROZEN DESSERTS

If you scream for ice cream, relax. We've found dozens of frozen desserts that have ditched the high fat, saturated fat, and cholesterol but kept the creamy texture and delicious taste you love.

On the pages that follow, you'll find nonfat and low-fat frozen yogurts, ice creams and ice milks, sherbets, sorbets, bars, and pops in all your favorite flavors.

Like all the other entries in this book, the frozen desserts entries that follow list sodium content. The AHA does not have criteria for sodium but recommends a total of no more than 3,000 mg a day.

If you find products that were introduced after this book went to press, use the following tables to help you evaluate them.

AHA Criteria for Frozen Desserts*

	Tot. Fat (g)	Sat. Fat (g)	Chol. (mg)
Frozen desserts, milk based, such as frozen dairy desserts, frozen yogurt, and sherbet	3	2	20
Frozen desserts, not milk based, such as fruit ices, ice pops, and sorbets	<0.5	<0.5	<2

*Per serving.

Frozen Desserts You'll Want to Limit

Some frozen desserts, like the examples below, are too high in fat, saturated fat, and/or cholesterol to meet AHA criteria. They aren't included in this book, and we recommend that you don't eat them often.

Compare the amounts of fat, saturated fat, cholesterol, sodium, and calories in these examples with the more healthful alternatives listed on the following pages.

Sample Frozen Desserts to Limit

	Tot. Fat (g)	Sat. Fat (g)	Chol. (mg)	Sod. (mg)	Cal.
Chocolate ice cream (½ cup)	7.3*	4.5*	22*	50	143
Chocolate soft-serve frozen yogurt (½ cup)	4.3*	2.6*	3	71	115
Vanilla ice cream, rich (½ cup)	12.0*	7.4*	45*	41	178

Adapted from USDA Handbook No. 8 series.

*These values exceed AHA criteria for frozen desserts.

	Tot. Fat (g)	Sat. Fat (g)	Chol. (mg)	Sod. (mg)	Cal.
BARS/POPS					
Chocolate Bars/Pops					
Chocolate Mousse Bar (1 bar)					
Weight Watchers (H.J. Heinz) . .	1.0	0.5	5	80	70
Chocolate Treat Bar (1 bar)					
Weight Watchers (H.J. Heinz) . .	1.0	0.0	10	150	100
No Sugar Added Chocolate Fudge Lites (2 bars)					
Wells' Blue Bunny Sweet Freedom (Wells' Dairy)	0.5	0.0	0	120	70
Fruit Pops					
Cherry Fruit Pops					
Cherry Freeze Bar (1 bar)					
Blue Bell (Blue Bell Creameries) .	0.0	0.0	0	5	70
Chunky Cherry Frozen Fruit Bar (1 bar)					
Frozfruit (Frozfruit Corp)	0.0	0.0	0	0	70
Lemon/Lime Fruit Pops					
Double Lemon Frozen Fruit Bar (1 bar)					
Frozfruit (Frozfruit Corp)	0.0	0.0	0	10	90
Double Lime Frozen Fruit Bar (1 bar)					
Frozfruit (Frozfruit Corp)	0.0	0.0	0	10	90
Mixed Fruit Pops					
Assorted Freezer Bars (2-oz bar)					
Mr. Freeze (Kraft General Foods)*	0.0	0.0	0	15	35
Assorted Freezer Bars (3 1-oz bars or 2 1.5-oz bars)					
Mr. Freeze (Kraft General Foods)*	0.0	0.0	0	20	50
No Sugar Added Assorted Pops (1 bar)					
Wells' Blue Bunny Sweet Freedom (Wells' Dairy)	0.0	0.0	0	10	10
No Sugar Added Bomb Pop, Jr. (1 bar)					
Wells' Blue Bunny Sweet Freedom (Wells' Dairy)	0.0	0.0	0	10	25
Orange Fruit Pops					
Chunky Orange Frozen Fruit Bar (1 bar)					
Frozfruit (Frozfruit Corp)	0.0	0.0	0	15	90

*Tobacco company, corporate subsidiary, or parent.

	Tot. Fat (g)	Sat. Fat (g)	Chol. (mg)	Sod. (mg)	Cal.
FRUIT POPS *(cont'd)*					
Orange Juice Bars (1 bar)					
Just Pik't (The Fresh Juice Company)	0.0	0.0	0	5	60
Other Fruit Pops					
Chunky Cantaloupe Frozen Fruit Bar (1 bar)					
Frozfruit (Frozfruit Corp)	0.0	0.0	0	5	60
Chunky Pineapple Frozen Fruit Bar (1 bar)					
Frozfruit (Frozfruit Corp)	0.0	0.0	0	0	80
Chunky Raspberry Frozen Fruit Bar (1 bar)					
Frozfruit (Frozfruit Corp)	0.0	0.0	0	5	80
Chunky Strawberry Frozen Fruit Bar (1 bar)					
Frozfruit (Frozfruit Corp)	0.0	0.0	0	20	80
Chunky Watermelon Frozen Fruit Bar (1 bar)					
Frozfruit (Frozfruit Corp)	0.0	0.0	0	0	50
No Sugar Added Citrus Lites (1 bar)					
Wells' Blue Bunny Sweet Freedom (Wells' Dairy)	0.0	0.0	0	10	20
ICE CREAM/ICE MILK BARS					
Cherry Cream Bar (1 bar)					
Blue Bell (Blue Bell Creameries)	2.0	1.0	10	20	110
Orange Cream Bar (1 bar)					
Blue Bell (Blue Bell Creameries)	2.0	1.0	10	25	100
Orange Vanilla Treat Bar (1 bar)					
Weight Watchers (H.J. Heinz)	1.0	0.5	1	80	70
YOGURT BARS/POPS					
Fruit Yogurt Bars/Pops					
Berries'n Creme Mousse Bar (3.5 fl oz)					
Weight Watchers (H.J. Heinz)	1.5	0.0	0	75	70
Frozen Nonfat Yogurt and Fruit Snacks Strawberry, Peach, and Burgundy Cherry Flavors (2 bars)					
Wells' Blue Bunny (Wells' Dairy)	0.0	0.0	0	50	90

	Tot. Fat (g)	Sat. Fat (g)	Chol. (mg)	Sod. (mg)	Cal.
Peach Fat-Free Frozen Fruit and Yogurt Bars (1 bar) Frozfruit (Frozfruit Corp)	0.0	0.0	0	95	100
Strawberry Banana Fat-Free Frozen Fruit and Yogurt Bars (1 bar) Frozfruit (Frozfruit Corp)	0.0	0.0	0	85	100
Strawberry Fat-Free Frozen Fruit and Yogurt Bars (1 bar) Frozfruit (Frozfruit Corp)	0.0	0.0	0	85	100
Other Bars/Pops					
Big Red (1 bar) Blue Bell (Blue Bell Creameries)	0.0	0.0	0	5	90
Big Shot (1 bar) Blue Bell (Blue Bell Creameries)	0.0	0.0	0	15	140
Box Tube Freeze Pops (1.5-oz stick) Delicious (Delicious Cookie Co)	0.0	0.0	0	0	30
Box Tube Freeze Pops (5-oz stick) Delicious (Delicious Cookie Co)	0.0	0.0	0	15	110
Buried Treasure (1 bar) Blue Bell (Blue Bell Creameries)	0.0	0.0	0	10	110
Flintstone Pushup (1 bar) Blue Bell (Blue Bell Creameries)	1.0	1.0	5	20	90
Frostbite (1 bar) Blue Bell (Blue Bell Creameries)	0.0	0.0	0	10	80
Giant Tube Freeze Pop (1 stick) Delicious (Delicious Cookie Co)	0.0	0.0	0	20	150
Rainbow Freeze (1 bar) Blue Bell (Blue Bell Creameries)	0.0	0.0	0	10	110
Rainbow Fruiti Freeze (1 bar) Blue Bell (Blue Bell Creameries)	0.0	0.0	0	10	120
Snow Cone (1 cone) Blue Bell (Blue Bell Creameries)	0.0	0.0	0	5	70
Sugar Free Freezer Bars (3 1-oz bars or 2 1.5-oz bars) Mr. Freeze (Kraft General Foods)*	0.0	0.0	0	45	20
Tropical Freezer Bars (3 1-oz bars or 2 1.5-oz bars) Mr. Freeze (Kraft General Foods)*	0.0	0.0	0	20	50

*Tobacco company, corporate subsidiary, or parent.

	Tot. Fat (g)	Sat. Fat (g)	Chol. (mg)	Sod. (mg)	Cal.
YOGURT BARS/POPS *(cont'd)*					
Twin Pop (1 bar)					
Blue Bell (Blue Bell Creameries)	0.0	0.0	0	5	80
FROZEN YOGURTS					
LOW-FAT FROZEN YOGURTS—*see also* NONFAT FROZEN YOGURTS, page 208					
Blueberry Low-Fat Frozen Yogurts					
Blueberry Cheesecake Low-Fat Frozen Yogurt (½ cup)					
Ben & Jerry's	2.0	1.5	10	90	150
Blueberry Low-Fat Frozen Yogurt (½ cup)					
Ben & Jerry's	2.0	1.0	10	60	160
Caramel Low-Fat Frozen Yogurts					
Caramel Fudge Sundae Low Fat Frozen Yogurt (½ cup)					
Colombo Shoppe Style (Colombo)	1.5	1.0	10	80	140
Cherry Low-Fat Frozen Yogurts					
Cherry Chocolate Cherry Hard Frozen Yogurt with Aspartame (½ cup)					
Dannon Pure Indulgence (The Dannon Company)	3.0	1.0	15	85	150
Cherry Garcia Low-Fat Frozen Yogurt (½ cup)					
Ben & Jerry's	3.0	2.0	10	70	170
Lowfat No Sugar Added Burgundy Cherry Frozen Yogurt (½ cup)					
Wells' Blue Bunny Sweet Freedom (Wells' Dairy)	1.5	1.0	10	50	70
Chocolate Low-Fat Frozen Yogurts—*see also* Cherry Low-Fat Frozen Yogurts, above					
Chocolate Frozen Yogurt (½ cup)					
Dreyer's (Dreyer's Grand Ice Cream)	3.0	1.5	10	30	100
Edy's (Edy's Grand Ice Cream)	3.0	1.5	10	30	100

	Tot. Fat (g)	Sat. Fat (g)	Chol. (mg)	Sod. (mg)	Cal.
Double Chocolate Chunk Lowfat Frozen Yogurt (½ cup)					
Blue Bell (Blue Bell Creameries)	3.0	2.0	5	75	130
Lowfat No Sugar Added Chocolate Frozen Yogurt (½ cup)					
Wells' Blue Bunny Sweet Freedom (Wells' Dairy)	1.5	1.0	10	65	80
Old World Chocolate Low Fat Frozen Yogurt (½ cup)					
Colombo Shoppe Style (Colombo)	2.0	1.0	10	75	130
Chocolate Swirl Low-Fat Frozen Yogurts—*see also* Vanilla Swirl Low-Fat Frozen Yogurts, page 207					
Chocolate Peanut Butter Twist Low Fat Frozen Yogurt (½ cup)					
Colombo Shoppe Style (Colombo)	3.0	1.0	5	65	140
Chocolate Raspberry Swirl Low-Fat Frozen Yogurt (½ cup)					
Ben & Jerry's	2.5	1.5	5	75	200
Marble Fudge Frozen Yogurt (½ cup)					
Dreyer's (Dreyer's Grand Ice Cream)	3.0	1.5	10	35	110
Edy's (Edy's Grand Ice Cream)	3.0	1.5	10	35	110
Cookies and Cream Low-Fat Frozen Yogurts					
Cookies N Cream Lowfat Frozen Yogurt (½ cup)					
Blue Bell (Blue Bell Creameries)	3.0	2.0	5	80	130
Mixed Fruit Low-Fat Frozen Yogurts					
Banana Strawberry Low-Fat Frozen Yogurt (½ cup)					
Ben & Jerry's	2.0	1.0	5	60	160
Citrus Heights Frozen Yogurt (½ cup)					
Dreyer's (Dreyer's Grand Ice Cream)	2.5	1.5	10	25	80
Edy's (Edy's Grand Ice Cream)	2.5	1.5	10	25	80

	Tot. Fat (g)	Sat. Fat (g)	Chol. (mg)	Sod. (mg)	Cal.
Low-Fat Frozen Yogurts *(cont'd)*					
Raspberry Peach Melba Low Fat Frozen Yogurt (½ cup) Colombo Shoppe Style (Colombo)	2.0	1.0	5	60	130
Orange Low-Fat Frozen Yogurts—*see* Vanilla Swirl Low-Fat Frozen Yogurts, page 207					
Peach Low-Fat Frozen Yogurts—*see also* Mixed Fruit Low-Fat Frozen Yogurts, page 205					
Lowfat No Sugar Added Peach Frozen Yogurt (½ cup) Wells' Blue Bunny Sweet Freedom (Wells' Dairy)	1.5	1.0	10	50	70
Perfectly Peach Frozen Yogurt (½ cup)					
Dreyer's (Dreyer's Grand Ice Cream)	2.5	1.5	10	25	100
Edy's (Edy's Grand Ice Cream)	2.5	1.5	10	25	100
Raspberry Low-Fat Frozen Yogurts—*see also* Chocolate Swirl Low-Fat Frozen Yogurts; Mixed Fruit Low-Fat Frozen Yogurts; Vanilla Swirl Low-Fat Frozen Yogurts, pages 205 and 207					
Raspberry Frozen Yogurt (½ cup)					
Dreyer's (Dreyer's Grand Ice Cream)	2.5	1.5	10	25	100
Edy's (Edy's Grand Ice Cream)	2.5	1.5	10	25	100
Strawberry Low-Fat Frozen Yogurts					
Lowfat No Sugar Added Strawberry Frozen Yogurt (½ cup) Wells' Blue Bunny Sweet Freedom (Wells' Dairy)	1.5	1.0	10	50	70
Strawberries 'N Cream Low Fat Frozen Yogurt (½ cup) Colombo Shoppe Style (Colombo)	2.0	1.0	5	65	130

	Tot. Fat (g)	Sat. Fat (g)	Chol. (mg)	Sod. (mg)	Cal.
Strawberry Cheesecake Low-Fat Frozen Yogurt (½ cup)					
Blue Bell (Blue Bell Creameries) .	2.0	1.0	5	135	120
Strawberry Frozen Yogurt (½ cup)					
Edy's (Edy's Grand Ice Cream) .	2.5	1.5	10	25	100
Vanilla Low-Fat Frozen Yogurts					
Lowfat No Sugar Added Vanilla Frozen Yogurt (½ cup)					
Wells' Blue Bunny Sweet Freedom (Wells' Dairy)	1.5	1.0	10	60	70
Simply Vanilla Low Fat Frozen Yogurt (½ cup)					
Colombo Shoppe Style (Colombo)	1.5	1.0	10	65	120
Vanilla Frozen Yogurt (½ cup)					
Dreyer's (Dreyer's Grand Ice Cream)	2.5	1.5	10	30	100
Edy's (Edy's Grand Ice Cream) .	2.5	1.5	10	30	100
Vanilla Hard Frozen Yogurt with Aspartame (½ cup)					
Dannon Pure Indulgence (The Dannon Company)	2.0	1.0	20	85	130
Vanilla Low-Fat Frozen Yogurt (½ cup)					
Blue Bell (Blue Bell Creameries) .	2.0	1.0	5	70	120
Vanilla Swirl Low-Fat Frozen Yogurts					
Boysenberry Vanilla Swirl Frozen Yogurt (½ cup)					
Dreyer's (Dreyer's Grand Ice Cream)	2.5	1.5	10	30	100
Orange Tango Frozen Yogurt & Sorbet (½ cup)					
Häagen-Dazs (Grand Metropolitan PLC)	1.0	0.5	20	25	130
Orange Vanilla Swirl Frozen Yogurt (½ cup)					
Dreyer's (Dreyer's Grand Ice Cream)	2.5	1.5	10	30	100
Edy's (Edy's Grand Ice Cream) .	2.5	1.5	10	30	100

	Tot. Fat (g)	Sat. Fat (g)	Chol. (mg)	Sod. (mg)	Cal.
LOW-FAT FROZEN YOGURTS *(cont'd)*					
Raspberry Rendezvous Frozen Yogurt & Sorbet (½ cup)					
Häagen-Dazs (Grand Metropolitan PLC)	1.5	0.5	20	25	130
Raspberry Vanilla Swirl Frozen Yogurt (½ cup)					
Dreyer's (Dreyer's Grand Ice Cream)	2.5	1.5	10	30	100
Edy's (Edy's Grand Ice Cream) .	2.5	1.5	10	30	100
Vanilla Chocolate Twist Low-Fat Frozen Yogurt (½ cup)					
Blue Bell (Blue Bell Creameries) .	2.0	1.0	5	65	120
Colombo Shoppe Style (Colombo)	1.5	1.0	10	70	120
Other Low-Fat Frozen Yogurts					
Apple Pie Low-Fat Frozen Yogurt (½ cup)					
Ben & Jerry's	3.0	2.0	10	85	170
Banana Split Low Fat Frozen Yogurt (½ cup)					
Colombo Shoppe Style (Colombo)	1.5	1.0	5	60	140
Pecan Pralines N Cream Low-Fat Frozen Yogurt (½ cup)					
Blue Bell (Blue Bell Creameries) .	2.0	1.0	10	80	140
NONFAT FROZEN YOGURTS—*see also* LOW-FAT FROZEN YOGURTS, page 204					
Banana Nonfat Frozen Yogurts—*see also* Mixed Fruit Nonfat Frozen Yogurts, page 210					
Banana Split Nonfat Frozen Yogurt (½ cup)					
Blue Bell (Blue Bell Creameries) .	0.0	0.0	0	55	110
Cappuccino/Coffee Nonfat Frozen Yogurts					
Cappuccino Frozen Yogurt (½ cup)					
Colombo Slender Scoops (Colombo)	0.0	0.0	0	75	80

	Tot. Fat (g)	Sat. Fat (g)	Chol. (mg)	Sod. (mg)	Cal.
Cappuccino Nonfat Hard Frozen Yogurt with Aspartame (½ cup)					
Dannon Light (The Dannon Company)	0.0	0.0	0	70	80
Cherry Nonfat Frozen Yogurts—*see also* Vanilla Swirl Nonfat Frozen Yogurts, page 213					
Black Cherry Chill Frozen Yogurt (½ cup)					
Colombo Slender Scoops (Colombo)	0.0	0.0	0	65	80
Burgundy Cherry Nonfat Frozen Yogurt (½ cup)					
Blue Bell (Blue Bell Creameries)	0.0	0.0	0	65	120
Nonfat Black Cherry Frozen Yogurt (½ cup)					
Yarnell's Guilt Free (Yarnell's Ice Cream Company)	0.0	0.0	4	80	80
Nonfat Burgundy Cherry Frozen Yogurt (½ cup)					
Wells' Blue Bunny (Wells' Dairy)	0.0	0.0	<5	55	100
Chocolate Nonfat Frozen Yogurts					
Chocolate Bliss Frozen Yogurt (½ cup)					
Colombo Slender Scoops (Colombo)	0.0	0.0	0	70	80
Chocolate Fat Free Frozen Yogurt (½ cup)					
Dreyer's (Dreyer's Grand Ice Cream)	0.0	0.0	0	60	90
Edy's (Edy's Grand Ice Cream)	0.0	0.0	0	60	90
Chocolate Fudge Fat Free Frozen Yogurt (½ cup)					
Dreyer's (Dreyer's Grand Ice Cream)	0.0	0.0	0	75	100
Edy's (Edy's Grand Ice Cream)	0.0	0.0	0	75	100
Chocolate Nonfat Frozen Yogurt (½ cup)					
Blue Bell (Blue Bell Creameries)	0.0	0.0	0	65	110

	Tot. Fat (g)	Sat. Fat (g)	Chol. (mg)	Sod. (mg)	Cal.
NONFAT FROZEN YOGURTS *(cont'd)*					
Chocolate Nonfat Hard Frozen Yogurt with Aspartame (½ cup) Dannon Light (The Dannon Company)	0.0	0.0	0	60	80
Chocolate Nonfat Soft Frozen Yogurt with Aspartame (½ cup) Dannon Light (The Dannon Company)	0.0	0.0	<5	60	70
Double Fudge Paradise Frozen Yogurt (½ cup) Colombo Slender Scoops (Colombo)	0.0	0.0	0	80	90
Nonfat Chocolate Frozen Yogurt (½ cup) Wells' Blue Bunny (Wells' Dairy)	0.0	0.0	<5	70	100
Nonfat Chocolate Fudge Frozen Yogurt (½ cup) Yarnell's Guilt Free (Yarnell's Ice Cream Company)	0.0	0.0	4	80	80
Chocolate Swirl Nonfat Frozen Yogurts—*see* Vanilla Swirl Nonfat Frozen Yogurts, page 213					
Coffee Nonfat Frozen Yogurts—*see* Cappuccino/Coffee Nonfat Frozen Yogurts, page 208					
Cookies and Cream Nonfat Frozen Yogurts					
Nonfat Cookies N Cream Frozen Yogurt (½ cup) Wells' Blue Bunny (Wells' Dairy)	0.0	0.0	<5	80	100
Mixed Fruit Nonfat Frozen Yogurts					
Banana Strawberry Fat Free Frozen Yogurt (½ cup) Dreyer's (Dreyer's Grand Ice Cream)	0.0	0.0	0	50	80

	Tot. Fat (g)	Sat. Fat (g)	Chol. (mg)	Sod. (mg)	Cal.
Fruit Cocktail Nonfat Frozen Yogurt (½ cup)					
Blue Bell (Blue Bell Creameries)	0.0	0.0	0	60	110
Mixed Berry Nonfat Soft Frozen Yogurt with Aspartame (½ cup)					
Dannon Light (The Dannon Company)	0.0	0.0	<5	60	70
Pine-Orange Paradise Fat Free Frozen Yogurt (½ cup)					
Dreyer's (Dreyer's Grand Ice Cream)	0.0	0.0	0	60	90
Edy's (Edy's Grand Ice Cream)	0.0	0.0	0	60	90
Lemon Nonfat Frozen Yogurts					
Lemon Chiffon Nonfat Hard Frozen Yogurt with Aspartame (½ cup)					
Dannon Light (The Dannon Company)	0.0	0.0	0	65	90
Neapolitan Nonfat Frozen Yogurts					
Nonfat Neapolitan Frozen Yogurt (½ cup)					
Wells' Blue Bunny (Wells' Dairy)	0.0	0.0	<5	65	90
Orange Nonfat Frozen Yogurts—*see* Mixed Fruit Nonfat Frozen Yogurts, page 210					
Peach Nonfat Frozen Yogurts					
Nonfat Peach Frozen Yogurt (½ cup)					
Yarnell's Guilt Free (Yarnell's Ice Cream Company)	0.0	0.0	4	60	70
Wells' Blue Bunny (Wells' Dairy)	0.0	0.0	<5	60	90
Peach Nonfat Hard Frozen Yogurt with Aspartame (½ cup)					
Dannon Light (The Dannon Company)	0.0	0.0	0	60	80
Pineapple Nonfat Frozen Yogurts—*see* Mixed Fruit Nonfat Frozen Yogurts, page 210					

	Tot. Fat (g)	Sat. Fat (g)	Chol. (mg)	Sod. (mg)	Cal.
NONFAT FROZEN YOGURTS *(cont'd)*					
Raspberry Nonfat Frozen Yogurts					
Raspberry Fat Free Frozen Yogurt (½ cup)					
Dreyer's (Dreyer's Grand Ice Cream)	0.0	0.0	0	50	80
Edy's (Edy's Grand Ice Cream)	0.0	0.0	0	50	80
Strawberry Nonfat Frozen Yogurts—*see also* Mixed Fruit Nonfat Frozen Yogurts, page 210					
Nonfat Strawberry Cheesecake Frozen Yogurt (½ cup)					
Wells' Blue Bunny (Wells' Dairy)	0.0	0.0	<5	60	100
Nonfat Strawberry Frozen Yogurt (½ cup)					
Wells' Blue Bunny (Wells' Dairy)	0.0	0.0	<5	55	90
Strawberry Fat Free Frozen Yogurt (½ cup)					
Dreyer's (Dreyer's Grand Ice Cream)	0.0	0.0	0	55	90
Edy's (Edy's Grand Ice Cream)	0.0	0.0	0	55	90
Strawberry Nonfat Frozen Yogurt (½ cup)					
Blue Bell (Blue Bell Creameries)	0.0	0.0	0	55	110
Strawberry Nonfat Hard Frozen Yogurt with Aspartame (½ cup)					
Dannon Light (The Dannon Company)	0.0	0.0	0	65	80
Vanilla Nonfat Frozen Yogurts—*see also* Cherry Nonfat Frozen Yogurts, page 209; Vanilla Swirl Nonfat Frozen Yogurts, page 213					
Nonfat Vanilla Frozen Yogurt (½ cup)					
Wells' Blue Bunny (Wells' Dairy)	0.0	0.0	<5	65	90
Yarnell's Guilt Free (Yarnell's Ice Cream Company)	0.0	0.0	4	60	80

	Tot. Fat (g)	Sat. Fat (g)	Chol. (mg)	Sod. (mg)	Cal.
Vanilla Fat Free Frozen Yogurt (½ cup)					
Dreyer's (Dreyer's Grand Ice Cream)	0.0	0.0	0	65	90
Edy's (Edy's Grand Ice Cream)	0.0	0.0	0	65	90
Vanilla Nonfat Hard Frozen Yogurt with Aspartame (½ cup)					
Dannon Light (The Dannon Company)	0.0	0.0	0	65	80
Vanilla Nonfat Soft Frozen Yogurt with Aspartame (½ cup)					
Dannon Light (The Dannon Company)	0.0	0.0	<5	60	70
Vanilla Silk Frozen Yogurt (½ cup)					
Colombo Slender Scoops (Colombo)	0.0	0.0	0	70	80
Vanilla Swirl Nonfat Frozen Yogurts					
Black Cherry Vanilla Swirl Fat Free Frozen Yogurt (½ cup)					
Dreyer's (Dreyer's Grand Ice Cream)	0.0	0.0	0	65	90
Edy's (Edy's Grand Ice Cream)	0.0	0.0	0	65	90
Cherry Vanilla Swirl Nonfat Hard Frozen Yogurt with Aspartame (½ cup)					
Dannon Light (The Dannon Company)	0.0	0.0	0	65	90
Nonfat Strawberry Swirl Frozen Yogurt (½ cup)					
Yarnell's Guilt Free (Yarnell's Ice Cream Company)	0.0	0.0	4	60	80
Vanilla Chocolate Swirl Fat Free Frozen Yogurt (½ cup)					
Dreyer's (Dreyer's Grand Ice Cream)	0.0	0.0	0	65	90
Edy's (Edy's Grand Ice Cream)	0.0	0.0	0	65	90

	Tot. Fat (g)	Sat. Fat (g)	Chol. (mg)	Sod. (mg)	Cal.
NONFAT FROZEN YOGURTS *(cont'd)*					
Vanilla Fudge Heaven Frozen Yogurt (½ cup)					
Colombo Slender Scoops (Colombo)	0.0	0.0	0	80	90
ICE CREAMS/ICE MILKS					
LOW-FAT ICE CREAMS/ICE MILKS					
Cappuccino/Coffee Low-Fat Ice Creams/Ice Milks					
Cappuccino Chocolate Chunk Ice Cream (½ cup)					
Healthy Choice (ConAgra)	2.0	1.0	10	60	120
Caramel Low-Fat Ice Creams/ Ice Milks					
Malt Caramel Cone Ice Cream (½ cup)					
Healthy Choice (ConAgra)	2.0	1.0	10	60	120
Praline & Caramel Ice Cream (½ cup)					
Healthy Choice (ConAgra)	2.0	0.5	<5	70	130
Cherry Low-Fat Ice Creams/ Ice Milks					
Black Forest Ice Cream (½ cup)					
Healthy Choice (ConAgra)	2.0	1.0	5	50	120
Bordeaux Cherry Chocolate Chip Ice Cream (½ cup)					
Healthy Choice (ConAgra)	2.0	1.5	<5	55	110
Cherry Vanilla Low Fat Ice Cream (½ cup)					
Borden	2.0	1.0	10	40	110
Chocolate Low-Fat Ice Creams/ Ice Milks—*see also* Cappuccino/ Coffee Low-Fat Ice Creams/ Ice Milks, above					
Chocolate Flavored Light Ice Cream (½ cup)					
Borden	3.0	2.0	15	60	110
Chocolate Low Fat Ice Cream (½ cup)					
Borden	2.0	1.0	10	50	110

	Tot. Fat (g)	Sat. Fat (g)	Chol. (mg)	Sod. (mg)	Cal.
Chocolate Revel Light Ice Cream (½ cup)					
Borden	2.0	1.0	10	55	100
Fudge Brownie Ice Cream (½ cup)					
Healthy Choice (ConAgra)	2.0	1.0	5	55	120
Lowfat Chocolate-Malt Milk Shake (1 cup)					
Milky Way (M & M/Mars)	3.0	2.0	10	135	220
Chocolate Swirl Low-Fat Ice Creams/Ice Milks					
Chocolate Marshmallow Swirl Low Fat Ice Cream (½ cup)					
Borden	2.0	1.5	10	50	110
Chocolate Swirl Low Fat Ice Cream (½ cup)					
Borden	2.0	1.0	10	45	110
Double Fudge Swirl Ice Cream (½ cup)					
Healthy Choice (ConAgra)	2.0	1.5	<5	50	120
Coffee Low-Fat Ice Creams/Ice Milks—*see* Cappuccino/Coffee Low-Fat Ice Creams/Ice Milks, page 214					
Cookies and Cream Low-Fat Ice Creams/Ice Milks					
Cookies 'N Cream Ice Cream (½ cup)					
Healthy Choice (ConAgra)	2.0	1.5	<5	90	120
Cookies 'N Cream Low Fat Ice Cream (½ cup)					
Borden	2.0	1.0	5	55	110
Mint Chocolate Chip Low-Fat Ice Creams/Ice Milks					
Mint Chocolate Chip Ice Cream (½ cup)					
Healthy Choice (ConAgra)	2.0	1.0	<5	50	120
Mixed Fruit Low-Fat Ice Creams/Ice Milks					
Orange Pineapple Light Ice Cream (½ cup)					
Borden	2.0	1.0	10	55	90

	Tot. Fat (g)	Sat. Fat (g)	Chol. (mg)	Sod. (mg)	Cal.
LOW-FAT ICE CREAMS/ICE MILKS *(cont'd)*					
Neapolitan Low-Fat Ice Creams/ Ice Milks					
Neapolitan Flavored Light Ice Cream (½ cup)					
Borden	2.0	1.5	10	55	90
Neapolitan Low Fat Ice Cream (½ cup)					
Borden	2.0	1.0	10	40	110
Orange Low-Fat Ice Creams/ Ice Milks—*see also* Mixed Fruit Low-Fat Ice Creams/Ice Milks, page 215					
Orange Sherbet N' Cream Low Fat Ice Cream (½ cup)					
Borden	2.0	1.0	10	35	100
Pineapple Low Fat Ice Creams/ Ice Milks—*see* Mixed Fruit Low-Fat Ice Creams/Ice Milks, page 215					
Rocky Road Low-Fat Ice Creams/Ice Milks					
Rocky Road Ice Cream (½ cup)					
Healthy Choice (ConAgra)	2.0	1.0	<5	60	140
Strawberry Low-Fat Ice Creams/ Ice Milks					
Strawberry Flavored Light Ice Cream (½ cup)					
Borden	1.5	1.0	10	50	80
Strawberry Low Fat Ice Cream (½ cup)					
Borden	2.0	1.0	10	40	100
Strawberry Revel Light Ice Cream (½ cup)					
Borden	2.0	1.5	10	55	90
Vanilla Low-Fat Ice Creams/ Ice Milks					
Vanilla Ice Cream (½ cup)					
Healthy Choice (ConAgra)	2.0	1.5	5	50	100

	Tot. Fat (g)	Sat. Fat (g)	Chol. (mg)	Sod. (mg)	Cal.
Vanilla Light Ice Cream (½ cup)					
Borden	1.5	1.0	10	55	80
Vanilla Low Fat Ice Cream (½ cup)					
Borden	2.0	1.0	10	40	100
Other Low-Fat Ice Creams/ Ice Milks					
Butter Pecan Crunch Ice Cream (½ cup)					
Healthy Choice (ConAgra)	2.0	1.0	<5	60	120
Chocolate Chip Cookie Dough Low Fat Ice Cream (½ cup)					
Borden	2.5	1.5	10	60	120
Peanut Butter Cookie Dough 'N Fudge Ice Cream (½ cup)					
Healthy Choice (ConAgra)	2.0	1.0	<5	60	120
NONFAT ICE CREAMS/ICE MILKS					
Banana Nonfat Ice Creams/ Ice Milks—*see also* Mixed Fruit Nonfat Ice Creams/Ice Milks, page 219					
Nonfat Banana Nut Crunch Ice Cream (½ cup)					
Yarnell's Guilt Free (Yarnell's Ice Cream Company)	0.0	0.0	5	85	80
Blueberry Nonfat Ice Creams/ Ice Milks—*see* Vanilla Swirl Nonfat Ice Creams/Ice Milks, page 221					
Cherry Nonfat Ice Creams/Ice Milks					
Black Cherry Fat Free Ice Cream (½ cup)					
Borden	0.0	0.0	0	45	90
Black Cherry Vanilla Grand Fat Free Ice Cream (½ cup)					
Dreyer's (Dreyer's Grand Ice Cream)	0.0	0.0	0	70	100
Edy's (Edy's Grand Ice Cream)	0.0	0.0	0	70	100

	Tot. Fat (g)	Sat. Fat (g)	Chol. (mg)	Sod. (mg)	Cal.
NONFAT ICE CREAMS/ICE MILKS *(cont'd)*					
Burgundy Cherry Nonfat Ice Cream (½ cup)					
Wells' Blue Bunny (Wells' Dairy)	0.0	0.0	0	60	110
Burgundy Cherry Nonfat No Added Sugar Ice Cream (½ cup)					
Wells' Blue Bunny Health Smart (Wells' Dairy)	0.0	0.0	0	70	70
Chocolate Nonfat Ice Creams/ Ice Milks					
Chocolate Diet Ice Cream (½ cup)					
Blue Bell (Blue Bell Creameries)	0.0	0.0	0	70	100
Chocolate Fat Free Ice Cream (½ cup)					
Borden	0.0	0.0	0	45	90
Chocolate Fudge Grand Fat Free Ice Cream (½ cup)					
Dreyer's (Dreyer's Grand Ice Cream)	0.0	0.0	0	75	100
Edy's (Edy's Grand Ice Cream)	0.0	0.0	0	75	100
Chocolate Nonfat Ice Cream (½ cup)					
Wells' Blue Bunny (Wells' Dairy)	0.0	0.0	<5	75	110
Chocolate Nonfat No Added Sugar Ice Cream (½ cup)					
Wells' Blue Bunny Health Smart (Wells' Dairy)	0.0	0.0	<5	70	70
Nonfat Chocolate Ice Cream (½ cup)					
Yarnell's Guilt Free (Yarnell's Ice Cream Company)	0.0	0.0	5	80	80
Nonfat Triple Chocolate Ice Cream (½ cup)					
Yarnell's Guilt Free (Yarnell's Ice Cream Company)	0.0	0.0	5	90	80
Chocolate Mint Nonfat Ice Creams/Ice Milks					
Mint Fudge Grand Fat Free Ice Cream (½ cup)					
Dreyer's (Dreyer's Grand Ice Cream)	0.0	0.0	0	75	100
Edy's (Edy's Grand Ice Cream)	0.0	0.0	0	75	100

	Tot. Fat (g)	Sat. Fat (g)	Chol. (mg)	Sod. (mg)	Cal.
Nonfat Mint Fudge Ice Cream (½ cup)					
Yarnell's Guilt Free (Yarnell's Ice Cream Company)	0.0	0.0	5	80	80
Chocolate Swirl Nonfat Ice Creams/Ice Milks—*see also* Vanilla Swirl Nonfat Ice Creams/ Ice Milks, page 221					
Marble Fudge Grand Fat Free Ice Cream (½ cup)					
Dreyer's (Dreyer's Grand Ice Cream)	0.0	0.0	0	75	100
Edy's (Edy's Grand Ice Cream)	0.0	0.0	0	75	100
Cookies and Cream Nonfat Ice Creams/Ice Milks					
Cookies & Cream Nonfat Ice Cream (½ cup)					
Wells' Blue Bunny (Wells' Dairy)	0.0	0.0	<5	80	120
Mixed Fruit Nonfat Ice Creams/ Ice Milks					
Banana Berry Diet Ice Cream (½ cup)					
Blue Bell (Blue Bell Creameries)	0.0	0.0	0	60	100
Diet Orange Pineapple Ice Cream (½ cup)					
Blue Bell (Blue Bell Creameries)	0.0	0.0	0	85	100
Neapolitan Nonfat Ice Creams/ Ice Milks					
Neapolitan Diet Ice Cream (½ cup)					
Blue Bell (Blue Bell Creameries)	0.0	0.0	0	75	100
Neapolitan Nonfat Ice Cream (½ cup)					
Wells' Blue Bunny (Wells' Dairy)	0.0	0.0	<5	65	110
Orange Nonfat Ice Creams/ Ice Milks—see Mixed Fruit Nonfat Ice Creams/Ice Milks, above					
Peach Nonfat Ice Creams/ Ice Milks					
Peach Fat Free Ice Cream (½ cup)					
Borden	0.0	0.0	0	45	90

	Tot. Fat (g)	Sat. Fat (g)	Chol. (mg)	Sod. (mg)	Cal.
Nonfat Ice Creams/Ice Milks *(cont'd)*					
Peach Nonfat Ice Cream (½ cup)					
Wells' Blue Bunny (Wells' Dairy)	0.0	0.0	0	55	100
Peach Nonfat No Added Sugar Ice Cream (½ cup)					
Wells' Blue Bunny Health Smart (Wells' Dairy)	0.0	0.0	0	70	70
Pineapple Nonfat Ice Creams/ Ice Milks—*see* Mixed Fruit Nonfat Ice Creams/Ice Milks, page 219					
Raspberry Nonfat Ice Creams/ Ice Milks—*see also* Vanilla Swirl Nonfat Ice Creams/Ice Milks, page 221					
Raspberry Nonfat No Added Sugar Ice Cream (½ cup)					
Wells' Blue Bunny Health Smart (Wells' Dairy)	0.0	0.0	0	70	70
Strawberry Nonfat Ice Creams/ Ice Milks					
Diet Strawberry Ice Cream (½ cup)					
Blue Bell (Blue Bell Creameries)	0.0	0.0	0	80	100
Nonfat Strawberry Ice Cream (½ cup)					
Yarnell's Guilt Free (Yarnell's Ice Cream Company)	0.0	0.0	5	80	80
Strawberry Fat Free Ice Cream (½ cup)					
Borden	0.0	0.0	0	45	80
Strawberry Grand Fat Free Ice Cream (½ cup)					
Dreyer's (Dreyer's Grand Ice Cream)	0.0	0.0	0	55	90
Edy's (Edy's Grand Ice Cream)	0.0	0.0	0	55	90
Strawberry Nonfat Ice Cream (½ cup)					
Wells' Blue Bunny (Wells' Dairy)	0.0	0.0	0	55	110

	Tot. Fat (g)	Sat. Fat (g)	Chol. (mg)	Sod. (mg)	Cal.
Strawberry Nonfat No Added Sugar Ice Cream (½ cup)					
Wells' Blue Bunny Health Smart (Wells' Dairy)	0.0	0.0	0	70	70
Vanilla Nonfat Ice Creams/ Ice Milks—*see also* Chocolate Swirl Nonfat Ice Creams/ Ice Milks, page 219					
Diet Vanilla Bean Ice Cream (½ cup)					
Blue Bell (Blue Bell Creameries)	0.0	0.0	0	85	100
Nonfat Vanilla Brownie Ice Cream (½ cup)					
Yarnell's Guilt Free (Yarnell's Ice Cream Company)	0.0	0.0	5	80	80
Nonfat Vanilla Ice Cream (½ cup)					
Yarnell's Guilt Free (Yarnell's Ice Cream Company)	0.0	0.0	5	70	80
Vanilla Fat Free Ice Cream (½ cup)					
Borden	0.0	0.0	0	45	80
Vanilla Flavored Nonfat Ice Cream (½ cup)					
Wells' Blue Bunny (Wells' Dairy)	0.0	0.0	<5	65	120
Vanilla Flavored Nonfat No Added Sugar Ice Cream (½ cup)					
Wells' Blue Bunny Health Smart (Wells' Dairy)	0.0	0.0	<5	75	80
Vanilla Grand Fat Free Ice Cream (½ cup)					
Dreyer's (Dreyer's Grand Ice Cream)	0.0	0.0	0	65	90
Edy's (Edy's Grand Ice Cream)	0.0	0.0	0	65	90
Vanilla Swirl Nonfat Ice Creams/ Ice Milks					
Nonfat Blueberry Swirl Ice Cream (½ cup)					
Yarnell's Guilt Free (Yarnell's Ice Cream Company)	0.0	0.0	5	80	80

	Tot. Fat (g)	Sat. Fat (g)	Chol. (mg)	Sod. (mg)	Cal.
NONFAT ICE CREAMS/ICE MILKS *(cont'd)*					
Nonfat Vanilla Fudge Ice Cream (½ cup)					
Yarnell's Guilt Free (Yarnell's Ice Cream Company)	0.0	0.0	5	80	80
Raspberry Vanilla Swirl Grand Fat Free Ice Cream (½ cup)					
Dreyer's (Dreyer's Grand Ice Cream)	0.0	0.0	0	35	70
Edy's (Edy's Grand Ice Cream)	0.0	0.0	0	35	70
Vanilla Chocolate Swirl Grand Fat Free Ice Cream (½ cup)					
Dreyer's (Dreyer's Grand Ice Cream)	0.0	0.0	0	45	80
Edy's (Edy's Grand Ice Cream)	0.0	0.0	0	45	80
Other Nonfat Ice Creams/ Ice Milks					
Nonfat Praline Pecan Crunch Ice Cream (½ cup)					
Yarnell's Guilt Free (Yarnell's Ice Cream Company)	0.0	0.0	5	85	80
ICE CREAM CONES					
CAKE CONES					
Assorted Color Cups (1 cup)					
Keebler	0.0	0.0	0	20	15
Cups (1 cone)					
Nabisco Comet (Nabisco Foods)*	0.0	0.0	0	20	20
Ice Creme Cups (1 cup)					
Keebler	0.0	0.0	0	20	15
Jumbo Cake Cup Cone (1 cone)					
Delicious (Delicious Cookie Co)	0.0	0.0	0	25	25
Rainbow Color Cup Cone (1 cone)					
Delicious (Delicious Cookie Co)	0.0	0.0	0	20	20
Vanilla Cake Cup Cone (1 cone)					
Delicious (Delicious Cookie Co)	0.0	0.0	0	20	20
SUGAR CONES					
Chocolate Cones (1 cone)					
Nabisco Oreo (Nabisco Foods)*	1.0	0.0	0	110	50

*Tobacco company, corporate subsidiary, or parent.

	Tot. Fat (g)	Sat. Fat (g)	Chol. (mg)	Sod. (mg)	Cal.
Cinnamon Cones (1 cone)					
Nabisco Teddy Grahams (Nabisco Foods)*	0.5	0.0	0	55	60
Sugar Cones (1 cone)					
Delicious (Delicious Cookie Co)	0.0	0.0	0	5	45
Keebler	0.5	0.0	0	35	50
Nabisco Comet (Nabisco Foods)*	0.0	0.0	0	40	50
Waffle Bowls (1 bowl)					
Keebler	1.0	0.0	0	25	50
Waffle Cones (1 cone)					
Keebler	1.0	0.0	0	25	50
Nabisco Comet (Nabisco Foods)*	0.5	0.0	0	30	70

ICE MILKS—*see* ICE CREAMS/ ICE MILKS, page 214

ICES/SHERBETS/SORBETS

BANANA ICES/SHERBETS/SORBETS—*see* MIXED FRUIT ICES/SHERBETS/ SORBETS, page 224

CHERRY ICES/SHERBETS/SORBETS

	Tot. Fat (g)	Sat. Fat (g)	Chol. (mg)	Sod. (mg)	Cal.
Cherry Italian Ice (3.5 fl oz)					
Mazzone's (Mazzone Enterprises)	0.0	0.0	0	0	70
Original Cherry Italian Ices (4 fl oz)					
Mama Tish's (Mama Tish's Italian Specialties)	0.0	0.0	0	0	100

LEMON ICES/SHERBETS/SORBETS—*see also* MIXED FRUIT ICES/ SHERBETS/SORBETS, page 224

	Tot. Fat (g)	Sat. Fat (g)	Chol. (mg)	Sod. (mg)	Cal.
Lemon Italian Ice (3.5 fl oz)					
Mazzone's (Mazzone Enterprises)	0.0	0.0	0	0	60
Lemon Sorbetto Molle Soft Italian Sorbet (4 fl oz)					
Mazzone's (Mazzone Enterprises)	0.0	0.0	0	10	113

*Tobacco company, corporate subsidiary, or parent.

	Tot. Fat (g)	Sat. Fat (g)	Chol. (mg)	Sod. (mg)	Cal.
LEMON ICES/SHERBETS/SORBETS *(cont'd)*					
No Sugar Added Lemon Italian Ices (4 fl oz)					
Mama Tish's (Mama Tish's Italian Specialties)	0.0	0.0	0	5	50
Original Lemon Italian Ices (4 fl oz)					
Mama Tish's (Mama Tish's Italian Specialties)	0.0	0.0	0	5	100
Zesty Lemon Sorbet (½ cup)					
Häagen-Dazs (Grand Metropolitan PLC)	0.0	0.0	0	5	120
LIME ICES/SHERBETS/SORBETS—see *also* MIXED FRUIT ICES/SHERBETS/SORBETS, below					
Lime Italian Ice (3.5 fl oz)					
Mazzone's (Mazzone Enterprises)	0.0	0.0	0	0	60
Lime Sherbet (½ cup)					
Blue Bell (Blue Bell Creameries)	1.0	1.0	5	30	130
Wells' Blue Bunny (Wells' Dairy)	1.0	0.5	<5	35	110
MIXED FRUIT ICES/SHERBETS/SORBETS					
Original Lemon-Lime Italian Ices (4 fl oz)					
Mama Tish's (Mama Tish's Italian Specialties)	0.0	0.0	0	0	90
Original Pineapple-Banana-Orange Italian Ices (4 fl oz)					
Mama Tish's (Mama Tish's Italian Specialties)	0.0	0.0	0	0	90
Original Tropical Italian Ices (4 fl oz)					
Mama Tish's (Mama Tish's Italian Specialties)	0.0	0.0	0	0	90
Piña Colada Sherbet (½ cup)					
Wells' Blue Bunny (Wells' Dairy)	1.5	0.5	<5	35	120
Rainbow Italian Ice (3.5 fl oz)					
Mazzone's (Mazzone Enterprises)	0.0	0.0	0	0	60
Rainbow Sherbet (½ cup)					
Blue Bell (Blue Bell Creameries)	1.0	1.0	5	30	130
Wells' Blue Bunny (Wells' Dairy)	1.0	0.5	<5	35	110

	Tot. Fat (g)	Sat. Fat (g)	Chol. (mg)	Sod. (mg)	Cal.
Tropical Fruit Sherbet (½ cup)					
Blue Bell (Blue Bell Creameries) .	1.0	1.0	5	25	120
Tropical Neapolitan Cooler Sherbet (½ cup)					
Wells' Blue Bunny (Wells' Dairy) .	1.0	0.5	<5	35	120
ORANGE ICES/SHERBETS/SORBETS—*see also* ICE CREAMS/ICE MILKS, Orange Low-Fat Ice Creams/Ice Milks, page 216; MIXED FRUIT ICES/SHERBETS/SORBETS, PAGE 224					
Fuzzy Navel Sherbet (½ cup)					
Wells' Blue Bunny (Wells' Dairy) .	1.0	0.5	<5	35	130
Ol' Fashion Premium Orange Sherbet (½ cup)					
Wells' Blue Bunny (Wells' Dairy) .	1.0	0.5	<5	35	110
Orange Italian Ice (3.5 fl oz)					
Mazzone's (Mazzone Enterprises)	0.0	0.0	0	0	60
Orange Sherbet (½ cup)					
Blue Bell (Blue Bell Creameries) .	1.0	1.0	5	30	130
Wells' Blue Bunny (Wells' Dairy) .	1.0	0.5	<5	35	110
PINEAPPLE ICES/SHERBETS/SORBETS—*see also* MIXED FRUIT ICES/SHERBETS/SORBETS, page 224					
Original Pineapple-Coconut Italian Ices (4 fl oz)					
Mama Tish's (Mama Tish's Italian Specialties)	0.0	0.0	0	0	90
Pineapple Sherbet (½ cup)					
Blue Bell (Blue Bell Creameries) .	1.0	1.0	5	30	120
Wells' Blue Bunny (Wells' Dairy) .	1.0	0.5	<5	35	110
RASPBERRY ICES/SHERBETS/SORBETS					
Ol' Fashion Premium Raspberry Sherbet (½ cup)					
Wells' Blue Bunny (Wells' Dairy) .	1.0	0.5	<5	35	110
Original Raspberry Italian Ices (4 fl oz)					
Mama Tish's (Mama Tish's Italian Specialties)	0.0	0.0	0	5	100
Raspberry Sherbet (½ cup)					
Wells' Blue Bunny (Wells' Dairy) .	1.0	0.5	<5	35	110

	Tot. Fat (g)	Sat. Fat (g)	Chol. (mg)	Sod. (mg)	Cal.
RASPBERRY ICES/SHERBETS/SORBETS *(cont'd)*					
Raspberry Sorbet (½ cup)					
Häagen-Dazs (Grand Metropolitan PLC)	0.0	0.0	0	0	120
Raspberry Sorbetto Molle Soft Italian Sorbet (4 fl oz)					
Mazzone's (Mazzone Enterprises)	0.0	0.0	0	5	83
STRAWBERRY ICES/SHERBETS/SORBETS					
No Sugar Added Strawberry Italian Ices (4 fl oz)					
Mama Tish's (Mama Tish's Italian Specialties)	0.0	0.0	0	10	40
Original Strawberry Italian Ices (4 fl oz)					
Mama Tish's (Mama Tish's Italian Specialties)	0.0	0.0	0	5	80
Strawberry Colada Sherbet (½ cup)					
Wells' Blue Bunny (Wells' Dairy)	1.0	0.5	<5	35	130
Strawberry Margarita Sherbet (½ cup)					
Wells' Blue Bunny (Wells' Dairy)	1.0	0.5	<5	35	130
Strawberry Sherbet (½ cup)					
Blue Bell (Blue Bell Creameries)	1.0	1.0	5	25	120
Wells' Blue Bunny (Wells' Dairy)	1.0	0.5	<5	35	110
Strawberry Sorbet (½ cup)					
Häagen-Dazs (Grand Metropolitan PLC)	0.0	0.0	0	0	130
Strawberry Sorbetto Molle Soft Italian Sorbet (4 fl oz)					
Mazzone's (Mazzone Enterprises)	0.0	0.0	0	15	116
WATERMELON ICES/SHERBETS/SORBETS					
Watermelon Italian Ice (3.5 fl oz)					
Mazzone's (Mazzone Enterprises)	0.0	0.0	0	0	60

	Tot. Fat (g)	Sat. Fat (g)	Chol. (mg)	Sod. (mg)	Cal.
Other Ices/Sherbets/Sorbets					
Mango Sorbet (½ cup)					
Häagen-Dazs (Grand Metropolitan PLC)	0.0	0.0	0	0	120
Original Chocolate Italian Ices (4 fl oz)					
Mama Tish's (Mama Tish's Italian Specialties)	0.0	0.0	0	125	100
Passion Fruit Sorbetto Molle Soft Italian Sorbet (4 fl oz)					
Mazzone's (Mazzone Enterprises)	0.0	0.0	0	5	101
Wildberry Crumble Sherbet (½ cup)					
Wells' Blue Bunny (Wells' Dairy)	1.5	0.5	<5	50	140
NONDAIRY FROZEN DESSERTS					
Black Leopard Nonfat Non-Dairy Frozen Dessert (½ cup)					
Sweet Nothings (Turtle Mountain)	0.0	0.0	0	5	100
Chocolate Mandarin Nonfat Non-Dairy Frozen Dessert (½ cup)					
Sweet Nothings (Turtle Mountain)	0.0	0.0	0	5	100
Chocolate Nonfat Non-Dairy Frozen Dessert (½ cup)					
Sweet Nothings (Turtle Mountain)	0.0	0.0	0	5	100
Espresso Fudge Nonfat Non-Dairy Frozen Dessert (½ cup)					
Sweet Nothings (Turtle Mountain)	0.0	0.0	0	5	110
Mango Raspberry Nonfat Non-Dairy Frozen Dessert (½ cup)					
Sweet Nothings (Turtle Mountain)	0.0	0.0	0	5	100
Raspberry Swirl Nonfat Non-Dairy Frozen Dessert (½ cup)					
Sweet Nothings (Turtle Mountain)	0.0	0.0	0	5	100

	Tot. Fat (g)	Sat. Fat (g)	Chol. (mg)	Sod. (mg)	Cal.
NONDAIRY FROZEN DESSERTS *(cont'd)*					
Tiger Stripes Nonfat Non-Dairy Frozen Dessert (½ cup)					
Sweet Nothings (Turtle Mountain)	0.0	0.0	0	5	110
Vanilla Nonfat Non-Dairy Frozen Dessert (½ cup)					
Sweet Nothings (Turtle Mountain)	0.0	0.0	0	5	110
Very Berry Blueberry Nonfat Non-Dairy Frozen Dessert (½ cup)					
Sweet Nothings (Turtle Mountain)	0.0	0.0	0	5	100

POPS—*see* BARS/POPS, page 201

SHERBETS—*see* ICES/ SHERBETS/SORBETS, page 223

SORBETS—*see* ICES/ SHERBETS/SORBETS, page 223

FRUITS

You'll go bananas over this chapter! That's because fruits are naturally low in fat, saturated fat, and cholesterol. From apples to watermelons, all fruits (except avocados, coconuts, and olives) meet AHA criteria for food nutrients.

You won't find name brand fresh fruits in this chapter. Instead, we list the fruits themselves. Fruits are low in fat and packed with vitamins and minerals. The three exceptions mentioned above contain fat. They're listed in the "Fats and Oils" chapter on page 188. Fruit-based snacks are listed in the "Snack Foods" chapter, page 340.

Although the sodium content of fruits is low, the amounts vary. The AHA does not have criteria for sodium but recommends a total of no more than 3,000 mg a day.

Following are the AHA criteria for fruits. You can use the table to evaluate any all-fruit product.

AHA Criteria for Fruits*

	Tot. Fat (g)	Sat. Fat (g)	Chol. (mg)
All fruit (except avocados, coconuts, olives, and those listed below)	3	<0.5	<2
Fruit used as ingredients, such as cranberries, lemons, and limes	<0.5	<0.5	<2

*Per serving.

	Tot. Fat (g)	Sat. Fat (g)	Chol. (mg)	Sod. (mg)	Cal.
APPLES					
DRIED					
Apples (½ cup)					
Most brands (USDA)	**0.1**	**0.0**	**0**	**38**	**105**
FRESH					
Apple (2¾" diam)	0.5	0.1	0	1	81
FROZEN					
Homestyle Cinnamon Scalloped Apples (½ cup)					
Campbell's Kitchen (Campbell Soup Co)	2.0	1.0	0	80	110
APPLESAUCE					
Applesauce, sweetened or cinnamon (½ cup)					
Most brands (USDA)	**0.2**	**0.0**	**0**	**4**	**97**
Applesauce, unsweetened (½ cup)					
Most brands (USDA)	**0.1**	**0.0**	**0**	**2**	**53**
Old Fashioned Unsweetened Apple Sauce (½ cup)					
America's Choice (A & P)	0.0	0.0	0	30	50
Original Apple Sauce (½ cup)					
America's Choice (A & P)	0.0	0.0	0	30	90
APRICOTS					
CANNED					
Apricots in heavy syrup (½ cup halves)					
Most brands (USDA)	**0.0**	**0.0**	**0**	**5**	**107**
Apricots in juice (½ cup halves)					
Most brands (USDA)	**0.0**	**0.0**	**0**	**5**	**60**
Apricots in light syrup (½ cup halves)					
Most brands (USDA)	**0.0**	**0.0**	**0**	**3**	**61**
Apricots in water (½ cup halves)					
Most brands (USDA)	**0.2**	**0.0**	**0**	**4**	**33**
Del Monte	0.0	0.0	0	10	40
Lite Apricot Halves in Extra Lite Syrup (½ cup)					
Del Monte	0.0	0.0	0	10	60

	Tot. Fat (g)	Sat. Fat (g)	Chol. (mg)	Sod. (mg)	Cal.
DRIED					
Apricots (10 halves)					
Most brands (USDA)	**0.2**	**0.0**	**0**	**3**	**83**
FRESH					
Apricots (4)	0.6	0.0	0	1	68
BANANAS					
FRESH					
Banana (8¾″ long)	0.6	0.2	0	1	105
BLACKBERRIES					
CANNED					
Blackberries in heavy syrup (½ cup)					
Most brands (USDA)	**0.1**	**0.0**	**0**	**3**	**118**
FRESH					
Blackberries, unsweetened (1 cup)	0.6	0.0	0	0	74
FROZEN					
Blackberries, unsweetened (1 cup)					
Most brands (USDA)	**0.7**	**0.0**	**0**	**2**	**97**
BLUEBERRIES					
CANNED					
Blueberries in heavy syrup (½ cup)					
Most brands (USDA)	**0.4**	**0.0**	**0**	**4**	**112**
FRESH					
Blueberries (1 cup)	0.6	0.0	0	9	82
FROZEN					
Blueberries, unsweetened (1 cup)					
Most brands (USDA)	**1.0**	**0.0**	**0**	**1**	**78**
BOYSENBERRIES					
CANNED					
Boysenberries in heavy syrup (½ cup)					
Most brands (USDA)	**0.2**	**0.0**	**0**	**4**	**113**
FROZEN					
Boysenberries, unsweetened (1 cup)					
Most brands (USDA)	**0.4**	**0.0**	**0**	**2**	**66**

	Tot. Fat (g)	Sat. Fat (g)	Chol. (mg)	Sod. (mg)	Cal.
CHERRIES					
CANNED					
Cherries, sweet, in heavy syrup (½ cup)					
Most brands (USDA)	**0.2**	**0.0**	**0**	**3**	**107**
Cherries, sweet, in juice (½ cup)					
Most brands (USDA)	**0.0**	**0.0**	**0**	**3**	**68**
Cherries, sweet, in light syrup (½ cup)					
Most brands (USDA)	**0.2**	**0.0**	**0**	**3**	**85**
Cherries, sweet, in water (½ cup)					
Most brands (USDA)	**0.2**	**0.0**	**0**	**2**	**57**
Dark Sweet Cherries, pitted (½ cup)					
Del Monte	0.0	0.0	0	10	100
Dark Sweet Cherries, whole (½ cup)					
Del Monte	0.0	0.0	0	10	90
Maraschino Cherries (1 cherry)					
America's Choice (A & P)	0.0	0.0	0	0	10
FRESH					
Cherries (1 cup)	1.4	0.3	0	0	104
CRABAPPLES					
FRESH					
Crabapple, sliced (1 cup)	0.3	0.1	0	1	83
CRANBERRIES					
CANNED					
Cranberry sauce, sweetened (½ cup)					
Most brands (USDA)	**0.2**	**0.0**	**0**	**40**	**209**
Jellied Cranberry Sauce (2¾ oz)					
Ocean Spray (Ocean Spray Cranberries)	0.0	0.0	0	5	110
Whole Berry Cranberry Sauce (2¾ oz)					
Ocean Spray (Ocean Spray Cranberries)	0.0	0.0	0	8	112
FRESH					
Cranberries, chopped (½ cup)	0.1	0.0	0	1	27

	Tot. Fat (g)	Sat. Fat (g)	Chol. (mg)	Sod. (mg)	Cal.
CURRANTS					
DRIED					
Currants (¼ cup)					
Most brands (USDA)	**0.1**	**0.0**	**0**	**3**	**102**
FRESH					
Currants, red or white (1 cup)	0.2	0.0	0	1	63
DATES					
DRIED					
Dates (5)					
Most brands (USDA)	**0.2**	**0.0**	**0**	**1**	**114**
Pitted Dates (¼ cup)					
Dole (Dole Dried Fruit & Nut)	0.0	0.0	0	10	120
FIGS					
CANNED					
Figs in heavy syrup (½ cup)					
Most brands (USDA)	**0.1**	**0.0**	**0**	**2**	**114**
Figs in light syrup (½ cup)					
Most brands (USDA)	**0.1**	**0.0**	**0**	**2**	**87**
Figs in water (½ cup)					
Most brands (USDA)	**0.1**	**0.0**	**0**	**2**	**65**
DRIED					
Figs (2)					
Most brands (USDA)	**0.4**	**0.1**	**0**	**4**	**95**
FRESH					
Figs (2 large)	0.4	0.0	0	2	94
FRUIT COCKTAIL					
CANNED					
Fruit Cocktail (in extra light syrup) (½ cup)					
Del Monte	0.0	0.0	0	10	60
Fruit Cocktail (in fruit juices from concentrate) (½ cup)					
Del Monte Fruit Naturals (Del Monte)	0.0	0.0	0	10	60
Fruit cocktail in heavy syrup (½ cup)					
Most brands (USDA)	**0.1**	**0.0**	**0**	**7**	**93**

	Tot. Fat (g)	Sat. Fat (g)	Chol. (mg)	Sod. (mg)	Cal.
CANNED *(cont'd)*					
Fruit cocktail in juice (½ cup)					
Most brands (USDA)	**0.0**	**0.0**	**0**	**4**	**56**
Fruit cocktail in light syrup (½ cup)					
Most brands (USDA)	**0.1**	**0.0**	**0**	**7**	**72**
Fruit cocktail in water (½ cup)					
Most brands (USDA)	**0.1**	**0.0**	**0**	**5**	**40**
GOOSEBERRIES					
FRESH					
Gooseberries (1 cup)	0.9	0.1	0	1	67
GRAPEFRUIT					
CANNED					
Grapefruit in juice (½ cup)					
Most brands (USDA)	**0.1**	**0.0**	**0**	**9**	**46**
Grapefruit in light syrup (½ cup)					
Most brands (USDA)	**0.1**	**0.0**	**0**	**2**	**76**
Grapefruit in water (½ cup)					
Most brands (USDA)	**0.1**	**0.0**	**0**	**2**	**44**
FRESH					
Grapefruit (½ of a 3¾″-diam grapefruit)	0.1	0.0	0	0	38
GRAPES					
FRESH					
Grapes (1 cup)	0.3	0.1	0	2	242
GUAVAS					
FRESH					
Guava (1)	0.5	0.2	0	2	45
KIWIFRUIT					
FRESH					
Kiwifruit (2 medium)	0.7	0.0	0	8	92
KUMQUATS					
FRESH					
Kumquats (7)	0.2	0.0	0	7	84

	Tot. Fat (g)	Sat. Fat (g)	Chol. (mg)	Sod. (mg)	Cal.
LEMONS					
FRESH					
Lemon (1 medium)	0.2	0.0	0	1	17
LIMES					
FRESH					
Lime (1)	0.1	0.0	0	1	20
LOGANBERRIES					
FRESH					
Loganberries (1 cup)	0.5	0.0	0	1	80
LOQUATS					
FRESH					
Loquats (9)	0.2	0.0	0	0	45
LYCHEES					
CANNED					
Lychees (in syrup, whole pitted) (15 pieces)					
Ka-me (Shaffer, Clarke & Co)	0.0	0.0	0	26	130
FRESH					
Lychees (9)	0.4	0.0	0	0	54
MANDARIN ORANGES					
CANNED					
Mandarin Oranges in Light Syrup (½ cup)					
Del Monte	0.0	0.0	0	10	80
MANGOS					
CANNED					
Mango (4 pieces)					
Ka-me (Shaffer, Clarke & Co)	0.0	0.0	0	10	102
FRESH					
Mango (½)	0.3	0.1	0	2	68
MELONS					
FRESH					
Cantaloupe, cubes (1 cup)	0.4	0.0	0	14	57
Casaba melon, cubes (1 cup)	0.1	0.0	0	20	45
Honeydew melon, cubes (1 cup)	0.2	0.0	0	17	60

	Tot. Fat (g)	Sat. Fat (g)	Chol. (mg)	Sod. (mg)	Cal.
FROZEN					
Melon balls (1 cup)					
Most brands (USDA)	**0.4**	**0.0**	**0**	**53**	**55**
MIXED FRUITS					
CANNED					
Chunky Mixed Fruit in Fruit Juices from Concentrate (½ cup)					
Del Monte Fruit Naturals (Del Monte)	0.0	0.0	0	10	60
Lite Chunky Mixed Fruit in Extra Light Syrup (½ cup)					
Del Monte	0.0	0.0	0	10	60
Lite Mixed Fruits in Extra Light Syrup (4½-oz can)					
Del Monte	0.0	0.0	0	10	60
Mixed Fruit in Heavy Syrup (1 fruit cup)					
America's Choice (A & P)	0.0	0.0	0	10	100
Mixed Fruits in Juice					
America's Choice Fruit Naturals (A & P) (1 fruit cup)	0.0	0.0	0	10	60
Del Monte Fruit Naturals (Del Monte) (4½-oz can)	0.0	0.0	0	10	60
Tropical Fruit Salad in Light Syrup with Passion Fruit Juice (½ cup)					
Del Monte	0.0	0.0	0	10	80
DRIED					
Mixed Dried Fruit (⅓ cup)					
Del Monte	0.0	0.0	0	50	110
MULBERRIES					
FRESH					
Mulberries (1 cup)	0.6	0.0	0	14	61
NECTARINES					
FRESH					
Nectarine (2½″ diam)	0.6	0.0	0	0	67

	Tot. Fat (g)	Sat. Fat (g)	Chol. (mg)	Sod. (mg)	Cal.
ORANGES					
Fresh					
Orange (2⅝" diam)	0.2	0.0	0	0	62
PAPAYAS					
Canned					
Papaya (¾ cup)					
Ka-me (Shaffer, Clarke & Co)	0.0	0.0	0	15	120
Fresh					
Papaya, cubes (1 cup)	0.4	0.1	0	8	54
PASSION FRUIT					
Fresh					
Passion fruit (8)	1.0	0.0	0	40	144
PEACHES					
Canned					
Diced Peaches (in peach juice)					
America's Choice Fruit Naturals (A & P) (1 fruit cup)	0.0	0.0	0	10	60
Del Monte Fruit Naturals (Del Monte) (4½-oz can)	0.0	0.0	0	10	60
Diced Peaches in Heavy Syrup (1 fruit cup)					
America's Choice (A & P)	0.0	0.0	0	10	100
Lite Diced Peaches in Extra Light Syrup (4½-oz can)					
Del Monte	0.0	0.0	0	10	60
Lite Diced Yellow Cling Peaches in Extra Light Syrup (4½-oz can)					
Del Monte	0.0	0.0	0	10	60
Lite Sliced Freestone Peaches in Extra Light Syrup (½ cup)					
Del Monte	0.0	0.0	0	10	60
Peaches in heavy syrup (½ cup)					
Most brands (USDA)	**0.1**	**0.0**	**0**	**8**	**95**
Peaches in juice (½ cup)					
Most brands (USDA)	**0.0**	**0.0**	**0**	**6**	**55**
Peaches in light syrup (½ cup)					
Most brands (USDA)	**0.0**	**0.0**	**0**	**7**	**68**

	Tot. Fat (g)	Sat. Fat (g)	Chol. (mg)	Sod. (mg)	Cal.
CANNED *(cont'd)*					
Peaches in water (½ cup)					
Most brands (USDA)	**0.1**	**0.0**	**0**	**4**	**29**
Sliced Yellow Cling Peaches (in peach juice from concentrate) (½ cup)					
Del Monte Fruit Naturals (Del Monte)	0.0	0.0	0	10	60
Yellow Cling Peaches in Extra Light Syrup (½ cup)					
Del Monte	0.0	0.0	0	10	60
DRIED					
Dried peaches (¼ cup halves)					
Most brands (USDA)	**0.3**	**0.0**	**0**	**3**	**192**
FRESH					
Peach (2½″ diam)	0.1	0.0	0	0	37
FROZEN					
Peaches, sliced, sweetened (½ cup)					
Most brands (USDA)	**0.1**	**0.0**	**0**	**8**	**118**
SPICED					
Spiced peaches in heavy syrup (½ cup)					
Most brands (USDA)	**0.1**	**0.0**	**0**	**5**	**90**
Whole Spiced Peaches (½ cup)					
Del Monte	0.0	0.0	0	10	100
PEARS					
CANNED					
Lite Pears in Extra Light Syrup (½ cup)					
Del Monte	0.0	0.0	0	10	60
Pears in heavy syrup (½ cup halves)					
Most brands (USDA)	**0.1**	**0.0**	**0**	**7**	**94**
Pears in juice (½ cup halves)					
Most brands (USDA)	**0.1**	**0.0**	**0**	**5**	**62**
Pears in light syrup (½ cup halves)					
Most brands (USDA)	**0.0**	**0.0**	**0**	**7**	**72**

	Tot. Fat (g)	Sat. Fat (g)	Chol. (mg)	Sod. (mg)	Cal.
Pears in Pear Juice from Concentrate (½ cup)					
Del Monte Fruit Naturals (Del Monte)	0.0	0.0	0	10	60
Pears in water (½ cup halves)					
Most brands (USDA)	**0.0**	**0.0**	**0**	**2**	**22**
DRIED					
Dried pears (¼ cup halves)					
Most brands (USDA)	**0.3**	**0.0**	**0**	**3**	**118**
FRESH					
Asian pear (2¼″ x 2½″ diam)	0.3	0.0	0	0	51
Pear (2½″ x 3½″ diam)	0.7	0.0	0	1	98
PERSIMMONS					
FRESH					
Japanese persimmon (2½″ x 3½″ diam)	0.3	0.0	0	3	118
Native persimmons (6)	0.6	0.0	0	0	192
PINEAPPLES					
CANNED					
Crushed Pineapple in juice (½ cup)					
Dole (Dole Food Company)	0.0	0.0	0	10	70
Pineapple Chunks in juice (½ cup)					
Dole (Dole Food Company)	0.0	0.0	0	10	60
Pineapple Slices in juice (2 slices)					
Dole (Dole Food Company)	0.0	0.0	0	10	60
Pineapple tidbits in heavy syrup (½ cup)					
Most brands (USDA)	**0.1**	**0.0**	**0**	**2**	**100**
Pineapple Tidbits in juice (½ cup)					
Most brands (USDA)	**0.1**	**0.0**	**0**	**2**	**75**
Dole (Dole Food Company)	0.0	0.0	0	10	60
Pineapple tidbits in light syrup (½ cup)					
Most brands (USDA)	**0.1**	**0.0**	**0**	**2**	**66**
Pineapple tidbits in water (½ cup)					
Most brands (USDA)	**0.1**	**0.0**	**0**	**2**	**40**

	Tot. Fat (g)	Sat. Fat (g)	Chol. (mg)	Sod. (mg)	Cal.
DRIED					
Dried Pineapple (30 pieces)					
Fisher (Procter & Gamble)	0.0	0.0	0	20	140
FRESH					
Pineapple, diced (1 cup)	0.7	0.1	0	1	134
FROZEN					
Pineapple, chunks, sweetened (½ cup)					
Most brands (USDA)	**0.1**	**0.0**	**0**	**2**	**104**
PLANTAINS					
FRESH					
Plantain (1)	0.7	0.0	0	7	218
PLUMS					
CANNED					
Plums in heavy syrup (½ cup)					
Most brands (USDA)	**0.1**	**0.0**	**0**	**25**	**115**
Plums in juice (½ cup)					
Most brands (USDA)	**0.0**	**0.0**	**0**	**1**	**73**
Plums in light syrup (½ cup)					
Most brands (USDA)	**0.1**	**0.0**	**0**	**25**	**79**
Plums in water (½ cup)					
Most brands (USDA)	**0.0**	**0.0**	**0**	**1**	**51**
FRESH					
Plums (2 2⅛″ diam)	0.8	0.1	0	0	72
POMEGRANATES					
FRESH					
Pomegranate (3⅜″ × 3¾″ diam)	0.5	0.0	0	5	104
PRICKLY PEARS					
Prickly pear (1)	0.5	0.0	0	6	42
PRUNES					
CANNED					
Prunes in heavy syrup (½ cup)					
Most brands (USDA)	**0.2**	**0.0**	**0**	**3**	**123**
DRIED					
Pitted Prunes (¼ cup)					
Dole (Dole Dried Fruit & Nut)	0.0	0.0	0	5	110

	Tot. Fat (g)	Sat. Fat (g)	Chol. (mg)	Sod. (mg)	Cal.
Prunes (5)					
Most brands (USDA)	**0.2**	**0.0**	**0**	**2**	**101**
PUMMELO					
Fresh					
Pummelo, sections (¾ cup)	0.1	0.0	0	2	53
QUINCE					
Fresh					
Quince (1)	0.1	0.0	0	4	53
RAISINS					
Golden Raisins (¼ cup)					
Del Monte	0.0	0.0	0	10	130
Raisins (¼ cup)					
Most brands (USDA)	**0.2**	**0.1**	**0**	**5**	**127**
Dole (Dole Dried Fruit & Nut)	0.0	0.0	0	10	130
RASPBERRIES					
Canned					
Raspberries in heavy syrup (½ cup)					
Most brands (USDA)	**0.2**	**0.0**	**0**	**4**	**117**
Fresh					
Raspberries (1 cup)	0.7	0.0	0	0	61
Frozen					
Raspberries, sweetened (½ cup)					
Most brands (USDA)	**0.2**	**0.0**	**0**	**1**	**128**
RHUBARB					
Fresh					
Rhubarb, diced (1 cup)	0.2	0.0	0	5	26
Frozen					
Rhubarb, uncooked (1 cup)					
Most brands (USDA)	**0.2**	**0.0**	**0**	**2**	**29**
STRAWBERRIES					
Canned					
Strawberries in heavy syrup (½ cup)					
Most brands (USDA)	**0.3**	**0.0**	**0**	**5**	**117**

	Tot. Fat (g)	Sat. Fat (g)	Chol. (mg)	Sod. (mg)	Cal.
FRESH					
Strawberries (1 cup)	0.6	0.0	0	2	45
FROZEN					
Strawberries, sweetened (½ cup)					
Most brands (USDA)	**0.0**	**0.0**	**0**	**2**	**100**
Strawberries, unsweetened (1 cup)					
Most brands (USDA)	**0.2**	**0.0**	**0**	**3**	**52**
TAMARINDS					
FRESH					
Tamarind, pulp only (1 cup)	0.7	0.3	0	33	287
TANGERINES					
CANNED					
Tangerines in juice (½ cup)					
Most brands (USDA)	**0.0**	**0.0**	**0**	**7**	**46**
Tangerines in light syrup (½ cup)					
Most brands (USDA)	**0.1**	**0.0**	**0**	**8**	**76**
FRESH					
Tangerine (2⅜″ diam)	0.2	0.0	0	1	37
WATERMELONS					
FRESH					
Watermelon, diced (1¾ cups)	1.2	0.0	0	5	88

GRAVIES AND SAUCES

Who doesn't love slathering hickory-flavored barbecue sauce over chicken on the grill and spooning spicy marinara over pasta?

The sauces and gravies on the following pages are low in total fat, saturated fat, and cholesterol as purchased or when prepared as indicated here.

Like all the other entries in this book, the gravies and sauces entries that follow list sodium content. The AHA does not have criteria for sodium but recommends a total of no more than 3,000 mg a day.

Generic Listings

By far, most of the foods in this book are brand name products. However, if a product is listed without a brand name, it means that most brands of that product contain about the same amount of fat, saturated fat, and cholesterol, and that these amounts are within the criteria cited below.

If you find products that were introduced after this book went to press, use the generic listings and the following tables to help you evaluate them.

AHA Criteria for Gravies and Sauces*

	Tot. Fat (g)	Sat. Fat (g)	Chol. (mg)
All gravies and sauces	3	<0.5	<2

*Per serving.

Sauces You'll Want to Limit

Some sauces, like the examples below, are too high in fat, saturated fat, and/or cholesterol to meet AHA criteria. They aren't included in this book, and we recommend that you don't eat them often.

Compare the amounts of fat, saturated fat, cholesterol, sodium, and calories in these examples with the more healthful alternatives listed on the following pages.

Sample Sauces to Limit

	Tot. Fat (g)	Sat. Fat (g)	Chol. (mg)	Sod. (mg)	Cal.
Bernaise sauce, made from mix with whole milk and butter (¼ cup)	17.1*	10.4*	47*	316	175
Cheese sauce, made from mix with whole milk (¼ cup)	4.3*	2.3*	13*	392	77
White sauce, made from mix with whole milk (¼ cup)	3.4	1.6*	9*	199	60

Adapted from USDA Handbook No. 8 series.

*These values exceed AHA criteria for sauces.

	Tot. Fat (g)	Sat. Fat (g)	Chol. (mg)	Sod. (mg)	Cal.
BARBECUE SAUCES					
Hickory Barbecue Sauces					
Hickory Barbecue Sauce (1 tbsp)					
Hunt's (Hunt-Wesson)	<1.0	0.0	0	160	20
Hickory Flavor BBQ Sauce (2 tbsp)					
Open Pit (Campbell Soup Co)	0.0	0.0	0	380	50
Hickory Smoke Barbecue Sauce (2 tbsp)					
Kraft (Kraft General Foods)*	0.0	0.0	0	440	40
Kraft Thick'N Spicy (Kraft General Foods)*	0.0	0.0	0	440	50
Hickory Smoke Onion Bits Barbecue Sauce (2 tbsp)					
Kraft (Kraft General Foods)*	0.0	0.0	0	340	50
Hickory Smoked Barbecue Sauce (2 tbsp)					
America's Choice (A & P)	0.0	0.0	0	380	45
Thick and Tangy Hickory BBQ Sauce (2 tbsp)					
Open Pit (Campbell Soup Co)	0.0	0.0	0	390	50
Honey Barbecue Sauces					
Dijon & Honey Barbecue Sauce (1 tbsp)					
Lawry's (Lawry's Foods)	1.0	0.0	0	750	60
Honey Barbecue Sauce (2 tbsp)					
Kraft (Kraft General Foods)*	0.0	0.0	0	320	50
Kraft Thick'N Spicy (Kraft General Foods)*	0.0	0.0	0	350	60
Hot Barbecue Sauces					
Hot Barbecue Sauce (2 tbsp)					
America's Choice (A & P)	0.0	0.0	0	380	45
Kraft (Kraft General Foods)*	0.0	0.0	0	540	40
Hot BBQ Sauce (2 tbsp)					
Open Pit (Campbell Soup Co)	0.0	0.0	0	380	50
Hot Hickory Smoke Barbecue Sauce (2 tbsp)					
Kraft (Kraft General Foods)*	0.0	0.0	0	360	40
Salsa Style Barbecue Sauce (2 tbsp)					
Kraft (Kraft General Foods)*	0.0	0.0	0	420	40

*Tobacco company, corporate subsidiary, or parent.

	Tot. Fat (g)	Sat. Fat (g)	Chol. (mg)	Sod. (mg)	Cal.
KANSAS CITY STYLE BARBECUE SAUCES					
Kansas City Style Barbecue Sauce					
Hunt's (Hunt-Wesson) (1 tbsp)	<1.0	0.0	0	85	20
Kraft (Kraft General Foods)* (2 tbsp)	0.0	0.0	0	280	45
Kraft Thick'N Spicy (Kraft General Foods)* (2 tbsp)	0.0	0.0	0	280	60
MESQUITE BARBECUE SAUCES					
Mesquite BBQ Sauce (2 tbsp)					
Open Pit (Campbell Soup Co)	1.0	0.0	0	440	50
Mesquite Smoke Barbecue Sauce (2 tbsp)					
Kraft (Kraft General Foods)*	0.0	0.0	0	410	40
Kraft Thick'N Spicy (Kraft General Foods)*	0.0	0.0	0	440	50
ONION BARBECUE SAUCES					
Onion Bits Barbecue Sauce (2 tbsp)					
Kraft (Kraft General Foods)*	0.0	0.0	0	340	50
Onion Flavor BBQ Sauce (2 tbsp)					
Open Pit (Campbell Soup Co)	0.0	0.0	0	480	50
Thick and Tangy Onion BBQ Sauce (2 tbsp)					
Open Pit (Campbell Soup Co)	0.0	0.0	0	380	50
ORIGINAL BARBECUE SAUCES					
Extra Rich Original Barbecue Sauce (2 tbsp)					
Kraft (Kraft General Foods)*	0.0	0.0	0	360	50
Original Barbecue Sauce					
America's Choice (A & P) (2 tbsp)	0.0	0.0	0	380	45
Hunt's (Hunt-Wesson) (1 tbsp)	<1.0	0.0	0	160	20
Kraft (Kraft General Foods)* (2 tbsp)	0.0	0.0	0	460	40
Kraft Thick'N Spicy (Kraft General Foods)* (2 tbsp)	0.0	0.0	0	440	50
Original BBQ Sauce (2 tbsp)					
Open Pit (Campbell Soup Co)	0.0	0.0	0	490	50
Original Flavor BBQ Sauce (2 tbsp)					
Open Pit (Campbell Soup Co)	0.0	0.0	0	450	50

*Tobacco company, corporate subsidiary, or parent.

	Tot. Fat (g)	Sat. Fat (g)	Chol. (mg)	Sod. (mg)	Cal.
OTHER BARBECUE SAUCES					
Char-Grill Barbecue Sauce (2 tbsp)					
Kraft (Kraft General Foods)*	1.0	0.0	0	440	60
Country Style Barbecue Sauce (1 tbsp)					
Hunt's (Hunt-Wesson)	<1.0	0.0	0	140	20
Garlic Original Barbecue Sauce (2 tbsp)					
Kraft (Kraft General Foods)*	0.0	0.0	0	420	40
Homestyle Barbecue Sauce (1 tbsp)					
Hunt's (Hunt-Wesson)	<1.0	0.0	0	170	20
Hong Kong Barbecue Sauce (1 tsp)					
House of Tsang (Hormel)	0.0	0.0	0	150	10
Italian Seasonings Barbecue Sauce (2 tbsp)					
Kraft (Kraft General Foods)*	0.5	0.0	0	280	45
New Orleans Style Barbecue Sauce (1 tbsp)					
Hunt's (Hunt-Wesson)	<1.0	0.0	0	150	20
Southern Style Barbecue Sauce (1 tbsp)					
Hunt's (Hunt-Wesson)	<1.0	0.0	0	170	20
Sweet Flavor BBQ Sauce (2 tbsp)					
Open Pit (Campbell Soup Co) . .	0.0	0.0	0	300	50
Teriyaki Barbecue Sauce (2 tbsp)					
Kraft (Kraft General Foods)*	1.0	0.0	0	430	60
Texas Style Barbecue Sauce (1 tbsp)					
Hunt's (Hunt-Wesson)	<1.0	0.0	0	150	25
Western Style Barbecue Sauce (1 tbsp)					
Hunt's (Hunt-Wesson)	<1.0	0.0	0	170	20

CHILI SAUCES—see "CONDIMENTS," CHILI/PICANTE/SALSA/TACO SAUCES, page 87

*Tobacco company, corporate subsidiary, or parent.

	Tot. Fat (g)	Sat. Fat (g)	Chol. (mg)	Sod. (mg)	Cal.
COOKING SAUCES—*see also* "CONDIMENTS," MARINADES, page 94, TOMATO PASTE, page103, TOMATO PUREE, page104; TERIYAKI SAUCES, page 259					
BOTTLED/CANNED COOKING SAUCES					
Bottled/Canned Italian Cooking Sauces					
Cacciatore (½ cup)					
Betty Crocker Recipe Sauces (General Mills)	0.0	0.0	0	620	50
Chicken Cacciatore Simmer Sauce (½ cup)					
Ragú Chicken Tonight (Van den Bergh Foods)	1.5	0.0	0	530	80
Italian Primavera Light Simmer Sauce (½ cup)					
Ragú Chicken Tonight (Van den Bergh Foods)	1.0	0.0	0	630	50
Parmigiana (½ cup)					
Betty Crocker Recipe Sauces (General Mills)	1.0	0.5	0	490	60
Skillet Lasagna Simmer Sauce (½ cup)					
Ragú Beef Tonight (Van den Bergh Foods)	2.0	1.0	<5	730	80
Bottled/Canned Mexican Cooking Sauces					
Chili Fixin's Sauce (5.3 oz)					
Hunt's Manwich (Hunt-Wesson)	<1.0	0.0	0	900	110
Fajitas Skillet Sauce (1 tbsp)					
Lawry's (Lawry's Foods)	0.0	0.0	0	600	15
Organic Mexican Chef Sauce (½ cup)					
Muir Glen	0.0	0.0	0	290	45
Original 7 Spice Chili Recipe (½ cup)					
Tabasco brand (McIlhenny Co)	0.5	0.0	0	115	50
Salsa Simmer Sauce (½ cup)					
Ragú Chicken Tonight (Van den Bergh Foods)	0.0	0.0	0	750	50

	Tot. Fat (g)	Sat. Fat (g)	Chol. (mg)	Sod. (mg)	Cal.
Spicy 7 Spice Chili Recipe (½ cup) Tabasco brand (McIlhenny Co)	0.5	0.0	0	115	60
Zesty Tomato Mexicali (½ cup) Campbell's Simmer Chef (Campbell Soup Co)	3.0	1.0	5	400	90
Bottled/Canned Oriental Cooking Sauces					
Oriental Simmer Sauce (½ cup) Ragú Chicken Tonight (Van den Bergh Foods)	0.5	0.0	0	750	60
Oriental Sweet and Sour (½ cup) Campbell's Simmer Chef (Campbell Soup Co)	1.0	0.0	0	280	110
Sweet & Sour (½ cup) Betty Crocker Recipe Sauces (General Mills)	0.0	0.0	0	350	160
Sweet & Sour Sauce (¼ cup) Chun King (Chun King Corp)	0.0	0.0	0	25	80
Sweet & Sour Simmer Sauce (½ cup) Ragú Chicken Tonight (Van den Bergh Foods)	0.0	0.0	0	320	120
Sweet & Spicy Light Simmer Sauce (½ cup) Ragú Chicken Tonight (Van den Bergh Foods)	1.0	0.0	0	330	60
Bottled/Canned Sandwich Cooking Sauces					
Extra Thick & Chunky Sauce (2.5 oz) Hunt's Manwich (Hunt-Wesson)	<1.0	0.0	0	640	60
Hickory Flavor Sloppy Joe Sauce (¼ cup) Del Monte	0.0	0.0	0	700	70
Italian Recipe Sloppy Joe Sauce (¼ cup) Del Monte	0.0	0.0	0	700	70
Mexican Sauce (2.5 oz) Hunt's Manwich (Hunt-Wesson)	1.0	0.0	0	460	35
Not-So-Sloppy-Joe Sauce (¼ cup) Hormel	0.0	0.0	0	720	70
Original Sloppy Joe Sauce (¼ cup) Del Monte	0.0	0.0	0	680	70

	Tot. Fat (g)	Sat. Fat (g)	Chol. (mg)	Sod. (mg)	Cal.
BOTTLED/CANNED COOKING SAUCES *(cont'd)*					
Sloppy Joe Sandwich Sauce (¼ cup)					
Green Giant (Grand Metropolitan PLC)	0.0	0.0	0	420	50
Sloppy Joe Sauce					
Hunt's Manwich (Hunt-Wesson) (2.5 oz)	<1.0	0.0	0	390	40
Libby's (Nestlé Food Company) (⅓ cup)	0.0	0.0	0	430	45
Other Bottled/Canned Cooking Sauces					
Barbecue Simmer Sauce (½ cup)					
Ragú Beef Tonight (Van den Bergh Foods)	0.5	0.0	0	800	110
Golden Honey Mustard Cooking Sauce (½ cup)					
Campbell's Simmer Chef (Campbell Soup Co)	2.0	0.0	0	400	150
Ham Glaze (2 tbsp)					
Chelten House (Chelten House Products)	0.0	0.0	0	20	50
Hearty Onion & Mushroom Cooking Sauce (½ cup)					
Campbell's Simmer Chef (Campbell Soup Co)	1.0	0.0	0	670	50
Honey Mustard Light Simmer Sauce (½ cup)					
Ragú Chicken Tonight (Van den Bergh Foods)	0.5	0.0	0	440	60
Hot Chicken Wing Sauce (2 tbsp)					
Chelten House (Chelten House Products)	0.0	0.0	0	135	20
Meatloaf Fixin's Tomato Sauce (2 oz)					
Hunt's (Hunt-Wesson)	<1.0	0.0	0	580	20
Organic Creole Chef Sauce (½ cup)					
Muir Glen	2.0	0.0	0	290	60
Raisin Sauce (2 tbsp)					
Chelten House (Chelten House Products)	0.0	0.0	0	15	60

	Tot. Fat (g)	Sat. Fat (g)	Chol. (mg)	Sod. (mg)	Cal.
Spanish Simmer Sauce (½ cup)					
Ragú Chicken Tonight (Van den Bergh Foods)	1.5	0.0	0	710	70
Spicy Simmer Sauce (½ cup)					
Newman's Own	3.0	0.0	0	600	70
DRY COOKING SAUCE MIXES					
Country Homestyle Sauce & Recipe Mix (2 tbsp)					
Village Saucerie (Alberto-Culver)	0.0	0.0	0	530	45
Garden Herb Sauce & Recipe Mix (2 tbsp)					
Village Saucerie (Alberto-Culver)	0.0	0.0	0	360	45
Garlic & Herb Sauce & Recipe Mix (2 tbsp)					
Village Saucerie (Alberto-Culver)	0.0	0.0	0	460	45
Lemon Butter Sauce Mix (1 tbsp)					
Weight Watchers (H.J. Heinz)	0.0	0.0	0	90	7
Southwest Sauce & Recipe Mix (2 tbsp)					
Village Saucerie (Alberto-Culver)	0.0	0.0	0	390	45
ENCHILADA SAUCES—*see also* "CONDIMENTS," CHILI/ PICANTE/SALSA/TACO SAUCES, page 87					
Enchilada Sauce Mix (2 tsp)					
Old El Paso (Pet)	0.0	0.0	0	540	10
Green Chile Enchilada Sauce (¼ cup)					
Las Palmas (Pet)	1.5	0.0	0	260	25
Green Enchilada Sauce (¼ cup)					
Old El Paso (Pet)	1.5	(0.2)	0	330	30
Hot Enchilada Sauce (¼ cup)					
Las Palmas (Pet)	0.5	0.0	0	330	20
Old El Paso (Pet)	1.5	(0.2)	0	190	30
Mild Enchilada Sauce (¼ cup)					
Old El Paso (Pet)	1.0	(0.2)	0	160	25
Original Enchilada Sauce (¼ cup)					
Las Palmas (Pet)	0.5	0.0	0	310	15

	Tot. Fat (g)	Sat. Fat (g)	Chol. (mg)	Sod. (mg)	Cal.
GRAVIES					
BOTTLED/CANNED GRAVIES					
Turkey Gravy (¼ cup)					
Franco-American (Campbell Soup Co)	1.0	0.0	0	290	25
DRY GRAVY MIXES					
Brown Dry Gravy Mixes					
Brown Gravy Mix, made with water (¼ cup)					
Pillsbury (Grand Metropolitan PLC)	0.0	0.0	0	270	10
Brown Gravy Mix, made with water (¼ cup)					
Weight Watchers (H.J. Heinz)	0.0	0.0	0	360	10
Brown Gravy Mix with Mushrooms, made with water (¼ cup)					
Weight Watchers (H.J. Heinz)	0.0	0.0	0	270	10
Brown Gravy Mix with Onions, made with water (¼ cup)					
Weight Watchers (H.J. Heinz)	0.0	0.0	0	310	10
Chicken Dry Gravy Mixes					
Chicken Gravy Mix, made with water (¼ cup)					
Weight Watchers (H.J. Heinz)	0.0	0.0	0	410	10
Chicken Style Gravy Mix, made with skim milk and water (¼ cup)					
Pillsbury (Grand Metropolitan PLC)	0.0	0.0	0	260	20
Other Dry Gravy Mixes					
Homestyle Gravy Mix, made with water (¼ cup)					
Pillsbury (Grand Metropolitan PLC)	0.0	0.0	0	270	10

HOT DOG SAUCES—*see* OTHER SAUCES, page 260

	Tot. Fat (g)	Sat. Fat (g)	Chol. (mg)	Sod. (mg)	Cal.
ORIENTAL DIPPING SAUCES—*see also* COOKING SAUCES, Other Bottled/Canned Cooking Sauces, page 250; TERIYAKI SAUCES, page 259					
SPICY ORIENTAL DIPPING SAUCES					
Hoisin Sauce					
House of Tsang (Hormel) (1 tsp)	0.0	0.0	0	105	15
Ka-me (Shaffer, Clarke & Co) (2 tbsp)	0.0	0.0	0	620	45
Hot Chili Sauce with Garlic (1 tbsp)					
Ka-me (Shaffer, Clarke & Co)	0.0	0.0	0	115	15
Spicy Brown Bean Sauce (1 tsp)					
House of Tsang (Hormel)	0.0	0.0	0	125	15
Szechuan Sauce (1 tbsp)					
Ka-me (Shaffer, Clarke & Co)	1.0	0.0	0	410	20
STIR-FRY DIPPING SAUCES					
Classic Stir Fry Sauce (1 tbsp)					
House of Tsang (Hormel)	1.0	0.0	0	570	25
Stir-Fry Sauce (1 tbsp)					
Ka-me (Shaffer, Clarke & Co)	0.0	0.0	0	570	10
Sweet & Sour Stir Fry Sauce (1 tbsp)					
House of Tsang (Hormel)	0.0	0.0	0	50	35
Szechuan Spicy Stir Fry Sauce (1 tbsp)					
House of Tsang (Hormel)	0.5	0.0	0	490	20
SWEET AND SOUR ORIENTAL DIPPING SAUCES—*see also* STIR-FRY DIPPING SAUCES, above					
Duck Sauce (2 tbsp)					
Ka-me (Shaffer, Clarke & Co)	0.0	0.0	0	480	80
Sweet & Pungent Duck Sauce (2 tbsp)					
Chelten House (Chelten House Products)	0.0	0.0	0	140	50
Sweet & Sour Concentrate (1 tsp)					
House of Tsang (Hormel)	0.0	0.0	0	15	10
Sweet & Sour Duck Sauce (1 tbsp)					
La Choy (Hunt-Wesson)	<1.0	0.0	0	40	25

	Tot. Fat (g)	Sat. Fat (g)	Chol. (mg)	Sod. (mg)	Cal.
SWEET AND SOUR ORIENTAL DIPPING SAUCES *(cont'd)*					
Sweet & Sour Sauce (1 tbsp)					
La Choy (Hunt-Wesson)	<1.0	0.0	0	40	25
Sweet & Sour Sauce with Ginger (2 tbsp)					
Ka-me (Shaffer, Clarke & Co)	0.0	0.0	0	270	50
Sweet 'N Sour Sauce (2 tbsp)					
Contadina (Nestlé Food Company)	1.0	0.0	0	110	40
Kraft (Kraft General Foods)*	0.5	0.0	0	180	80
Woody's (Reily Foods Co)	0.0	0.0	0	610	70
Sweet'n Sour Sauce (2 tbsp)					
Kraft Sauceworks (Kraft General Foods)*	0.0	0.0	0	125	60
OTHER ORIENTAL DIPPING SAUCES					
Black Bean Sauce (1 tbsp)					
Ka-me (Shaffer, Clarke & Co)	0.0	0.0	0	550	10
Fish Sauce (1 tbsp)					
Ka-me (Shaffer, Clarke & Co)	0.0	0.0	0	1300	10
Lemon Sauce (1 tbsp)					
Ka-me (Shaffer, Clarke & Co)	0.0	0.0	0	125	45
Mandarin Orange Sauce (2 tbsp)					
Ka-me (Shaffer, Clarke & Co)	0.0	0.0	0	430	80
Oyster Flavored Sauce (1 tbsp)					
Ka-me (Shaffer, Clarke & Co)	0.0	0.0	0	460	10
Plum Sauce (2 tbsp)					
Ka-me (Shaffer, Clarke & Co)	0.0	0.0	0	420	80
Tempura Sauce (2 tbsp)					
Ka-me (Shaffer, Clarke & Co)	0.0	0.0	0	1790	15
PASTA/SPAGHETTI SAUCES					
CHUNKY PASTA/SPAGHETTI SAUCES					
Chunky Garden Style Spaghetti Sauce (½ cup)					
Pritikin (Quaker Oats Company)	0.5	0.0	0	30	50
Chunky Spaghetti Sauce (4 oz)					
Hunt's (Hunt-Wesson)	<1.0	0.0	0	470	50
Chunky Tomato with Basil Sauce (½ cup)					
DiGiorno Light Varieties (Kraft General Foods)*	0.0	0.0	0	290	70

*Tobacco company, corporate subsidiary, or parent.

	Tot. Fat (g)	Sat. Fat (g)	Chol. (mg)	Sod. (mg)	Cal.
Organic Low Fat Chunky Style Pasta Sauce (½ cup) Muir Glen	2.0	0.0	0	300	80
GARDEN VEGETABLE PASTA/ SPAGHETTI SAUCES					
Garden Medley Pasta Sauce (½ cup) Ragú Fino Italian (Van den Bergh Foods)	3.0	0.0	0	580	90
Light Pasta Sauce (½ cup) Ragú Garden Harvest (Van den Bergh Foods)	0.0	0.0	0	410	50
GARLIC PASTA/SPAGHETTI SAUCES					
Extra Garlic & Onion Spaghetti Sauce (½ cup) Campbell's (Campbell Soup Co)	1.0	0.0	0	370	60
Garlic & Basil Pasta Sauce (½ cup) Ragú Fino Italian (Van den Bergh Foods)	3.0	0.0	0	580	90
Organic Fat Free Garlic and Onion Pasta Sauce (½ cup) Muir Glen	0.0	0.0	0	300	60
Spaghetti Sauce with Garlic and Onions (½ cup) Del Monte	1.0	0.0	0	440	70
MEAT-FLAVORED PASTA/SPAGHETTI SAUCES					
Spaghetti Sauce with Meat					
Hunt's (Hunt-Wesson) (4 oz)	2.0	0.3	2	570	70
Weight Watchers (H.J. Heinz) (½ cup)	1.0	0.0	0	430	60
MUSHROOM PASTA/SPAGHETTI SAUCES					
Chunky Mushroom Light Pasta Sauce (½ cup) Ragú (Van den Bergh Foods)	0.0	0.0	0	410	50
Homestyle Spaghetti Sauce with Mushrooms (4 oz) Hunt's (Hunt-Wesson)	1.0	0.2	0	530	50
Mushroom Spaghetti Sauce (½ cup) Campbell's (Campbell Soup Co)	1.0	0.0	0	390	60

	Tot. Fat (g)	Sat. Fat (g)	Chol. (mg)	Sod. (mg)	Cal.
MUSHROOM PASTA/SPAGHETTI SAUCES *(cont'd)*					
Mushroom Thick & Hearty Pasta Sauce (½ cup)					
Ragú (Van den Bergh Foods) . . .	3.0	0.5	0	580	120
Organic Mushrooms and Green Peppers Pasta Sauce (½ cup)					
Muir Glen	2.0	0.0	0	300	70
Sliced Mushroom Pasta Sauce (½ cup)					
Ragú Fino Italian (Van den Bergh Foods)	3.0	0.0	0	580	90
Spaghetti Sauce with Mushrooms					
Del Monte (½ cup)	1.5	0.0	0	520	80
Hunt's (Hunt-Wesson) (4 oz) . . .	2.0	0.3	0	560	70
Newman's Own (½ cup)	2.0	0.0	0	700	60
Weight Watchers (H.J. Heinz) (½ cup)	0.0	0.0	0	420	60
PLAIN/REGULAR PASTA/SPAGHETTI SAUCES					
Homestyle Spaghetti Sauce					
Campbell's (Campbell Soup Co) (½ cup)	0.0	0.0	0	410	70
Hunt's (Hunt-Wesson) (4 oz) . . .	2.0	0.3	0	530	60
Italian Style Spaghetti Sauce (½ cup)					
Campbell's (Campbell Soup Co)	0.0	0.0	0	410	50
Marinara Sauce (½ cup)					
Pritikin (Quaker Oats Company) .	0.0	0.0	0	260	60
Marinara Spaghetti Sauce (½ cup)					
Campbell's (Campbell Soup Co)	0.0	0.0	0	410	70
Original Spaghetti Sauce (½ cup)					
Pritikin (Quaker Oats Company) .	0.5	0.0	0	30	60
Plum Tomato & Mushroom Sauce (½ cup)					
DiGiorno (Kraft General Foods)*	0.0	0.0	0	310	70
Spaghetti Sauce (½ cup)					
Newman's Own	2.0	0.0	0	700	60
Tomato & Herb Light Pasta Sauce (½ cup)					
Ragú (Van den Bergh Foods) . . .	0.0	0.0	0	410	50

*Tobacco company, corporate subsidiary, or parent.

	Tot. Fat (g)	Sat. Fat (g)	Chol. (mg)	Sod. (mg)	Cal.
Tomato & Herb Pasta Sauce (½ cup)					
Ragú Fino Italian (Van den Bergh Foods)	3.0	0.0	0	580	90
Traditional Spaghetti Sauce					
Campbell's (Campbell Soup Co) (½ cup)	2.0	0.0	0	590	100
Del Monte (½ cup)	1.0	0.0	0	470	80
Hunt's (Hunt-Wesson) (4 oz)	2.0	0.3	0	530	70
OTHER PASTA/SPAGHETTI SAUCES					
No Sugar Added Light Pasta Sauce (½ cup)					
Ragú (Van den Bergh Foods)	1.5	0.0	0	410	60
Organic Fat Free Italian Herb Pasta Sauce (½ cup)					
Muir Glen	0.0	0.0	0	300	60
Organic Fat Free Tomato Basil Pasta Sauce (½ cup)					
Muir Glen	0.0	0.0	0	300	60
Sockarooni Sauce (½ cup)					
Newman's Own	2.0	0.0	0	700	60
Zesty Tomato Pasta Sauce (½ cup)					
Ragú Fino Italian (Van den Bergh Foods)	3.0	0.0	0	580	90
PICANTE SAUCES—*see* "CONDIMENTS," CHILI/PICANTE/SALSA/TACO SAUCES, page 87					
PIZZA SAUCES					
Chunky Mushroom Sauce (¼ cup)					
Ragú Pizza Quick (Van den Bergh Foods)	1.5	0.0	0	340	40
Chunky Tomato Sauce (¼ cup)					
Ragú Pizza Quick (Van den Bergh Foods)	1.5	0.0	0	300	40
Garlic & Basil Sauce (¼ cup)					
Ragú Pizza Quick (Van den Bergh Foods)	1.5	0.0	0	340	40

	Tot. Fat (g)	Sat. Fat (g)	Chol. (mg)	Sod. (mg)	Cal.
PIZZA SAUCES *(cont'd)*					
Pizza Sauce (¼ cup)					
Contadina (Nestlé Food Company)	1.5	0.0	0	350	35
Progresso (Pet)	1.0	0.0	0	140	35
Pizza Sauce with Italian Cheeses (¼ cup)					
Contadina (Nestlé Food Company)	1.5	0.0	0	420	40
Pizza Squeeze (¼ cup)					
Contadina (Nestlé Food Company)	1.5	0.0	0	350	35
Traditional Pizza Sauce (¼ cup)					
Prego (Campbell Soup Co)	2.0	0.0	0	230	40
Traditional Sauce (¼ cup)					
Ragú Pizza Quick (Van den Bergh Foods)	1.5	0.0	0	340	40
SALSAS—*see* "CONDIMENTS," CHILI/PICANTE/SALSA/TACO SAUCES, page 87					
SANDWICH SAUCES—*see* COOKING SAUCES, page 248					
SPAGHETTI SAUCES—*see* PASTA/SPAGHETTI SAUCES, page 254					
SWEET AND SOUR SAUCES—*see* COOKING SAUCES, page 248; ORIENTAL DIPPING SAUCES, page 253					
TACO SAUCES—*see* "CONDIMENTS," CHILI/PICANTE/SALSA/TACO SAUCES, page 87					
TARTAR SAUCES					
Nonfat Tartar Sauce (2 tbsp)					
Kraft (Kraft General Foods)*	0.0	0.0	0	210	25

*Tobacco company, corporate subsidiary, or parent.

	Tot. Fat (g)	Sat. Fat (g)	Chol. (mg)	Sod. (mg)	Cal.
Reduced Fat Tartar Sauce (2 tbsp)					
Best Foods	4.5	0.5	0	340	60
Hellmann's (Best Foods)	4.5	0.5	0	340	60
TERIYAKI SAUCES					
Korean Teriyaki (1 tbsp)					
House of Tsang (Hormel)	0.5	0.0	0	430	30
Lite Teriyaki Sauce (1 tbsp)					
Chun King (Chun King Corp)	0.0	0.0	0	470	15
Teriyaki Sauce (1 tbsp)					
Chun King (Chun King Corp)	0.0	0.0	0	700	15
Teriyaki Sauce and Marinade (1 tbsp)					
Ka-me (Shaffer, Clarke & Co)	0.0	0.0	0	480	10
TOMATO SAUCES—*see also* "CONDIMENTS," TOMATO PASTE, page 103, TOMATO PUREE, page 104					
Fresh Tomato Sauce (¼ cup)					
America's Choice (A & P)	0.0	0.0	0	300	20
Herb Flavored Tomato Sauce (4 oz)					
Hunt's (Hunt-Wesson)	2.0	0.6	<1	470	70
Italian Tomato Sauce					
Contadina (Nestlé Food Company) (¼ cup)	0.0	0.0	0	320	15
Hunt's (Hunt-Wesson) (4 oz)	2.0	0.5	<1	460	60
No Salt Added Tomato Sauce (¼ cup)					
Del Monte	0.0	0.0	0	20	20
Organic Tomato Sauce (¼ cup)					
Muir Glen	0.0	0.0	0	190	20
Special Tomato Sauce (4 oz)					
Hunt's (Hunt-Wesson)	<1.0	0.0	0	280	35
Thick & Zesty Tomato Sauce (¼ cup)					
Contadina (Nestlé Food Company)	0.0	0.0	0	330	15
Tomato Sauce with Bits (4 oz)					
Hunt's (Hunt-Wesson)	<1.0	0.0	0	620	30

	Tot. Fat (g)	Sat. Fat (g)	Chol. (mg)	Sod. (mg)	Cal.
TOMATO SAUCES *(cont'd)*					
Tomato Sauce with Garlic (4 oz)					
Hunt's (Hunt-Wesson)	2.0	0.3	0	480	70
Tomato Sauce with Mushrooms (4 oz)					
Hunt's (Hunt-Wesson)	<1.0	0.0	0	710	25
Tomato Sauce with Onions (4 oz)					
Hunt's (Hunt-Wesson)	<1.0	0.0	0	650	40
Tomatoes & Green Chilies Sauce (¼ cup)					
Old El Paso (Pet)	0.0	0.0	0	310	10
Tomatoes & Jalapeños Sauce (¼ cup)					
Old El Paso (Pet)	0.0	0.0	0	290	15
OTHER SAUCES					
Chili Hot Dog Sauce (1 tbsp)					
Wolf Brand (Quaker Oats Company)	1.0	0.0	0	90	15

JUICES

If you think that apples upset your applecart and peaches are the pits, you can still get the nutrition of fruits and vegetables by drinking the juice. Fruit and vegetable juices are loaded with vitamins and minerals and contain little if any fat, saturated fat, and cholesterol. They can be high in sodium, however, so check the listings that follow or read package labels carefully. Like all the other entries in this book, the juices entries that follow list sodium content. The AHA does not have criteria for sodium but recommends a total of no more than 3,000 mg a day.

Generic Listings

Only a few of the juices in this book are brand name products. That's because most brands of pure fruit juice contain about the same amount of fat, saturated fat, and cholesterol and these amounts are within the criteria cited below.

If you find products that were introduced after this book went to press, use the generic listings and the following tables to help you evaluate them.

AHA Criteria for Juices*

	Tot. Fat (g)	Sat. Fat (g)	Chol. (mg)
All juices	<0.5	<0.5	<2

*Per serving.

	Tot. Fat (g)	Sat. Fat (g)	Chol. (mg)	Sod. (mg)	Cal.
CLAM JUICE					
Clam Juice (300 g)					
Gorton's (General Mills)	0.0	0.0	0	740	0
FRUIT JUICES					
APPLE JUICES					
Ready-to-Serve					
Acrobat Apple Squeezit 100 (1 bottle)					
Betty Crocker (General Mills) ...	0.0	0.0	0	20	110
Apple Juice (8 fl oz)					
Most brands (USDA)	**0.3**	**0.0**	**0**	**7**	**116**
Hansen (Hansen Beverage Co) .	0.0	0.0	0	15	100
Apple Juice 100% Juice (10 fl oz)					
Dole (Dole Food Company)	0.0	0.0	0	25	160
100% Pure Apple Juice Fresh Pressed (8 fl oz)					
Just Pik't (The Fresh Juice Company)	0.0	0.0	0	60	120
Reconstituted from Frozen					
Apple Juice, made with water (8 fl oz)					
Ocean Spray (Ocean Spray Cranberries)	0.0	0.0	0	35	110
APRICOT JUICES					
Apricot nectar (8 fl oz)					
Most brands (USDA)	**0.2**	**0.0**	**0**	**9**	**141**
BERRY JUICES					
Ready-to-Serve					
Berry Squeezit 100 (1 bottle)					
Betty Crocker (General Mills) ...	0.0	0.0	0	20	100
Boysenberry Naturally 100% Fruit Juice (8 fl oz)					
Smucker's (The J.M. Smucker Co)	0.0	0.0	0	10	120
Country Raspberry 100% Juice (8 fl oz)					
Dole (Dole Food Company)	0.0	0.0	0	30	140

	Tot. Fat (g)	Sat. Fat (g)	Chol. (mg)	Sod. (mg)	Cal.
Red Raspberry Naturally 100% Fruit Juice (8 fl oz) Smucker's (The J.M. Smucker Co)	0.0	0.0	0	10	120
Reconstituted from Frozen					
Country Raspberry 100% Juice, made with water (8 fl oz) Dole (Dole Food Company)	0.0	0.0	0	30	140
CHERRY JUICES					
Ready-to-Serve					
Black Cherry Naturally 100% Fruit Juice (8 fl oz) Smucker's (The J.M. Smucker Co)	0.0	0.0	0	10	130
Mountain Cherry 100% Juice (8 fl oz) Dole (Dole Food Company)	0.0	0.0	0	30	120
Reconstituted from Frozen					
Mountain Cherry 100% Juice, made with water (8 fl oz) Dole (Dole Food Company)	0.0	0.0	0	30	120
GRAPE JUICES					
Ready-to-Serve					
Caped Grape Squeezit 100 (1 bottle) Betty Crocker (General Mills)	0.0	0.0	0	20	100
Grape juice (8 fl oz) **Most brands** (USDA)	**0.2**	**0.1**	**0**	**7**	**155**
GRAPEFRUIT JUICES					
Ready-to-Serve					
Fresh Squeezed Grapefruit Juice (8 fl oz) Just Pik't (The Fresh Juice Company)	0.0	0.0	0	0	100
Grapefruit Juice (8 fl oz) Ocean Spray (Ocean Spray Cranberries)	0.0	0.0	0	35	100
Grapefruit juice, sweetened (8 fl oz) **Most brands** (USDA)	**<1.0**	**0.2**	**0**	**4**	**116**
Grapefruit juice, unsweetened (8 fl oz) **Most brands** (USDA)	**0.2**	**0.0**	**0**	**3**	**93**

	Tot. Fat (g)	Sat. Fat (g)	Chol. (mg)	Sod. (mg)	Cal.
GRAPEFRUIT JUICES *(cont'd)*					
Ruby Red Premium Grapefruit Juice (8 fl oz)					
Florida's Natural (Citrus World) . .	0.0	0.0	0	0	100
Sun Ripe Grapefruit 100% Juice (10 fl oz)					
Dole (Dole Food Company)	0.0	0.0	0	45	160
LEMON/LIME JUICES					
Lemon juice (1 tsp)					
Most brands (USDA)	**0.0**	**0.0**	**0**	**1**	**1**
Lime juice (1 tsp)					
Most brands (USDA)	**0.0**	**0.0**	**0**	**0**	**1**
MIXED FRUIT JUICES					
Ready-to-Serve					
Apple-Cranberry Naturally 100% Fruit Juice (8 fl oz)					
Smucker's (The J.M. Smucker Co)	0.0	0.0	0	10	120
Orange/Grapefruit juice (8 fl oz)					
Most brands (USDA)	**0.2**	**0.0**	**0**	**8**	**107**
Pilot Punch Squeezit 100 (1 bottle)					
Betty Crocker (General Mills) . . .	0.0	0.0	0	20	100
Pine-Orange Banana 100% Juice (8 fl oz)					
Dole (Dole Food Company)	0.0	0.0	0	20	130
Pine-Passion Banana 100% Juice (8 fl oz)					
Dole (Dole Food Company)	0.0	0.0	0	20	120
Premium Orange Pineapple Juice (8 fl oz)					
Florida's Natural (Citrus World) . .	0.0	0.0	0	0	130
Tropical Fruit 100% Juice (8 fl oz)					
Dole (Dole Food Company)	0.0	0.0	0	30	140
Reconstituted from Frozen					
Pine-Passion Banana 100% Juice, made with water (8 fl oz)					
Dole (Dole Food Company)	0.0	0.0	0	20	120
Pineapple Orange 100% Juice, made with water (8 fl oz)					
Dole (Dole Food Company)	0.0	0.0	0	20	120

	Tot. Fat (g)	Sat. Fat (g)	Chol. (mg)	Sod. (mg)	Cal.
Tropical Fruit 100% Juice, made with water (8 fl oz)					
Dole (Dole Food Company)	0.0	0.0	0	30	140
ORANGE JUICES					
Ready-to-Serve					
Fresh Squeezed Orange Juice (8 fl oz)					
Just Pik't (The Fresh Juice Company)	0.0	0.0	0	0	120
Home Squeezed Style Premium Orange Juice (8 fl oz)					
Florida's Natural (Citrus World) ..	0.0	0.0	0	0	120
Orange Blend (10 oz)					
Minute Maid (Coca-Cola Foods)	0.0	0.0	0	0	150
Orange juice (8 fl oz)					
Most brands (USDA)	**0.4**	**0.0**	**0**	**6**	**104**
Premium Orange Juice (8 fl oz)					
Florida's Natural (Citrus World) ..	0.0	0.0	0	0	120
Reconstituted from Frozen Orange Juice, made with water (8 fl oz)					
Most brands (USDA)	**0.1**	**0.0**	**0**	**2**	**112**
Ocean Spray (Ocean Spray Cranberries)	0.0	0.0	0	35	120
PAPAYA JUICES					
Papaya nectar (8 fl oz)					
Most brands (USDA)	**0.4**	**0.1**	**0**	**14**	**142**
PASSION FRUIT JUICES					
Passion fruit juice, purple (8 fl oz)					
Most brands (USDA)	**0.1**	**0.0**	**0**	**18**	**126**
Passion fruit juice, yellow (8 fl oz)					
Most brands (USDA)	**0.4**	**0.0**	**0**	**15**	**149**
PEACH JUICES					
Ready-to-Serve					
Orchard Peach 100% Juice (8 fl oz)					
Dole (Dole Food Company)	0.0	0.0	0	30	140
Peach Naturally 100% Fruit Juice (8 fl oz)					
Smucker's (The J.M. Smucker Co)	0.0	0.0	0	10	120

	Tot. Fat (g)	Sat. Fat (g)	Chol. (mg)	Sod. (mg)	Cal.
PEACH JUICES *(cont'd)*					
Peach nectar (8 fl oz)					
Most brands (USDA)	**0.1**	**0.0**	**0**	**17**	**134**
Reconstituted from Frozen					
Orchard Peach 100% Juice, made with water (8 fl oz)					
Dole (Dole Food Company)	0.0	0.0	0	30	140
PEAR JUICES					
Pear nectar (8 fl oz)					
Most brands (USDA)	**0.0**	**0.0**	**0**	**9**	**149**
PINEAPPLE JUICES					
Ready-to-Serve					
Pineapple juice (8 fl oz)					
Most brands (USDA)	**0.2**	**0.0**	**0**	**2**	**139**
Pineapple Juice 100% Juice (8 fl oz)					
Dole (Dole Food Company)	0.0	0.0	0	20	130
Pineapple Juice 100% Unsweetened (8 fl oz)					
Dole (Dole Food Company)	0.0	0.0	0	10	120
Reconstituted from Frozen					
Pineapple Juice 100% Juice, made with water (8 fl oz)					
Dole (Dole Food Company)	0.0	0.0	0	20	130
PRUNE JUICE					
Ready-to-Serve					
Prune Juice (6 fl oz)					
Most brands (USDA)	**0.1**	**0.0**	**0**	**11**	**181**
Del Monte	0.0	0.0	0	20	170
TANGERINE JUICES					
Ready-to-Serve					
Mandarin Tangerine 100% Juice (8 fl oz)					
Dole (Dole Food Company)	0.0	0.0	0	30	140
Tangerine juice, sweetened, canned (8 fl oz)					
Most brands (USDA)	**0.5**	**0.0**	**0**	**2**	**125**
Reconstituted from Frozen					
Tangerine Juice, made with water (8 fl oz)					
Minute Maid (Coca-Cola Foods)	0.0	0.0	0	0	120

	Tot. Fat (g)	Sat. Fat (g)	Chol. (mg)	Sod. (mg)	Cal.
TOMATO JUICES					
Low Sodium Tomato Juice with Enhanced Tomato Flavor (8 fl oz)					
Campbell's (Campbell Soup Co)	0.0	0.0	0	140	50
No-salt-added tomato juice (8 fl oz)					
Most brands (USDA)	**0.1**	**0.0**	**0**	**24**	**42**
Snap-E-Tom (8 fl oz)					
Del Monte	0.0	0.0	0	670	50
Tomato Del Mar (8 fl oz)					
Campbell's (Campbell Soup Co)	1.0	1.0	0	880	110
Tomato Juice (8 fl oz)					
Most brands (USDA)	**0.1**	**0.0**	**0**	**882**	**42**
America's Choice (A & P)	0.0	0.0	0	550	40
Campbell's (Campbell Soup Co)	0.0	0.0	0	860	50
VEGETABLE JUICES					
CARROT JUICES					
Carrot Juice (5.5 fl oz)					
Most brands (USDA)	**0.4**	**0.0**	**0**	**72**	**98**
Just Pik't (The Fresh Juice Company)	0.0	0.0	0	0	44
MIXED VEGETABLE JUICES					
Hearty Hot & Spicy Vegetable Juice (8 fl oz)					
Smucker's (The J.M. Smucker Co)	0.1	0.0	0	650	58
Hearty Vegetable Juice (8 fl oz)					
Smucker's (The J.M. Smucker Co)	0.1	0.0	0	714	58
Light in Sodium and Tangy 100% Vegetable Juice (1 cup)					
V8 (Campbell Soup Co)	0.0	0.0	0	340	60
Low Sodium Vegetable Juice (8 fl oz)					
V8 (Campbell Soup Co)	0.0	0.0	0	140	60
100% Vegetable Juice (8 fl oz)					
V8 (Campbell Soup Co)	0.0	0.0	0	620	50
Picante Vegetable Juice (8 fl oz)					
V8 (Campbell Soup Co)	0.0	0.0	0	690	50

	Tot. Fat (g)	Sat. Fat (g)	Chol. (mg)	Sod. (mg)	Cal.
MIXED VEGETABLE JUICES *(cont'd)*					
Spicy Hot 100% Vegetable Juice (8 fl oz)					
V8 (Campbell Soup Co)	0.0	0.0	0	780	50
Vegetable Cocktail (8 oz)					
Del Monte	0.0	0.0	0	490	50
Vegetable juice cocktail (8 fl oz)					
Most brands (USDA)	**0.2**	**0.0**	**0**	**884**	**44**
SAUERKRAUT JUICES					
Sauerkraut Juice (8 fl oz)					
Bush's (Bush Brothers)	0.5	0.0	0	1670	14

TOMATO JUICES—*see* FRUIT JUICES, TOMATO JUICES, page 267

MAIN DISHES AND MEAL-TYPE PRODUCTS

You're running late again. It's time to reach into the pantry or freezer for a prepared meal. Fortunately, grocery stores today offer a wide variety of scrumptious main dishes and meal-type products that are also healthful. The products on the following pages are low in fat, saturated fat, and cholesterol as purchased or when prepared according to package directions.

The AHA criteria for these products, shown below, are figured per 100 grams, or about 3½ ounces. That means the actual amounts of fat, saturated fat, and cholesterol in a manufacturer's serving of a food depend on the total *weight* of that serving. For example, if you are going to eat a 10½-ounce product, you'll need to use the criteria given for total fat, saturated fat, and cholesterol in the chart and multiply by 3. That means the 10½-ounce portion (3 × 3½ ounces, or 300 grams total) can have a maximum of 9 grams of fat (3 × 3 grams), 3 grams of saturated fat (3 × 1 gram), and 60 milligrams of cholesterol (3 × 20 milligrams) and still qualify for inclusion in this book.

Like all the other entries in this book, the main dishes and meal-type products entries that follow list sodium content. The AHA does not have criteria for sodium but recommends a total of no more than 3,000 mg a day.

If you find products that were introduced after this book went to press, use the generic listings and the following tables to help you evaluate them.

AHA Criteria for Main Dishes and Meal-Type Products*

	Tot. Fat (g)	Sat. Fat (g)	Chol. (mg)
All main dishes and meal-type products	3 g per 100-g serving** *and* 30% or less of calories from fat	1 g per 100-g serving** *and* less than 10% of calories from fat	20 mg per 100-g serving**

*See also following table.

**100 g = about 3½ oz.

AHA Criteria for Main Dishes and Meal-Type Products at Various Weights

Weight (oz)	Tot. Fat (g)	Sat. Fat (g)	Chol. (mg)
6	5	2	35
7	6	2	40
8	7	2	45
9	8	3	50
10	9	3	55
11	9	3	60
12	10	3	70
13	11	4	75

Meal-Type Products You'll Want to Limit

Some main dishes and meal-type products, like the examples below, are too high in fat, saturated fat, and/or cholesterol to meet AHA criteria. They aren't included in this book, and we recommend that you don't eat them often.

Compare the amounts of fat, saturated fat, cholesterol, sodium, and calories in these examples with the more healthful alternatives listed on the following pages.

Sample Meal-Type Products to Limit

	Tot. Fat (g)	Sat. Fat (g)	Chol. (mg)	Sod. (mg)	Cal.
Beef enchilada dinner (12 oz)	29.0*	14.6*	81*	2270	750
Beef stroganoff dinner (10 oz)	14.0*	5.6*	76*	1075	320
Chicken and noodles dinner (12 oz)	17.6*	6.6*	96*	611	400
Macaroni and cheese dinner (12¾ oz)	15.8*	7.1*	33	990	382

Adapted from Nutrition Data System, University of Minnesota, Minneapolis.

*These values exceed AHA criteria for meal-type products.

	Tot. Fat (g)	Sat. Fat (g)	Chol. (mg)	Sod. (mg)	Cal.
CANNED AND SHELF-STABLE ENTRÉES/DINNERS					
BEEF ENTRÉES/DINNERS, CANNED AND SHELF STABLE—*see also* Beef Pasta-Based Entrées/Dinners, Canned and Shelf Stable, page 275; ORIENTAL ENTRÉES/ DINNERS, CANNED AND SHELF STABLE, page 274					
Chunky Beef Stew (7.5 oz)					
Weight Watchers (H.J. Heinz) . .	2.0	1.0	20	450	120
Roast Beef with Gravy					
Hormel (2 oz)	2.0	1.0	30	280	60
Libby's (Nestlé Food Company) (⅔ cup)	3.0	1.5	70	800	140
CHICKEN ENTRÉES/DINNERS, CANNED AND SHELF STABLE—*see also* CHILI ENTRÉES/DINNERS, CANNED AND SHELF STABLE, below; Chicken Pasta-Based Entrées/Dinners, Canned and Shelf Stable, page 275					
Chicken Cacciatore Two Minute Entree (1 bowl)					
Hormel Top Shelf (Hormel)	2.5	1.0	45	850	210
CHILI ENTRÉES/DINNERS, CANNED AND SHELF STABLE					
Black Bean Chili, made with onions, tomato sauce, and chilies (bag) (1 cup)					
Buckeye Beans & Herbs	1.3	0.0	0	1248	260
Black Bean Chili, made with onions, tomato sauce, and chilies (box) (1 cup)					
Buckeye Beans & Herbs	1.3	0.0	0	1248	240
Chicken Chili, made with onions, chicken, and green chilies (1 cup)					
Aunt Patsy's Pantry (Buckeye Beans & Herbs)	5.2	1.2	69	1488	440

	Tot. Fat (g)	Sat. Fat (g)	Chol. (mg)	Sod. (mg)	Cal.
Fat-Free Mild Black Bean Chili (½ cup) Health Valley (Health Valley Foods)	0.0	0.0	0	160	80
Fat-Free Spicy Black Bean Chili (½ cup) Health Valley (Health Valley Foods)	0.0	0.0	0	160	80
Fat-Free 3 Bean Chili (½ cup) Health Valley (Health Valley Foods)	0.0	0.0	0	160	80
Lentil Chili, made with onions and tomato sauce (1 cup) Aunt Patsy's Pantry (Buckeye Beans & Herbs)	1.3	0.0	0	1104	220
Mild Vegetarian Chili with Beans (½ cup) Health Valley (Health Valley Foods)	0.0	0.0	0	100	80
Mild Vegetarian Chili with Lentils (½ cup) Health Valley (Health Valley Foods)	0.0	0.0	0	100	80
No Salt Mild Vegetarian Chili with Beans (½ cup) Health Valley (Health Valley Foods)	0.0	0.0	0	35	80
No Salt Mild Vegetarian Chili with Lentils (½ cup) Health Valley (Health Valley Foods)	0.0	0.0	0	50	80
No Salt Spicy Vegetarian Chili with Beans (½ cup) Health Valley (Health Valley Foods)	0.0	0.0	0	35	80
Souper Black Bean Chili, made with onions, tomato sauce, and green chilies (1 cup) Aunt Patsy's Pantry (Buckeye Beans & Herbs)	1.3	0.0	0	1248	230

	Tot. Fat (g)	Sat. Fat (g)	Chol. (mg)	Sod. (mg)	Cal.
CHILI ENTRÉES/DINNERS, CANNED AND SHELF STABLE *(cont'd)*					
Spicy Vegetarian Chili with Beans (½ cup)					
Health Valley (Health Valley Foods)	0.0	0.0	0	100	80
Three Bean Chili (½ cup)					
Pritikin (Quaker Oats Company)	0.5	0.0	0	170	90
White Chicken Chili, made with onions, chicken, and chilies (1 cup)					
Buckeye Beans & Herbs	4.6	1.2	69	984	430
MEATLESS ENTRÉES/DINNERS, CANNED AND SHELF STABLE—*see also* Meatless Pasta-Based Entrées/Dinners, Canned and Shelf Stable, page 275; ORIENTAL ENTRÉES/DINNERS, CANNED AND SHELF STABLE, BELOW					
Amaranth Garden Vegetable (1 cup)					
Health Valley Vegetarian Cuisine (Health Valley Foods)	0.0	0.0	0	290	160
Lentil Garden Vegetable (1 cup)					
Health Valley Vegetarian Cuisine (Health Valley Foods)	1.0	0.0	0	240	160
Tofu Baked Beans (1 cup)					
Health Valley Vegetarian Cuisine (Health Valley Foods)	1.0	0.0	0	270	170
Tofu Black Bean (1 cup)					
Health Valley Vegetarian Cuisine (Health Valley Foods)	1.0	0.0	0	290	170
Tofu Lentil (1 cup)					
Health Valley Vegetarian Cuisine (Health Valley Foods)	1.0	0.0	0	290	160
Western Black Bean (1 cup)					
Health Valley Vegetarian Cuisine (Health Valley Foods)	1.0	0.0	0	230	230
ORIENTAL ENTRÉES/DINNERS, CANNED AND SHELF STABLE					
Beef Chow Mein Entree (¾ cup)					
La Choy (Hunt-Wesson)	2.0	0.8	16	960	40

	Tot. Fat (g)	Sat. Fat (g)	Chol. (mg)	Sod. (mg)	Cal.
Meatless Chow Mein Entree (¾ cup)					
La Choy (Hunt-Wesson)	<1.0	0.0	0	860	25
PASTA-BASED ENTRÉES/DINNERS, CANNED AND SHELF STABLE					
Beef Pasta-Based Entrées/ Dinners, Canned and Shelf Stable					
Spaghetti & Meatballs (7.75 oz)					
Libby's Diner (Nestlé Food Company)	5.0	2.0	20	940	190
Chicken Pasta-Based Entrées/ Dinners, Canned and Shelf Stable					
Pasta Spirals & Chicken (7.75 oz)					
Libby's Diner (Nestlé Food Company)	4.0	1.0	15	980	130
Meatless Pasta-Based Entrées/ Dinners, Canned and Shelf Stable					
Cheese & Garlic Ravioli (1 cup)					
DiGiorno Light Varieties (Kraft General Foods)*	2.0	1.0	5	580	270
Cheese Ravioli (1 cup)					
Progresso (Pet)	2.0	1.0	<5	930	220
Elbows'n Tomato Sauce (1 container)					
Lunch Bucket (Dial Corp)	2.0	0.5	0	830	160
Light Italian Pasta Salad, made as directed on box (¾ cup)					
Kraft (Kraft General Foods)*	2.0	1.0	<5	660	190
Spaghetti (1 cup)					
Bush's (Bush Brothers)	3.0	1.0	0	1450	180
Spaghetti in Tomato Sauce with Cheese (7¾ oz)					
Franco-American (Campbell Soup Co)	2.0	1.0	5	890	180
Spaghetti Pasta in Tomato & Cheese Sauce (1 cup)					
Franco-American (Campbell Soup Co)	2.0	1.0	5	1020	210
Spaghetti Rings (1 cup)					
Bush's (Bush Brothers)	2.5	1.0	0	1500	170

*Tobacco company, corporate subsidiary, or parent.

	Tot. Fat (g)	Sat. Fat (g)	Chol. (mg)	Sod. (mg)	Cal.
PASTA-BASED ENTRÉES/DINNERS, CANNED AND SHELF STABLE *(cont'd)*					
SpaghettiOs Garfield PizzaOs Pasta in Pizza Sauce (1 cup) Franco-American (Campbell Soup Co)	3.0	1.0	5	910	210
SpaghettiOs Pasta in Tomato & Cheese Sauce					
Franco-American (Campbell Soup Co) (7½-oz can)	2.0	1.0	5	840	160
Franco-American (Campbell Soup Co) (1 cup)	2.0	1.0	5	990	190
FROZEN ENTRÉES/DINNERS					
BEEF ENTRÉES/DINNERS, FROZEN—*see also* Beef Italian Entrées/Dinners, Frozen, page 281; Beef Mexican Entrées/Dinners, Frozen, page 286; Beef Oriental Entrées/Dinners, Frozen, page 287; Beef Pasta-Based Entrées/Dinners, Frozen, page 289					
Barbecue Beef Entrées/Dinners, Frozen					
Mesquite Beef Barbecue (11 oz) Healthy Choice (ConAgra)	4.0	1.5	45	490	310
Beef Tips Entrées/Dinners, Frozen					
Beef Tips Francais (9.5 oz) Healthy Choice (ConAgra)	5.0	1.5	30	520	280
Beef Tips with BBQ Sauce (11 oz) Healthy Choice (ConAgra)	6.0	2.5	40	270	290
Traditional Beef Tips (11.25 oz) Healthy Choice (ConAgra)	5.0	2.0	40	390	260
Roast Beef Entrées/Dinners, Frozen					
Beef Pot Roast with Whipped Potatoes (9 oz) Stouffer's Lean Cuisine (Stouffer's)	7.0	1.5	40	570	210

	Tot. Fat (g)	Sat. Fat (g)	Chol. (mg)	Sod. (mg)	Cal.
Yankee Pot Roast (11 oz) Healthy Choice (ConAgra)	5.0	2.0	45	460	280
Yankee Pot Roast Dinner (16 oz) Swanson Hungry Man (Campbell Soup Co)	11.0	3.0	45	910	400
Yankee Pot Roast Light and Healthy Dinner (10.5 oz) The Budget Gourmet (Kraft General Foods)*	7.0	2.5	30	430	270
Salisbury Steak Entrées/Dinners, Frozen					
Beef Sirloin Salisbury Steak Light and Healthy Entree (9 oz) The Budget Gourmet (Kraft General Foods)*	5.0	2.0	40	550	240
Beef Sirloin Salisbury Steak with Red Skinned Potatoes Light and Healthy Dinner (11 oz) The Budget Gourmet (Kraft General Foods)*	8.0	3.0	35	430	260
Salisbury Steak (11 oz) Healthy Choice (ConAgra)	6.0	2.5	30	500	260
Traditional Salisbury Steak (11.5 oz) Healthy Choice (ConAgra)	6.0	3.0	45	470	320
Other Beef Entrées/Dinners, Frozen					
Beef Macaroni Casserole (8.5 oz) Healthy Choice (ConAgra)	1.0	0.5	15	450	200
Beef Sirloin Meatballs and Gravy Light and Healthy Dinner (11 oz) The Budget Gourmet (Kraft General Foods)*	8.0	3.0	35	540	310
Meatloaf and Whipped Potatoes (9⅜ oz) Stouffer's Lean Cuisine (Stouffer's)	7.0	2.0	45	570	250
Sirloin Beef Peppercorn (8¾ oz) Stouffer's Lean Cuisine Cafe Classics (Stouffer's)	7.0	1.5	25	480	210

*Tobacco company, corporate subsidiary, or parent.

	Tot. Fat (g)	Sat. Fat (g)	Chol. (mg)	Sod. (mg)	Cal.
BEEF ENTRÉES/DINNERS, FROZEN *(cont'd)*					
Sirloin of Beef in Wine Sauce Light and Healthy Dinner (11 oz) The Budget Gourmet (Kraft General Foods)*	6.0	2.0	40	460	270
Special Recipe Sirloin of Beef Light and Healthy Dinner (11 oz) The Budget Gourmet (Kraft General Foods)*	7.0	3.0	25	550	310
Stuffed Pepper (10 oz) Stouffer's	8.0	1.5	25	900	200
CHICKEN ENTRÉES/DINNERS, FROZEN—*see also* Chicken Italian Entrées/Dinners, Frozen, page 281; Chicken Mexican Entrées/ Dinners, Frozen, page 286; Chicken Oriental Entrées/ Dinners, Frozen, page 287					
Baked Chicken Entrées/Dinners, Frozen					
Baked Chicken (8 oz) Stouffer's Lean Cuisine (Stouffer's)	5.0	0.5	35	480	240
Calypso Chicken (8½ oz) Stouffer's Lean Cuisine Cafe Classics (Stouffer's)	6.0	2.0	40	590	280
Barbecue Chicken Entrées/ Dinners, Frozen					
Barbecue Glazed Chicken (7.4 oz) Weight Watchers (H.J. Heinz)	3.5	1.0	20	340	190
Chicken in Honey Barbecue Sauce (8¾ oz) Stouffer's Lean Cuisine (Stouffer's)	4.5	1.0	50	560	250
Chicken in Mesquite Barbecue Sauce Light and Healthy Dinner (11 oz) The Budget Gourmet (Kraft General Foods)*	6.0	2.0	40	480	280

*Tobacco company, corporate subsidiary, or parent.

	Tot. Fat (g)	Sat. Fat (g)	Chol. (mg)	Sod. (mg)	Cal.
Mesquite Chicken BBQ (10.5 oz) Healthy Choice (ConAgra)	2.0	0.5	35	290	320
Smoky Chicken Barbecue (12.75 oz) Healthy Choice (ConAgra)	5.0	1.5	50	450	380
Chicken with Vegetables Entrées/Dinners, Frozen					
Chicken and Vegetables (10½ oz) Stouffer's Lean Cuisine (Stouffer's)	5.0	1.0	35	520	240
Chicken & Vegetables Marsala (11.5 oz) Healthy Choice (ConAgra)	1.0	0.0	30	440	220
Dijon/Honey Mustard Chicken Entrées/Dinners, Frozen					
Chicken Dijon (11 oz) Healthy Choice (ConAgra)	4.0	1.5	30	410	280
Honey Mustard Chicken Healthy Choice (ConAgra) (9.5 oz)	2.0	0.0	30	550	260
Weight Watchers Smart Ones (H.J. Heinz) (7.5 oz)	1.0	0.5	15	340	140
Honey Mustard Chicken Breast Light and Healthy Dinner (11 oz) The Budget Gourmet (Kraft General Foods)*	6.0	1.5	50	540	310
Glazed Chicken Entrées/Dinners, Frozen					
Country Glazed Chicken (8.5 oz) Healthy Choice (ConAgra)	1.5	0.5	30	480	200
Grilled Glazed Chicken (8 oz) Weight Watchers Smart Ones (H.J. Heinz)	1.0	0.0	10	460	130
Orange Glazed Chicken Breast Light and Healthy Entree (9 oz) The Budget Gourmet (Kraft General Foods)*	2.0	1.0	30	920	300
Roast Glazed Chicken (8.9 oz) Weight Watchers (H.J. Heinz) ..	5.0	2.5	15	510	200
Southwestern Glazed Chicken (12.5 oz) Healthy Choice (ConAgra)	3.0	1.0	45	430	300

*Tobacco company, corporate subsidiary, or parent.

	Tot. Fat (g)	Sat. Fat (g)	Chol. (mg)	Sod. (mg)	Cal.
CHICKEN ENTRÉES/DINNERS, FROZEN *(cont'd)*					
Herb Chicken Entrées/Dinners, Frozen					
Country Herb Chicken (11.5 oz) Healthy Choice (ConAgra)	4.0	1.5	35	340	270
Herb Roasted Chicken (8 oz) Stouffer's Lean Cuisine Cafe Classics (Stouffer's)	5.0	1.0	40	430	210
Herbed Chicken Breast with Fettucini Light and Healthy Dinner (11 oz) The Budget Gourmet (Kraft General Foods)*	8.0	3.0	65	620	300
Lemon Herb Chicken Piccata (7.5 oz) Weight Watchers Smart Ones (H.J. Heinz)	1.0	0.0	15	520	170
Roast Chicken Breast with Herb Gravy Light and Healthy Dinner (11 oz) The Budget Gourmet (Kraft General Foods)*	7.0	2.0	35	660	240
Orange Chicken Entrées/ Dinners, Frozen					
Chicken A L'Orange (8 oz) Weight Watchers Smart Ones (H.J. Heinz)	1.0	0.0	15	320	200
Chicken à l'Orange (9 oz) Stouffer's Lean Cuisine (Stouffer's)	2.5	0.5	40	260	260
Other Chicken Entrées/Dinners, Frozen					
Chicken Cordon Bleu (9 oz) Weight Watchers (H.J. Heinz)	6.0	2.0	20	500	220
Chicken Francais (8.5 oz) Weight Watchers Smart Ones (H.J. Heinz)	1.0	0.0	10	390	150
Chicken Francesca (12.5 oz) Healthy Choice (ConAgra)	5.0	2.0	30	500	360

*Tobacco company, corporate subsidiary, or parent.

	Tot. Fat (g)	Sat. Fat (g)	Chol. (mg)	Sod. (mg)	Cal.
Chicken Imperial (9 oz)					
Healthy Choice (ConAgra)	4.0	1.0	40	470	230
Chicken Marsala (8 oz)					
Weight Watchers Smart Ones (H.J. Heinz)	1.0	0.0	10	340	110
Chicken Mirabella (9.2 oz)					
Weight Watchers Smart Ones (H.J. Heinz)	1.0	0.0	10	480	160
CHILI ENTRÉES/DINNERS, FROZEN					
Three-Bean Chili (9 oz)					
Stouffer's Lean Cuisine (Stouffer's)	6.0	2.0	10	460	210
ITALIAN ENTRÉES/DINNERS, FROZEN					
Beef Italian Entrées/Dinners, Frozen					
Lasagna with Meat Sauce					
Stouffer's Lean Cuisine (Stouffer's) (10¼ oz)	6.0	2.5	25	560	270
Weight Watchers (H.J. Heinz) (10.3 oz)	6.0	2.0	5	510	270
Rigatoni (9 oz)					
Stouffer's Lean Cuisine (Stouffer's)	4.0	1.5	20	560	180
Spaghetti Bolognese (10 oz)					
Healthy Choice (ConAgra)	3.0	1.0	15	470	260
Spaghetti with Chunky Tomato and Meat Sauce (10 oz)					
The Budget Gourmet (Kraft General Foods)*	7.0	2.5	5	470	320
Spaghetti with Meat Sauce					
Stouffer's Lean Cuisine (Stouffer's) (11½ oz)	6.0	1.5	20	550	290
Weight Watchers (H.J. Heinz) (10 oz)	7.0	1.5	5	490	240
Spaghetti with Meatballs (9½ oz)					
Stouffer's Lean Cuisine (Stouffer's)	7.0	2.0	30	520	290
Chicken Italian Entrées/Dinners, Frozen					
Cacciatore Chicken (12.5 oz)					
Healthy Choice (ConAgra)	3.0	0.5	25	510	260

*Tobacco company, corporate subsidiary, or parent.

	Tot. Fat (g)	Sat. Fat (g)	Chol. (mg)	Sod. (mg)	Cal.
Italian Entrées/Dinners, Frozen *(cont'd)*					
Cheese Lasagna with Chicken Scaloppini (10 oz) Stouffer's Lean Cuisine Cafe Classics (Stouffer's)	8.0	2.5	40	560	290
Chicken Broccoli Alfredo (12.1 oz) Healthy Choice (ConAgra)	8.0	3.0	45	470	370
Chicken Cacciatore (10⅞ oz) Stouffer's Lean Cuisine (Stouffer's)	7.0	2.0	45	570	280
Chicken Carbonara (9 oz) Stouffer's Lean Cuisine Cafe Classics (Stouffer's)	8.0	2.0	40	540	290
Chicken Fettucini (9 oz) Stouffer's Lean Cuisine (Stouffer's)	6.0	2.5	45	580	270
Chicken Fettuccine Alfredo (8.5 oz) Healthy Choice (ConAgra)	3.0	1.0	30	370	250
Chicken Fettucini with Broccoli (10¼ oz) Stouffer's Lean Cuisine Lunch Express (Stouffer's)	8.0	3.5	40	570	290
Chicken Italiano (9 oz) Stouffer's Lean Cuisine (Stouffer's)	6.0	1.5	40	560	270
Chicken Marsala with Vegetables (8⅛ oz) Stouffer's Lean Cuisine (Stouffer's)	4.0	1.0	60	470	180
Chicken Mediterranean (10⅛ oz) Stouffer's Lean Cuisine Cafe Classics (Stouffer's)	4.0	1.0	30	570	250
Chicken Parmesan (10⅞) Stouffer's Lean Cuisine (Stouffer's)	5.0	1.5	50	530	220
Chicken Parmigiana (11.5 oz) Healthy Choice (ConAgra)	1.5	0.5	35	490	300
Chicken Picata (9 oz) Stouffer's Lean Cuisine Cafe Classics (Stouffer's)	6.0	1.5	30	540	290

	Tot. Fat (g)	Sat. Fat (g)	Chol. (mg)	Sod. (mg)	Cal.
Italian Style Vegetables and Chicken Light and Healthy Special Selection (10 oz) The Budget Gourmet (Kraft General Foods)*	7.0	2.0	25	660	280
Pasta and Chicken Marinara (9⅛ oz) Stouffer's Lean Cuisine Lunch Express (Stouffer's)	6.0	1.5	20	540	270
Rigatoni in Cream Sauce with Broccoli and Chicken Light and Healthy Special Selection (10.8 oz) The Budget Gourmet (Kraft General Foods)*	6.0	2.5	15	670	310
Meatless Italian Entrées/ Dinners, Frozen					
Angel Hair Pasta (10 oz) Stouffer's Lean Cuisine (Stouffer's)	4.0	1.0	0	420	210
Baked Cheese Ravioli (9 oz) Weight Watchers (H.J. Heinz)	6.0	2.0	15	560	280
Cheese Lasagna Casserole (9½ oz) Stouffer's Lean Cuisine Lunch Express (Stouffer's)	7.0	2.5	15	590	270
Cheese Ravioli Parmigiana (9 oz) Healthy Choice (ConAgra)	4.0	2.0	20	290	250
Cheese Tortellini with Tomato Sauce (9 oz) Weight Watchers (H.J. Heinz)	4.0	2.0	25	510	290
Classic Cheese Lasagna (11½ oz) Stouffer's Lean Cuisine (Stouffer's)	6.0	3.0	30	560	290
Fettuccine Alfredo (8 oz) Healthy Choice (ConAgra)	5.0	2.0	10	430	240
Fettucini Primavera (10 oz) Stouffer's Lean Cuisine (Stouffer's)	8.0	2.5	35	580	260
Garden Lasagna (11 oz) Weight Watchers (H.J. Heinz)	5.0	1.0	5	460	230
Italian Cheese Lasagna (11 oz) Weight Watchers (H.J. Heinz)	8.0	3.0	25	560	300

*Tobacco company, corporate subsidiary, or parent.

	Tot. Fat (g)	Sat. Fat (g)	Chol. (mg)	Sod. (mg)	Cal.
ITALIAN ENTRÉES/DINNERS, FROZEN *(cont'd)*					
Lasagna Florentine (10 oz)					
Weight Watchers Smart Ones (H.J. Heinz)	1.0	0.5	10	420	190
Lasagna Roma (13.5 oz)					
Healthy Choice (ConAgra)	5.0	2.0	15	550	390
Macaroni and Cheese and Broccoli (9¾ oz)					
Stouffer's Lean Cuisine Lunch Express (Stouffer's)	6.0	3.0	15	460	240
Marinara Twist (10 oz)					
Stouffer's Lean Cuisine (Stouffer's)	3.0	1.0	5	440	240
Pasta Italiano (12 oz)					
Healthy Choice (ConAgra)	4.0	1.0	10	360	340
Pasta Portafino (9.5 oz)					
Weight Watchers Smart Ones (H.J. Heinz)	1.0	0.0	0	270	150
Pasta Shells Marinara (12 oz)					
Healthy Choice (ConAgra)	3.0	1.5	25	390	360
Ravioli Florentine (8.5 oz)					
Weight Watchers Smart Ones (H.J. Heinz)	1.0	0.0	10	530	170
Vegetable Pasta Italiano (10 oz)					
Healthy Choice (ConAgra)	1.0	0.0	0	340	220
Vegetable Pizza (⅕ pizza)					
Tombstone Light (Kraft General Foods)*	7.0	2.5	10	500	240
Zucchini Lasagna					
Healthy Choice (ConAgra) (14 oz)	1.5	1.0	10	310	330
Stouffer's Lean Cuisine (Stouffer's) (11 oz)	4.0	1.5	15	470	240
Pizza Italian Entrées/Dinners, Frozen					
Deluxe French Bread Pizza (6⅛ oz)					
Stouffer's Lean Cuisine (Stouffer's)	6.0	2.5	30	560	330

*Tobacco company, corporate subsidiary, or parent.

	Tot. Fat (g)	Sat. Fat (g)	Chol. (mg)	Sod. (mg)	Cal.
Original Canadian Style Bacon Pizza (¼ pizza)					
Tombstone (Kraft General Foods)*	15.0	7.0	40	920	360
Pepperoni French Bread Pizza (5¼ oz)					
Stouffer's Lean Cuisine (Stouffer's)	7.0	3.0	25	590	330
Supreme Pizza (⅕ pizza)					
Tombstone Light (Kraft General Foods)*	9.0	3.5	20	710	270
Seafood Italian Entrées/ Dinners, Frozen					
Pasta and Tuna Casserole (9¾ oz)					
Stouffer's Lean Cuisine Lunch Express (Stouffer's)	6.0	2.0	20	590	280
Shrimp Marinara					
Healthy Choice (ConAgra) (10.5 oz)	0.5	0.0	50	220	220
Weight Watchers Smart Ones (H.J. Heinz) (8 oz)	1.0	0.0	25	400	150
Turkey Italian Entrées/Dinners, Frozen					
Pasta and Turkey Dijon (9⅞ oz)					
Stouffer's Lean Cuisine Lunch Express (Stouffer's)	6.0	1.5	30	570	270
Turkey Fettuccine alla Crema (12.5 oz)					
Healthy Choice (ConAgra)	4.0	1.5	30	370	350
Other Italian Entrées/Dinners, Frozen					
Penne Pasta with Chunky Tomato Sauce and Italian Sausage Light and Healthy Special Selection (10 oz)					
The Budget Gourmet (Kraft General Foods)*	8.0	2.5	10	530	330

*Tobacco company, corporate subsidiary, or parent.

	Tot. Fat (g)	Sat. Fat (g)	Chol. (mg)	Sod. (mg)	Cal.
MEATLESS ENTRÉES/DINNERS, FROZEN—*see* Meatless Italian Entrées/Dinners, Frozen, page 283; Meatless Mexican Entrées/ Dinners, Frozen, page 287; Meatless Pasta-Based Entrées/ Dinners, Frozen, page 289; VEGETABLE ENTRÉES/DINNERS, FROZEN, page 291					
MEXICAN ENTRÉES/DINNERS, FROZEN					
Beef Mexican Entrées/Dinners, Frozen					
Beef Enchiladas Rio Grande (13.4 oz)					
Healthy Choice (ConAgra)	8.0	3.0	15	480	410
Chicken Mexican Entrées/ Dinners, Frozen					
Chicken Enchilada Suiza					
Stouffer's Lean Cuisine (Stouffer's) (9 oz)	5.0	2.0	25	530	290
Chicken Enchiladas Suiza					
Healthy Choice (ConAgra) (10 oz)	4.0	2.0	25	440	270
Weight Watchers (H.J. Heinz) (9 oz)	7.0	1.5	40	530	230
Chicken Picante (11.3 oz)					
Healthy Choice (ConAgra)	2.0	1.5	35	330	220
Fiesta Chicken					
Stouffer's Lean Cuisine (Stouffer's) (8½ oz)	5.0	1.0	45	590	240
Weight Watchers Smart Ones (H.J. Heinz) (8 oz)	1.0	0.5	15	460	200
Fiesta Chicken Fajitas (7 oz)					
Healthy Choice (ConAgra)	4.0	1.0	30	410	260
Grilled Chicken Salsa (8⅞ oz)					
Stouffer's Lean Cuisine Cafe Classics (Stouffer's)	6.0	1.5	40	550	240
Grilled Chicken Suiza (8.6 oz)					
Weight Watchers (H.J. Heinz)	6.0	2.0	35	590	240

	Tot. Fat (g)	Sat. Fat (g)	Chol. (mg)	Sod. (mg)	Cal.
Mexican Style Rice with Chicken (9 oz)					
Stouffer's Lean Cuisine Lunch Express (Stouffer's)	8.0	1.5	20	590	270
Tex-Mex Chicken (8.3 oz)					
Weight Watchers (H.J. Heinz)	4.0	1.5	35	430	260
Meatless Mexican Entrées/ Dinners, Frozen					
Nacho Cheese Enchiladas (8.9 oz)					
Weight Watchers (H.J. Heinz)	6.0	2.5	25	520	250
ORIENTAL ENTRÉES/DINNERS, FROZEN					
Beef Oriental Entrées/Dinners, Frozen					
Beef & Peppers Cantonese (11.5 oz)					
Healthy Choice (ConAgra)	5.0	2.5	35	560	270
Beef Broccoli Beijing (12 oz)					
Healthy Choice (ConAgra)	3.0	1.0	20	500	330
Beef Pepper Steak Oriental (9.5 oz)					
Healthy Choice (ConAgra)	4.0	1.5	35	470	250
Green Pepper Steak (10½ oz)					
Stouffer's	9.0	3.0	35	650	330
Teriyaki Beef Light and Healthy Dinner (10.75 oz)					
The Budget Gourmet (Kraft General Foods)*	6.0	2.0	45	600	310
Chicken Oriental Entrées/ Dinners, Frozen					
Chicken Bangkok (9.5 oz)					
Healthy Choice (ConAgra)	4.0	.5	45	390	270
Chicken Cantonese (11.3 oz)					
Healthy Choice (ConAgra)	0.5	0.0	30	360	210
Chicken Chow Mein (9 oz)					
Weight Watchers Smart Ones (H.J. Heinz)	1.0	0.0	20	480	200
Chicken Chow Mein with Rice					
Stouffer's Lean Cuisine (Stouffer's) (9 oz)	5.0	1.0	35	510	210
Stouffer's Lunch Express (Stouffer's) (10⅝ oz)	4.0	1.0	30	940	260

*Tobacco company, corporate subsidiary, or parent.

Main Dishes and Meal-Type Products

	Tot. Fat (g)	Sat. Fat (g)	Chol. (mg)	Sod. (mg)	Cal.
ORIENTAL ENTRÉES/DINNERS, FROZEN *(cont'd)*					
Chicken in Peanut Sauce (9 oz)					
Stouffer's Lean Cuisine (Stouffer's)	6.0	1.0	45	590	280
Chicken Oriental (9 oz)					
Stouffer's Lean Cuisine (Stouffer's)	6.0	1.0	45	530	260
Chicken Oriental Light and Healthy Entree (9 oz)					
The Budget Gourmet (Kraft General Foods)*	6.0	2.0	20	700	300
Chicken Teriyaki (12.25 oz)					
Healthy Choice (ConAgra)	2.0	0.5	40	420	270
Ginger Chicken Hunan (12.6 oz)					
Healthy Choice (ConAgra)	2.5	0.5	25	430	350
Mandarin Chicken					
Healthy Choice (ConAgra) (10 oz)	2.5	0.0	25	520	280
Stouffer's Lean Cuisine Lunch Express (Stouffer's) (9¾ oz)	6.0	1.0	30	520	270
Mandarin Chicken Light and Healthy Entree (10 oz)					
The Budget Gourmet (Kraft General Foods)*	5.0	1.0	45	850	250
Sesame Chicken Shanghai (12 oz)					
Healthy Choice (ConAgra)	5.0	1.0	30	460	310
Spring Vegetables with Teriyaki Chicken (9 oz)					
Weight Watchers (H.J. Heinz)	2.0	1.0	20	440	150
Sweet & Sour Chicken (11.5 oz)					
Healthy Choice (ConAgra)	5.0	1.0	50	250	310
Sweet and Sour Chicken Original Entree (10 oz)					
The Budget Gourmet (Kraft General Foods)*	5.0	1.0	40	700	330
Sweet and Sour Chicken with Vegetables and Rice (10⅜ oz)					
Stouffer's Lean Cuisine (Stouffer's)	2.5	1.0	45	440	260

*Tobacco company, corporate subsidiary, or parent.

	Tot. Fat (g)	Sat. Fat (g)	Chol. (mg)	Sod. (mg)	Cal.
Teriyaki Chicken Breast with Oriental Style Vegetables Light and Healthy Dinner (11 oz)					
The Budget Gourmet (Kraft General Foods)*	6.0	1.0	35	800	290
Teriyaki Stir-Fry (9 oz)					
Stouffer's Lean Cuisine Lunch Express (Stouffer's)	5.0	1.0	30	550	260
Other Oriental Entrées/Dinners, Frozen					
Sweet & Sour Stir Fry Kit (10 oz)					
Gorton's (General Mills)	1.5	0.0	50	550	270
Teriyaki Stir Fry Kit (10 oz)					
Gorton's (General Mills)	1.5	0.0	50	1470	290
PASTA-BASED ENTRÉES/DINNERS, FROZEN—*see also* ITALIAN ENTRÉES/ DINNERS, FROZEN, page 281					
Beef Pasta-Based Entrées/ Dinners, Frozen					
Macaroni and Beef					
Stouffer's Lean Cuisine (Stouffer's) (10 oz)	8.0	2.0	25	550	280
Weight Watchers (H.J. Heinz) (9.5 oz)	5.0	1.5	15	540	230
Meatless Pasta-Based Entrées/ Dinners, Frozen					
Angel Hair Pasta (8.55 oz)					
Weight Watchers Smart Ones (H.J. Heinz)	1.0	0.0	5	320	150
Cheddar Bake (9 oz)					
Stouffer's Lean Cuisine (Stouffer's)	6.0	2.0	20	560	220
Macaroni & Cheese (9 oz)					
Healthy Choice (ConAgra)	5.0	2.0	15	580	290
Weight Watchers (H.J. Heinz)	6.0	2.0	20	550	260
One Serving Broccoli, Carrots & Rotini in Cheese Flavored Sauce (5.5 oz)					
Green Giant (Grand Metropolitan PLC)	2.0	<1.0	5	440	100

*Tobacco company, corporate subsidiary, or parent.

	Tot. Fat (g)	Sat. Fat (g)	Chol. (mg)	Sod. (mg)	Cal.
PASTA-BASED ENTRÉES/DINNERS, FROZEN *(cont'd)*					
Right for Lunch Tortellini Provencale (9.5 oz) Green Giant Garden Gourmet (Grand Metropolitan PLC)	6.0	2.0	15	840	260
SEAFOOD ENTRÉES/DINNERS, FROZEN—*see also* SEAFOOD ITALIAN ENTRÉES/DINNERS, FROZEN, page 285					
Lemon Pepper Fish (10.7 oz) Healthy Choice (ConAgra)	5.0	1.0	25	360	290
Shrimp and Vegetables Maria (12.5 oz) Healthy Choice (ConAgra)	2.0	0.5	35	540	260
Shrimp Mariner Light and Healthy Dinner (11 oz) The Budget Gourmet (Kraft General Foods)*	6.0	2.0	60	540	260
Tuna Noodle Casserole (9.5 oz) Weight Watchers (H.J. Heinz)	7.0	2.5	15	580	240
TURKEY ENTRÉES/DINNERS, FROZEN—*see also* TURKEY ITALIAN ENTRÉES/DINNERS, FROZEN, page 285					
Country Inn Roast Turkey (10 oz) Healthy Choice (ConAgra)	4.0	1.0	30	530	250
Country Roast Turkey with Mushrooms (8.5 oz) Healthy Choice (ConAgra)	4.0	1.0	25	440	220
Country Turkey and Pasta (12.6 oz) Healthy Choice (ConAgra)	4.0	2.0	35	450	300
Glazed Turkey Light and Healthy Entree (9 oz) The Budget Gourmet (Kraft General Foods)*	4.0	2.0	30	730	250
Homestyle Turkey (9⅜ oz) Stouffer's Lean Cuisine (Stouffer's)	6.0	1.5	50	590	230

*Tobacco company, corporate subsidiary, or parent.

	Tot. Fat (g)	Sat. Fat (g)	Chol. (mg)	Sod. (mg)	Cal.
Homestyle Turkey with Vegetables (9.5 oz)					
Healthy Choice (ConAgra)	2.0	0.5	35	490	260
Roast Turkey Medallions (8.5 oz)					
Weight Watchers Smart Ones (H.J. Heinz)	1.0	0.0	15	490	190
Roasted Turkey Breast (9¾ oz)					
Stouffer's Lean Cuisine (Stouffer's)	4.0	1.0	25	530	290
Stuffed Turkey Breast Light and Healthy Dinner (11 oz)					
The Budget Gourmet (Kraft General Foods)*	6.0	2.0	35	660	260
Traditional Breast of Turkey (10.5 oz)					
Healthy Choice (ConAgra)	3.0	1.0	45	460	280
Turkey Dinner (Mostly White Meat) (11½ oz)					
Swanson Hungry Man (Campbell Soup Co)	7.0	2.0	35	970	310
VEGETABLE ENTRÉES/DINNERS, FROZEN—*see also* MEATLESS ITALIAN ENTRÉES/DINNERS, FROZEN, page 283					
Broccoli and Cheese Baked Potato (10 oz)					
Weight Watchers (H.J. Heinz)	7.0	2.0	10	510	230
Cheddar Broccoli Potatoes (10 oz)					
Healthy Choice (ConAgra)	5.0	2.0	10	550	310
Garden Potato Casserole (9.25 oz)					
Healthy Choice (ConAgra)	4.0	1.5	10	520	200
Right for Lunch Asparagus Pilaf (9.5 oz)					
Green Giant Garden Gourmet (Grand Metropolitan PLC)	4.0	2.0	10	610	190
Stuffed Cabbage (9½ oz)					
Stouffer's Lean Cuisine (Stouffer's)	7.0	1.5	25	460	220

*Tobacco company, corporate subsidiary, or parent.

MEAT, POULTRY, SEAFOOD, AND MEAT SUBSTITUTES

If you're looking for an easy way to cut the fat, saturated fat, and cholesterol from your diet, you've come to the right chapter. Most Americans eat too much protein. It's a good idea to eat only about 6 ounces a day. By reducing the amount of protein you eat and choosing lean meat and poultry without skin, you'll cut out a lot of the fat.

In the grocery, you'll find that the meats lowest in fat are labeled "select," higher-fat meats are "choice," and the meats highest in fat are "prime." To cut your fat intake, choose "select," "lean," or "extra lean" meats. Also, trim the fat before cooking. And choose seafood often. Most seafood is naturally low in total fat and saturated fat. (Different kinds of seafood have varying amounts of cholesterol, however.)

Like all the other entries in this book, the meat, poultry, seafood, and meat substitutes entries that follow list sodium content. The AHA does not have criteria for sodium but recommends a total of no more than 3,000 mg a day.

Generic Listings

By far, most of the foods in this book are brand name products. However, if a product is listed without a brand name, it means that most brands of that product contain about the same amount of fat, saturated fat, and cholesterol and that these amounts are within the criteria cited below.

If you find products that were introduced after this book went to press, use the generic listings and the following tables to help you evaluate them.

AHA Criteria for Meat, Poultry, Seafood, and Meat Substitutes*

	Tot. Fat (g)	Sat. Fat (g)	Chol. (mg)
Seafood and game, cooked (3 oz)	5	2	95
Seafood and poultry, canned (2 oz)	3	1	20
Luncheon meat, processed, including hot dogs and sausage (2 oz)	6	2	55
Meat and poultry, cooked (3 oz)	9	3	80
Meat, canned	6	2	55
Meat substitutes (2 oz)	3	1	<2

*Per serving.

Meat, Poultry, Seafood, and Meat Substitutes You'll Want to Limit

Some meat, poultry, seafood, and meat substitutes, like the examples below, are too high in fat, saturated fat, and/or cholesterol to meet AHA criteria. They aren't included in this book, and we recommend that you don't eat them often.

Compare the amounts of fat, saturated fat, cholesterol, sodium, and calories in these examples with the more healthful alternatives listed on the following pages.

Sample Meat, Poultry, Seafood, and Meat Substitutes to Limit

	Tot. Fat (g)	Sat. Fat (g)	Chol. (mg)	Sod. (mg)	Cal.
Bacon, broiled (1 oz)	34.9*	4.9*	24	451	162
Beef bologna (1 oz)	8.1*	3.4*	16	278	88
Beef liver, braised (3 oz)	4.2	1.6	331*	59	137
Chicken, dark meat with skin, stewed (3 oz)	12.4*	3.4*	69	59	197
Duck, domesticated, without skin, roasted (3 oz)	9.5*	3.5*	76	55	171
Ground beef (regular), pan-fried (3 oz)	19.2*	7.5*	75	71	260
Link pork sausage (2 oz, or about 3½ sml links, 2″ long and ¾″ in diam)	18.0*	6.4*	38	851	221
Picnic ham, lean and fat, roasted (3 oz)	18.2*	6.5*	49	912	238
Prime rib of beef, lean and fat, fat trimmed to ¼″ (3 oz)	29.6*	12.3*	72	54	348
Shrimp, boiled, shells removed (3 oz)	0.9	0.2	166*	190	84

Adapted from USDA Handbook No. 8 series.

*These values exceed AHA criteria for meat, poultry, and seafood.

	Tot. Fat (g)	Sat. Fat (g)	Chol. (mg)	Sod. (mg)	Cal.
BEEF—*see also* LUNCHEON MEAT, BEEF LUNCHEON MEAT, page 299					
CANNED BEEF					
Sliced Dried Beef					
Armour Star (Dial Corp) (7 slices)	1.5	0.5	25	1370	60
Hormel (10 slices)	1.5	0.5	25	1240	50
FRESH OR FROZEN BEEF					
Ground Beef, Fresh or Frozen					
Ground beef, 7% fat, with carrageenan or oat bran, no added salt, cooked (3 oz)	7.0	(2.5)	64	(53)	149
Ground beef, 7% fat, with carrageenan or oat bran, salt added, cooked (3 oz)	7.0	(2.5)	64	(238)	149
Steak, Fresh or Frozen					
Beef bottom round, choice, lean only					
Trimmed to 0″ fat, roasted (3 oz)	6.6	2.2	66	56	164
Trimmed to ¼″ fat, roasted (3 oz)	7.1	2.4	66	56	168
Beef bottom round, select, lean only					
Trimmed to 0″ fat, roasted (3 oz)	4.6	1.5	66	56	146
Trimmed to ¼″ fat, roasted (3 oz)	5.3	1.8	66	56	152
Beef eye of round, select, lean only					
Trimmed to 0″ fat, roasted (3 oz)	3.0	1.1	59	53	132
Trimmed to ¼″ fat, roasted (3 oz)	3.4	1.2	59	53	136
Beef tenderloin, select, lean only					
Trimmed to 0″ fat, broiled (3 oz) .	7.5	2.8	71	54	170
Trimmed to ¼″ fat, broiled (3 oz)	7.4	2.8	71	54	169
Beef top round, choice, lean only					
Trimmed to 0″ fat, roasted (3 oz)	5.4	1.9	69	55	153
Trimmed to ¼″ fat, roasted (3 oz)	6.2	2.2	69	55	160

	Tot. Fat (g)	Sat. Fat (g)	Chol. (mg)	Sod. (mg)	Cal.
Fresh or Frozen Beef *(cont'd)*					
Beef top round, select, lean only					
Trimmed to 0″ fat, roasted (3 oz)	4.5	1.6	69	55	145
Trimmed to ¼″ fat, roasted (3 oz)	5.4	1.9	69	55	153
Beef top loin, choice, lean only					
Trimmed to 0″ fat, broiled (3 oz)	8.2	3.1	65	58	177
Beef top loin, select, lean only					
Trimmed to 0″ fat, broiled (3 oz)	5.9	2.2	65	58	157
Trimmed to ¼″ fat, broiled (3 oz)	6.6	2.5	65	58	164
Beef top round, choice, lean only					
Trimmed to 0″ fat, braised (3 oz)	4.9	1.7	76	38	176
Trimmed to ¼″ fat, braised (3 oz)	5.5	1.9	76	38	181
Trimmed to ¼″ fat, broiled (3 oz)	5.0	1.7	71	52	160
Beef top round, select, lean only					
Trimmed to 0″ fat, braised (3 oz)	3.4	1.2	76	38	162
Trimmed to ¼″ fat, braised (3 oz)	3.9	1.3	76	38	166
Trimmed to ¼″ fat, broiled (3 oz)	3.1	1.1	71	52	143
Beef top sirloin, choice, lean only					
Trimmed to 0″ fat, broiled (3 oz)	6.6	2.6	76	56	170
Trimmed to ¼″ fat, broiled (3 oz)	6.8	2.7	76	56	172
Beef top sirloin, select, lean only					
Trimmed to 0″ fat, broiled (3 oz)	4.8	1.9	76	56	153
Trimmed to ¼″ fat, broiled (3 oz)	5.3	2.1	76	56	158
Other Beef, Fresh or Frozen					
Beef ribs, small end, select, lean only					
Trimmed to 0″ fat, broiled (3 oz)	7.4	3.0	68	59	168
Trimmed to ¼″ fat, broiled (3 oz)	8.2	3.3	68	59	176
Trimmed to ¼″ fat, roasted (3 oz)	8.3	3.3	67	61	172
Beef shank, crosscuts, choice, lean only					
Trimmed to ¼″ fat, simmered (3 oz)	5.4	1.9	54	66	171
Beef tripe, raw (3 oz)	3.4	1.7	80	39	84

	Tot. Fat (g)	Sat. Fat (g)	Chol. (mg)	Sod. (mg)	Cal.
Preseasoned Beef					
Teriyaki Seasoned Boneless Beef Rib Eye Steaks (7 oz raw) Menu Maker by Rymer (Rymer Foods)	10.0	4.0	95	560	240
CHICKEN—*see also* LUNCHEON MEAT, Chicken Luncheon Meat, page 300					
Canned Chicken					
Premium Chunk White Chicken in Water (¼ cup) Swanson (Campbell Soup Co)	1.0	1.0	15	240	80
Fresh or Frozen Chicken					
Dark Meat Chicken, Fresh or Frozen					
Chicken dark meat					
Without skin, roasted (3 oz)	8.3	2.3	79	79	174
Without skin, stewed (3 oz)	7.6	2.1	75	63	163
Chicken drumstick					
Without skin, roasted (1.6 oz)	2.5	0.7	41	42	76
Without skin, stewed (1.6 oz)	2.6	0.7	40	37	78
Chicken thigh					
Without skin, stewed (2 oz)	5.6	1.5	50	42	110
White Meat Chicken, Fresh or Frozen					
Chicken breast					
Meat and skin, roasted (3 oz)	6.6	1.9	72	60	167
Meat and skin, stewed (3 oz)	6.3	1.8	64	53	156
Without skin, roasted (3 oz)	3.1	0.9	73	63	142
Without skin, stewed (3 oz)	2.6	0.7	65	52	129
Chicken light meat					
With skin, stewed (3 oz)	8.4	2.4	63	54	171
Without skin, roasted (3 oz)	3.8	1.1	72	66	147
Without skin, stewed (3 oz)	3.4	1.0	65	55	135
Chicken wing					
Without skin, roasted (¾ oz)	1.7	0.5	18	19	43
Without skin, stewed (1 oz)	2.0	0.6	21	21	50
Preseasoned Chicken					
Butter Seasoned Boneless, Skinless Chicken Breasts (3.5 oz) Menu Maker by Rymer (Rymer Foods)	2.0	1.0	50	430	110

	Tot. Fat (g)	Sat. Fat (g)	Chol. (mg)	Sod. (mg)	Cal.
PRESEASONED CHICKEN *(cont'd)*					
Lemon Herb Boneless, Skinless Chicken Breasts (3.5 oz) Menu Maker by Rymer (Rymer Foods)	1.0	0.0	50	290	110
Southern Style Breaded Boneless, Skinless Chicken Breasts (3.5 oz) Menu Maker by Rymer (Rymer Foods)	1.0	0.0	40	1070	130
Teriyaki Seasoned Boneless, Skinless Chicken Breasts (3.5 oz) Menu Maker by Rymer (Rymer Foods)	1.0	0.0	50	400	110
FISH—*see* SEAFOOD, page 311					
GAME					
Beefalo, roasted (3 oz)	5.4	2.3	49	70	160
Deer, roasted (3 oz)	2.7	1.1	95	46	134
Elk, roasted (3 oz)	1.6	0.6	62	52	124
Goat, roasted (3 oz)	2.6	0.8	64	73	122
Moose, roasted (3 oz)	0.8	0.3	66	58	114
Rabbit, domesticated, stewed (3 oz)	7.2	2.1	73	31	175
Squirrel, roasted (3 oz)	3.1	0.4	80	80	116
HAM—*see* LUNCHEON MEAT, HAM (DELI TYPE) LUNCHEON MEAT, page 301; PORK, HAM, page 309					
HOT DOGS—*see* LUNCHEON MEAT, GAME LUNCHEON MEAT, page 300; TURKEY LUNCHEON MEAT, page 308					
LAMB					
Lamb, cubed for stew or kebab (leg and shoulder), lean only, broiled (3 oz)	6.2	2.2	77	65	158
Lamb, leg, shank half, choice, lean only roasted (3 oz)	5.7	2.0	74	56	153

	Tot. Fat (g)	Sat. Fat (g)	Chol. (mg)	Sod. (mg)	Cal.
Lamb, loin, choice, lean only					
Broiled (3 oz)	8.3	3.0	80	71	183
Roasted (3 oz)	8.3	3.2	74	56	171
Lamb loin chops, lean only, broiled (3 oz)	8.3	3.0	80	71	183
Lamb, shoulder, arm, choice, lean only					
Broiled (3 oz)	7.7	2.9	78	70	170
Roasted (3 oz)	7.9	3.1	73	57	163
LUNCHEON MEAT					
BEEF LUNCHEON MEAT—*see also* BEEF, page 295					
Beef and Pork Luncheon Meat					
Honey Loaf (1 slice)					
Oscar Mayer (Oscar Mayer Foods)*	1.0	0.0	15	380	35
Beef Bologna Luncheon Meat					
Bologna (2 slices)					
Oscar Mayer Healthy Favorites (Oscar Mayer Foods)*	1.0	0.0	15	510	45
Beef Pastrami Luncheon Meat					
Pastrami 97% Fat Free (2 oz)					
Healthy Choice (Armour Swift-Eckrich)	1.5	0.5	30	500	60
Corned Beef Luncheon Meat					
Corned Roast Beef 97% Fat Free (2 oz)					
Healthy Choice (Armour Swift-Eckrich)	1.5	1.0	30	460	60
Roast Beef Luncheon Meat					
Medium Roast Beef 98% Fat Free (2 oz)					
Healthy Choice (Armour Swift-Eckrich)	1.5	1.0	25	450	60
Roast Beef (4 slices)					
Oscar Mayer Deli-Thin (Oscar Mayer Foods)*	1.5	0.5	25	530	60
Structured Roast Beef 98% Fat Free (2 oz)					
Healthy Choice (Armour Swift-Eckrich)	1.0	0.5	25	480	50

*Tobacco company, corporate subsidiary, or parent.

	Tot. Fat (g)	Sat. Fat (g)	Chol. (mg)	Sod. (mg)	Cal.
BEEF LUNCHEON MEAT *(cont'd)*					
Sausage Luncheon Meat					
New England Brand Sausage (2 slices)					
Oscar Mayer (Oscar Mayer Foods)*	2.5	1.0	25	570	60
CHICKEN LUNCHEON MEAT—*see also* CHICKEN, page 297					
Roasted Chicken Luncheon Meat					
Deluxe Oven Roasted Chicken Breast (1 slice)					
Louis Rich (Louis Rich Co)*	1.0	0.0	15	330	30
Oven Roasted Chicken Breast (4 slices)					
Louis Rich Deli-Thin (Louis Rich Co)*	1.5	0.5	25	620	60
Oscar Mayer Healthy Favorites (Oscar Mayer Foods)*	0.0	0.0	25	620	40
Oven Roasted White Chicken (1 slice)					
Louis Rich (Louis Rich Co)*	2.5	0.5	15	350	40
Skinless Fat Free Chicken Breast (2 oz)					
Healthy Choice (Armour Swift-Eckrich)	0.0	0.0	25	460	45
Smoked Chicken Luncheon Meat					
Hickory Smoked Chicken Breast (1 slice)					
Louis Rich (Louis Rich Co)*	1.0	0.0	15	360	30
Other Chicken Luncheon Meat					
Chicken roll, light (3 oz)					
Most brands (USDA)	**6.3**	**1.7**	**42**	**497**	**135**
Honey Glazed Chicken Breast (4 slices)					
Oscar Mayer Deli-Thin (Oscar Mayer Foods)*	1.0	0.0	25	740	60
GAME LUNCHEON MEAT—*see also* GAME, page 298					
Beefalo Beef Franks (1 hot dog)					
Errot's Blue Ridge (Blue Ridge Beefalo)	5.0	2.0	na	na	90

*Tobacco company, corporate subsidiary, or parent.

	Tot. Fat (g)	Sat. Fat (g)	Chol. (mg)	Sod. (mg)	Cal.
HAM (DELI TYPE) LUNCHEON MEAT—					
see also **PORK, HAM, page 309**					
Baked/Roasted Ham Luncheon Meat					
Baked Cooked Ham 98% Fat Free with Natural Juices (1 slice)					
Hafnia Lean & Low (International Trading Co)	0.5	0.0	15	380	30
Baked Ham, water added					
Oscar Mayer (Oscar Mayer Foods)* (3 slices)	1.0	0.5	30	720	60
Oscar Mayer Healthy Favorites (Oscar Mayer Foods)* (4 slices)	1.0	0.0	25	600	50
Baked Ham with Natural Juices (2 slices)					
Louis Rich Carving Board Meats (Louis Rich Co)*	1.0	0.0	25	510	45
Boiled Ham Luncheon Meat					
Boiled Ham, water added					
Oscar Mayer (Oscar Mayer Foods)* (3 slices)	2.5	1.0	30	820	60
Oscar Mayer Deli-Thin (Oscar Mayer Foods)* (4 slices)	2.0	0.5	25	680	50
Chopped Ham Luncheon Meat					
Chopped Ham 95% Fat Free with Natural Juices (1 slice)					
Hafnia Lean & Low (International Trading Co)	1.0	0.0	15	380	35
Cooked Ham Luncheon Meat					
Cooked Ham 97% Fat Free (2 oz)					
Healthy Choice (Armour Swift-Eckrich)	1.5	0.5	25	460	60
96% Fat Free Cooked Ham Water Added (1 slice)					
Continental Lean & Low (International Trading Co)	1.0	0.0	15	380	30
Danish Ham Luncheon Meat					
Danish Ham 98% Fat Free with Natural Juices (1 slice)					
Hafnia Lean & Low (International Trading Co)	0.5	0.0	15	380	25

*Tobacco company, corporate subsidiary, or parent.

	Tot. Fat (g)	Sat. Fat (g)	Chol. (mg)	Sod. (mg)	Cal.
Ham (Deli Type) Luncheon Meat *(cont'd)*					
98% Fat Free Danish Ham with Natural Juices (2 oz) Hafnia Lean & Low (International Trading Co)	1.0	0.0	26	760	50
97% Fat Free Danish Ham Water Added (2 oz) Hafnia Lean & Low (International Trading Co)	1.5	0.5	26	760	60
Thin Sliced Danish Ham 98% Fat Free with Natural Juices (2 slices) Hafnia Lean & Low (International Trading Co)	1.0	0.0	25	760	50
Honey Ham Luncheon Meat					
Honey Ham 97% Fat Free (Deli) (2 oz) Healthy Choice (Armour Swift-Eckrich)	1.5	0.5	25	580	60
Honey Ham, water added					
Oscar Mayer (Oscar Mayer Foods)* (3 slices)	2.5	1.0	30	760	70
Oscar Mayer Deli-Thin (Oscar Mayer Foods)* (4 slices)	2.0	0.5	25	630	60
Oscar Mayer Healthy Favorites (Oscar Mayer Foods)* (4 slices)	1.5	0.5	25	630	50
Honey Ham with Natural Juices, Thin Carved (6 slices) Louis Rich Carving Board Meats (Louis Rich Co)*	2.0	1.0	35	760	70
Honey Ham with Natural Juices, Traditional Carved (2 slices) Louis Rich Carving Board Meats (Louis Rich Co)*	1.5	0.5	25	530	50
98% Fat Free Honey Ham with Natural Juices (2 oz) Hafnia Lean & Low (International Trading Co)	0.5	0.0	25	760	50

*Tobacco company, corporate subsidiary, or parent.

	Tot. Fat (g)	Sat. Fat (g)	Chol. (mg)	Sod. (mg)	Cal.
Lower-Salt Ham Luncheon Meat					
Less Sodium Boneless Cooked Ham (2 oz)					
Alpine Lace (Alpine Lace Brands)	2.0	1.0	25	380	60
Lower Sodium Ham 98% Fat Free with Natural Juices (1 slice)					
Hafnia Lean & Low (International Trading Co)	0.5	0.0	15	240	25
Lower Sodium Ham, water added (3 slices)					
Oscar Mayer (Oscar Mayer Foods)*	2.5	1.0	30	520	70
98% Fat Free Lower Sodium Ham with Natural Juices (2 oz)					
Hafnia Lean & Low (International Trading Co)	1.0	0.0	25	480	50
Smoked Ham Luncheon Meat					
Smoked Cooked Ham, water added					
Oscar Mayer (Oscar Mayer Foods)* (3 slices)	2.5	1.0	30	750	60
Oscar Mayer Deli-Thin (Oscar Mayer Foods)* (4 slices)	2.0	0.5	25	620	50
Oscar Mayer Healthy Favorites (Oscar Mayer Foods)* (4 slices)	1.5	0.5	25	620	50
Smoked Ham Cooked with Natural Juices (2 slices)					
Louis Rich Carving Board Meats (Louis Rich Co)*	1.5	0.5	25	560	50
Smoked Ham 97% Fat Free (2 oz)					
Healthy Choice (Armour Swift-Eckrich)	1.5	0.5	30	390	60
Other Ham Luncheon Meat					
98% Fat Free Ham Water Added (1 slice)					
Continental Lean & Low (International Trading Co)	0.5	0.0	15	380	25
Hafnia Lean & Low (International Trading Co)	0.5	0.0	15	380	25

*Tobacco company, corporate subsidiary, or parent.

	Tot. Fat (g)	Sat. Fat (g)	Chol. (mg)	Sod. (mg)	Cal.
HAM (DELI TYPE) LUNCHEON MEAT *(cont'd)*					
98% Fat Free Ham with Natural Juices (1 slice)					
Hafnia Lean & Low (International Trading Co)	0.5	0.0	15	380	25
97% Fat Free Ham Water Added (1 slice)					
Continental Lean & Low (International Trading Co)	1.0	0.0	15	380	30
Hafnia Lean & Low (International Trading Co)	1.0	0.0	15	380	30
97% Fat Free Ham with Natural Juices (1 slice)					
Hafnia Lean & Low (International Trading Co)	0.5	0.0	15	380	30
Virginia Brand 97% Fat Free Ham (2 oz)					
Healthy Choice (Armour Swift-Eckrich)	1.5	0.5	25	510	60
PORK LUNCHEON MEAT—*see also* LUNCHEON MEAT, BEEF AND PORK, page 299; PORK, page 309					
Canadian Bacon—*see* PORK, CANADIAN BACON, page 309					
Ham Luncheon Meat—*see* LUNCHEON MEAT, HAM (DELI TYPE), page 301; PORK, HAM, page 309					
Hot Dogs—*see* LUNCHEON MEAT, GAME, page 300; Turkey, below					
TURKEY LUNCHEON MEAT—*see also* TURKEY, page 310					
Honey Turkey Breast Luncheon Meat					
Honey Roasted & Smoked Fat Free Turkey Breast (2 oz)					
Healthy Choice (Armour Swift-Eckrich)	0.0	0.0	25	410	60

	Tot. Fat (g)	Sat. Fat (g)	Chol. (mg)	Sod. (mg)	Cal.
Honey Roasted & Smoked Skinless Turkey Breast (2 oz)					
Butterball (Armour Swift-Eckrich)	0.0	0.0	25	490	60
Honey Roasted Breast of Turkey Dinner Slices (1 slice)					
Louis Rich (Louis Rich Co)*	1.0	0.5	35	940	80
Honey Roasted Turkey Breast (1 slice)					
Louis Rich (Louis Rich Co)*	1.0	0.0	10	320	30
Smoked Honey Roasted Turkey (4 slices)					
Oscar Mayer Deli-Thin (Oscar Mayer Foods)*	1.0	0.0	20	520	60
Roasted Turkey Breast Luncheon Meat					
Fat Free Oven Roasted Turkey Breast					
Louis Rich (Louis Rich Co)* (1 slice)	0.0	0	10	310	25
Louis Rich Deli-Thin (Louis Rich Co)* (4 slices)	0.0	0	15	610	40
Oven Roasted Breast of Turkey Dinner Slices (1 slice)					
Louis Rich (Louis Rich Co)*	1.0	0.0	35	910	70
Oven Roasted Low Sodium Skinless Turkey Breast (2 oz)					
Butterball (Armour Swift-Eckrich)	0.0	0.0	25	310	50
Oven Roasted Skinless Turkey Breast (2 oz)					
Butterball (Armour Swift-Eckrich)	0.0	0.0	20	440	50
Oven Roasted Turkey Breast					
Louis Rich (Louis Rich Co)* (1 slice)	0.5	0.0	10	310	30
Louis Rich Deli-Thin (Louis Rich Co)* (4 slices)	1.0	0.0	20	580	50
Oscar Mayer Healthy Favorites (Oscar Mayer Foods)* (4 slices) .	0.0	0.0	15	610	40
Oven Roasted Turkey Breast, Thin Carved (6 slices)					
Louis Rich Carving Board Meats (Louis Rich Co)*	0.5	0	25	740	60

*Tobacco company, corporate subsidiary, or parent.

	Tot. Fat (g)	Sat. Fat (g)	Chol. (mg)	Sod. (mg)	Cal.
TURKEY LUNCHEON MEAT *(cont'd)*					
Oven Roasted Turkey Breast, Traditional Carved (2 slices)					
Louis Rich Carving Board Meats (Louis Rich Co)*	0.5	0	20	560	40
Roast Turkey (4 slices)					
Oscar Mayer Deli-Thin (Oscar Mayer Foods)*	1.0	0.0	20	580	50
Smoked Turkey Breast Luncheon Meat					
Fat Free Hickory Smoked Turkey Breast (1 slice)					
Louis Rich (Louis Rich Co)*	0.0	0	10	300	25
Hickory Smoked Breast of Turkey Dinner Slices (1 slice)					
Louis Rich (Louis Rich Co)*	1.0	0.0	35	1060	80
Smoked Fat Free Turkey Breast (2 oz)					
Healthy Choice (Armour Swift-Eckrich)	0.0	0.0	25	410	50
Smoked Skinless Turkey Breast (2 oz)					
Butterball (Armour Swift-Eckrich)	0.0	0.0	25	430	50
Smoked Turkey Breast					
Louis Rich (Louis Rich Co)* (1 slice)	0.5	0.0	10	260	25
Louis Rich Carving Board Meats (Louis Rich Co)* (2 slices)	0.5	0	20	560	40
Louis Rich Deli-Thin (Louis Rich Co)* (4 slices)	1.0	0.0	20	490	50
Oscar Mayer Healthy Favorites (Oscar Mayer Foods)* (4 slices)	0.0	0.0	15	550	40
Smoked White Turkey (1 slice)					
Louis Rich (Louis Rich Co)*	1.0	0.0	15	290	30
Other Turkey Breast Luncheon Meat					
Browned 99% Fat Free Turkey Breast (2 oz)					
Healthy Choice (Armour Swift-Eckrich)	0.5	0.0	25	420	50

*Tobacco company, corporate subsidiary, or parent.

	Tot. Fat (g)	Sat. Fat (g)	Chol. (mg)	Sod. (mg)	Cal.
98% Fat Free Turkey Breast (1 slice)					
Hafnia Lean & Low (International Trading Co)	0.5	0.0	15	380	25
97% Fat Free Turkey Breast (1 slice)					
Continental Lean & Low (International Trading Co)	1.0	0.0	15	380	25
Skinless Fat Free Turkey Breast (2 oz)					
Healthy Choice (Armour Swift-Eckrich)	0.0	0.0	20	380	45
Turkey Ham Luncheon Meat					
Chopped Turkey Ham, 10% water added (1 slice)					
Louis Rich (Louis Rich Co)*	2.5	1.0	20	290	40
Hickory Cured Turkey Ham, 10% water added (3 slices)					
Louis Rich (Louis Rich Co)*	2.0	0.5	45	660	15
95% Fat Free Turkey Ham Cured Turkey Thigh Meat 15% Water Added (1 slice)					
Continental Lean & Low (International Trading Co)	1.0	0.0	15	380	30
Hafnia Lean & Low (International Trading Co)	1.0	0.0	15	380	30
Turkey Ham (2 oz)					
Louis Rich (Louis Rich Co)*	2.0	1.0	40	640	60
Turkey ham, cured, thigh meat (3 oz)					
Most brands (USDA)	**4.3**	**1.5**	**(16)**	**848**	**110**
Turkey Ham, 15% water added (2 oz)					
Louis Rich (Louis Rich Co)*	3.0	1.0	45	640	70
Turkey Ham, 10% water added					
Louis Rich (Louis Rich Co)* (1 round slice)	1.0	1.0	20	300	35
Louis Rich (Louis Rich Co)* (3 square slices)	2.5	0.5	45	710	70
Louis Rich Deli-Thin (Louis Rich Co)* (4 slices)	1.5	0.5	35	580	60

*Tobacco company, corporate subsidiary, or parent.

	Tot. Fat (g)	Sat. Fat (g)	Chol. (mg)	Sod. (mg)	Cal.
TURKEY LUNCHEON MEAT *(cont'd)*					
Turkey Hot Dogs					
Hot Dogs made with Turkey and Beef (1 link)					
Oscar Mayer Healthy Favorites (Oscar Mayer Foods)*	1.5	0.5	25	570	60
Turkey Pastrami Luncheon Meat					
Turkey Pastrami					
Most brands (USDA) (1 oz)	**1.8**	**0.5**	**15**	**297**	**40**
Louis Rich (Louis Rich Co)* (2 square slices)	1.5	0.0	30	520	45
Louis Rich (Louis Rich Co)* (2 oz)	2.0	1.0	40	590	70
Turkey Salami Luncheon Meat					
Turkey Cotto Salami (1 slice)					
Louis Rich (Louis Rich Co)*	2.5	1.0	25	290	40
Turkey Salami (1 slice)					
Louis Rich (Louis Rich Co)*	2.5	1.0	20	290	45
Turkey Sausage Luncheon Meat					
Ground Turkey Sausage (2.5 oz)					
Louis Rich (Louis Rich Co)*	6.0	2.5	50	580	110
Turkey & Cheddar Smoked Sausage (2 oz)					
Louis Rich (Louis Rich Co)*	5.0	2.0	35	550	90
Turkey Polska Kielbasa (2 oz)					
Louis Rich (Louis Rich Co)*	4.5	1.5	35	510	80
Turkey Sausage Links (2 links)					
Louis Rich (Louis Rich Co)*	6.0	1.5	45	470	90
Turkey Smoked Sausage (2 oz)					
Louis Rich (Louis Rich Co)*	5.0	1.5	35	510	90
Other Turkey Luncheon Meat					
Turkey roll, light and dark meat (3 oz)					
Most brands (USDA)	**5.9**	**1.7**	**47**	**498**	**126**
MEAT SUBSTITUTES					
Italian Style Harvest Burgers (1 burger)					
Green Giant (Grand Metropolitan PLC)	4.5	1.5	0	370	140

*Tobacco company, corporate subsidiary, or parent.

	Tot. Fat (g)	Sat. Fat (g)	Chol. (mg)	Sod. (mg)	Cal.
Original Flavor Harvest Burgers (1 burger)					
Green Giant (Grand Metropolitan PLC)	4.0	1.5	0	380	140
Sausage Style Breakfast Patties (1 patty)					
Green Giant (Grand Metropolitan PLC)	3.0	1.0	0	230	90
Southwestern Style Harvest Burgers (1 burger)					
Green Giant (Grand Metropolitan PLC)	4.0	1.5	0	370	140
Vegi-Patties (1 patty)					
Lifestream Natural Foods	3.0	0.0	0	440	140
PORK—*see also* LUNCHEON MEAT, HAM (DELI TYPE), page 301					
CANADIAN BACON					
Canadian bacon, grilled (3 oz)					
Most brands (USDA)	**7.2**	**2.4**	**49**	**1316**	**157**
Canadian Style Bacon (2 slices)					
Oscar Mayer (Oscar Mayer Foods)*	2.0	1.0	25	600	50
FRESH OR FROZEN PORK					
Fresh pork, boneless loin chops, lean only, broiled (3 oz)	6.6	2.3	68	55	173
Fresh pork, boneless loin roasts, lean only, roasted (3 oz)	6.4	2.4	66	38	165
Fresh pork, boneless sirloin chops,					
Lean and fat, broiled (3 oz)	7.3	2.5	78	47	177
Lean only, broiled (3 oz)	5.7	1.9	78	48	164
Fresh pork, loin chops, lean only, broiled (3 oz)	6.9	2.5	70	51	171
HAM					
Baked Cooked Ham Dinner Slices, water added (1 slice)					
Louis Rich (Louis Rich Co)*	1.5	0.5	40	1150	80
Boneless extra lean ham, canned, roasted (3 oz)					
Most brands (USDA)	**4.1**	**1.4**	**25**	**966**	**116**

*Tobacco company, corporate subsidiary, or parent.

	Tot. Fat (g)	Sat. Fat (g)	Chol. (mg)	Sod. (mg)	Cal.
HAM *(cont'd)*					
Boneless extra lean ham, roasted (3 oz)					
Most brands (USDA)	**4.7**	**1.5**	**45**	**1023**	**123**
Chunk Ham (2 oz)					
Hormel	6.0	2.0	30	600	90
Dinner Ham Slice, water added (3 oz)					
Oscar Mayer (Oscar Mayer Foods)*	3.0	1.0	45	1030	90
Dinner Ham Steak (1 slice)					
Hafnia Lean & Low (International Trading Co)	2.0	0.5	45	1520	100
Dinner Ham Steak, water added (1 steak)					
Oscar Mayer (Oscar Mayer Foods)*	2.0	0.5	30	750	60
OTHER PORK					
Pickled Pigs Feet (2 oz)					
Hormel	6.0	2.0	45	530	80
TURKEY—*see also* LUNCHEON MEAT, TURKEY LUNCHEON MEAT, page 304					
CANNED TURKEY					
Premium Chunk White Turkey in Water (¼ cup)					
Swanson (Campbell Soup Co)	2.0	1.0	35	220	90
COOKED TURKEY					
Barbecued Skinless Breast of Turkey (2 oz)					
Louis Rich (Louis Rich Co)*	1.0	0	25	680	60
Hickory Smoked Skinless Breast of Turkey (2 oz)					
Louis Rich (Louis Rich Co)*	0.5	0	25	760	60
Honey Roasted Skinless Breast of Turkey (2 oz)					
Louis Rich (Louis Rich Co)*	0.5	0	25	690	60
Oven Roasted Skinless Breast of Turkey (2 oz)					
Louis Rich (Louis Rich Co)*	0.5	0	25	650	50

*Tobacco company, corporate subsidiary, or parent.

	Tot. Fat (g)	Sat. Fat (g)	Chol. (mg)	Sod. (mg)	Cal.
Oven Roasted Turkey Breast (2 oz)					
Louis Rich (Louis Rich Co)*	1.5	0.5	25	640	60
Fresh or Frozen Turkey					
Ground Turkey (3 oz)					
Louis Rich (Louis Rich Co)*	9.0	2.5	70	105	140
Turkey, dark meat, without skin, roasted (3 oz)	6.1	2.1	72	67	159
Turkey, light meat, meat only, roasted (3 oz)	2.7	0.9	59	54	133
Turkey, young toms, dark meat without skin, roasted (3 oz)	5.9	2.0	75	70	158
Turkey, young toms, light meat only, roasted (3 oz)	2.5	0.8	59	58	129
Turkey, young toms, light meat with skin, roasted (3 oz)	6.5	1.8	64	57	163
Turkey, young toms, meat only, roasted (3 oz)	4.0	1.3	66	63	143
SEAFOOD					
Canned Seafood					
Clams					
Minced Clams					
Crown-Prince (about ⅓ cup)	0.0	0.0	15	310	45
Progresso (Pet) (¼ cup)	0.0	0.0	10	250	25
Ocean Chopped and Minced Clams, undrained (¼ cup)					
Gorton's (General Mills)	0.0	0.0	10	360	20
Mackerel					
Mackerel, drained solids (3 oz)					
Most brands (USDA)	**5.4**	**1.5**	**67**	**322**	**132**
Salmon					
Chum salmon, drained solids with bone (3 oz)					
Most brands (USDA)	**4.7**	**1.3**	**33**	**414**	**120**
Tuna					
Light tuna in water, drained solids (3 oz)					
Most brands (USDA)	**0.4**	**0.1**	**(20)**	**303**	**111**

*Tobacco company, corporate subsidiary, or parent.

	Tot. Fat (g)	Sat. Fat (g)	Chol. (mg)	Sod. (mg)	Cal.
FRESH OR FROZEN SEAFOOD					
Bass—*see* Sea Bass, page 313					
Cod					
Atlantic cod, cooked, dry heat (3 oz)	0.7	0.1	47	66	89
Cod Cakes (4 oz)					
Gorton's (General Mills)	0.5	0	15	640	100
Pacific cod, cooked, dry heat (3 oz) .	0.7	0.1	40	77	89
Crab, imitation					
Imitation Alaska king crab, made from surimi (3 oz)					
Most brands (USDA)	**1.1**	**(0.2)**	**17**	**715**	**87**
Flounder					
Flounder, cooked, dry heat (3 oz) . . .	1.3	0.3	58	89	99
Natural Flounder Fillets (1 fillet)					
Van de Kamp's (Pet)	2.0	0.0	45	105	110
Grouper					
Grouper, cooked, dry heat (3 oz) . . .	1.1	0.3	40	45	100
Haddock					
Haddock, cooked, dry heat (3 oz) . .	0.8	0.1	63	74	95
Halibut					
Halibut, cooked, dry heat (3 oz)	2.5	0.4	35	59	119
Ocean Perch					
Ocean perch, cooked, dry heat (3 oz)	1.8	0.3	46	82	103
Octopus					
Octopus, common, cooked, moist heat (3 oz)	1.8	0.4	82	(50)	140
Orange Roughy					
Orange roughy, cooked, dry heat (3 oz)	0.8	0.0	22	69	75
Pike					
Northern pike, cooked, dry heat (3 oz)	0.8	0.1	43	42	96
Pollack, Walleye					
Walleye pollack, cooked, dry heat (3 oz)	1.0	0.2	82	98	96
Red Snapper—*see* Snapper, page 313					
Redfish—*see* Ocean Perch, above					

	Tot. Fat (g)	Sat. Fat (g)	Chol. (mg)	Sod. (mg)	Cal.
Rockfish					
Rockfish, cooked, dry heat (3 oz)	1.7	0.4	38	65	103
Salmon					
Chinook salmon, smoked (3 oz)	3.7	0.8	20	666	99
Chum salmon, cooked, dry heat (3 oz)	4.1	0.9	81	54	131
Pink salmon, cooked, dry heat (3 oz)	3.8	0.6	57	73	127
Scallops, Imitation					
Imitation scallops, made from surimi (3 oz)					
Most brands (USDA)	**0.4**	**0.1**	**18**	**676**	**84**
Scrod—*see* Atlantic Cod, page 312					
Sea Bass					
Bass, freshwater, cooked, dry heat (3 oz)	4.0	0.9	74	87	124
Sea bass, cooked, dry heat (3 oz)	2.2	0.6	45	74	105
Shrimp, Imitation					
Shrimp, imitation, made from surimi (3 oz)					
Most brands (USDA)	**1.3**	**0.3**	**31**	**599**	**86**
Snapper					
Snapper, cooked, dry heat (3 oz)	1.5	0.3	40	48	109
Sole					
Natural Sole Fillets (1 fillet)					
Van de Kamp's (Pet)	1.5	0.0	50	125	110
Seafood Stuffed Sole (1 portion)					
Gorton's (General Mills)	2.0	0.5	40	500	150
Select Sole Country Herb (2 portions)					
Gorton's (General Mills)	3.0	0.5	75	320	110
Surimi—*see* Crab, Imitation, page 312; Scallops, Imitation, above; Shrimp, Imitation, above					
Swordfish					
Swordfish, cooked, dry heat (3 oz)	4.4	1.2	43	98	132
Trout					
Rainbow trout, cooked, dry heat (3 oz)	3.7	0.7	62	29	129

	Tot. Fat (g)	Sat. Fat (g)	Chol. (mg)	Sod. (mg)	Cal.
FRESH OR FROZEN SEAFOOD *(cont'd)*					
Tuna					
Bluefin tuna, fresh, cooked, dry heat (3 oz)	5.3	1.4	42	43	157
Yellowfin tuna, fresh, cooked, dry heat (3 oz)	1.0	0.3	49	40	118
Whiting					
Whiting, cooked, dry heat (3 oz)	1.4	0.3	71	113	98
Other Fresh or Frozen Seafood					
Beach Haven Breaded Fish Sticks (4 sticks)					
Mrs. Paul's (Campbell Soup Co)	3.0	2.0	20	350	170
Breaded Fish Fillets					
Mrs. Paul's Healthy Treasures (Campbell Soup Co) (3-oz fillet) .	3.0	1.0	25	220	130
Mrs. Paul's Healthy Treasures (Campbell Soup Co) (4-oz fillet) .	3.0	2.0	30	290	170
Breaded Fish Sticks (3 oz)					
Mrs. Paul's Healthy Treasures (Campbell Soup Co)	3.0	2.0	20	350	170
Crisp & Healthy Breaded Fish Fillets (2 fillets)					
Van de Kamp's (Pet)	2.5	0.5	30	380	150
Crisp & Healthy Breaded Fish Sticks (6 sticks)					
Van de Kamp's (Pet)	3.0	0.5	25	440	180
Kitchen Fillets in Sauce (1 fillet)					
Mrs. Paul's (Campbell Soup Co)	5.0	2.0	25	450	120
SMOKED SEAFOOD					
Smoked whitefish (3 oz)					
Most brands (USDA)	**0.8**	**0.2**	**28**	**866**	**92**

PASTA, RICE, AND OTHER GRAIN PRODUCTS

Some people think that pasta and rice are high in calories and fat. But that's not true.

The good news is that pasta, rice, and other grains are reasonably low in calories and contain little if any total fat, saturated fat, and cholesterol. For example, pasta made without egg yolks has less than 1 gram of fat per cup, and it's under 200 calories. It's what you put on top—the rich cream and oily pesto sauces—that adds the fat and calories.

When buying pasta, look for products made without egg yolks, because egg yolks add cholesterol.

Like all the other entries in this book, the pasta, rice, and other grain products entries that follow list sodium content. The AHA does not have criteria for sodium but recommends a total of no more than 3,000 mg a day.

Generic Listings

By far, most of the foods in this book are brand name products. However, if a product is listed without a brand name, it means that most brands of that product contain about the same amount of fat, saturated fat, and cholesterol and that these amounts are within the criteria cited below.

If you find products that were introduced after this book went to press, use the generic listings and the following tables to help you evaluate them.

AHA Criteria for Pasta, Rice, and Other Grain Products*

	Tot. Fat (g)	Sat. Fat (g)	Chol. (mg)
Pasta, rice, and other grain products	3	<0.5	<2
Pasta salad	3	1	<2

*Per serving.

Pasta, Rice, and Other Grain Products You'll Want to Limit

Some pasta, rice, and other grain products, like the examples below, are too high in fat, saturated fat, and/or cholesterol to meet AHA criteria. They aren't included in this book, and we recommend that you don't eat them often.

Compare the amounts of fat, saturated fat, cholesterol, sodium, and calories in these examples with the more healthful alternatives listed on the following pages.

Sample Rice and Other Grain Products to Limit

	Tot. Fat (g)	Sat. Fat (g)	Chol. (mg)	Sod. (mg)	Cal.
Chinese chow mein noodles (0.9 oz)	7.7*	1.1*	0	110	132
Rice made from commercial seasoned mix with margarine (5 oz)	6.0*	1.4*	1	833	189

Adapted from USDA Handbook No. 8 series.

*These values exceed AHA criteria for rice and other grain products.

	Tot. Fat (g)	Sat. Fat (g)	Chol. (mg)	Sod. (mg)	Cal.
BULGUR					
Bulgur (¼ cup dry)					
Arrowhead Mills (Arrowhead Mills)	0.5	0.0	0	0	150
COUSCOUS					
Couscous (1 cup cooked)					
Most brands (USDA)	**<1.0**	**0.0**	**0**	**9**	**201**
PASTA/NOODLES					
MACARONI—*see also* NOODLES, below					
Cooked Macaroni					
Macaroni (1 cup)					
Most brands (USDA)	**1.0**	**<1.0**	**0**	**1**	**197**
Vegetable macaroni (1 cup)					
Most brands (USDA)	**<1.0**	**0.0**	**0**	**9**	**171**
Whole wheat macaroni (1 cup)					
Most brands (USDA)	**1.0**	**<1.0**	**0**	**4**	**174**
Dry Macaroni					
Macaroni (2 oz)					
Most brands (USDA)	**1.0**	**0.0**	**0**	**0**	**210**
Spiral Pasta (⅔ cup)					
Pritikin (Quaker Oats Co)	1.0	0.0	0	10	190
Tri-Colored Rotini (2 oz)					
Creamette (Borden)	1.0	0.0	0	20	210
Tri-Colored Shells (2 oz)					
Creamette (Borden)	1.0	0.0	0	20	210
Tricolor Twists (2 oz)					
Mueller's (Best Foods)	1.0	0.0	0	10	210
NOODLES—*see also* MACARONI, above					
Cooked Noodles					
Noodles, Japanese soba (1 cup)					
Most brands (USDA)	**<1.0**	**0.0**	**0**	**68**	**113**
Noodles, Japanese somen (1 cup)					
Most brands (USDA)	**<1.0**	**0.0**	**0**	**284**	**230**

	Tot. Fat (g)	Sat. Fat (g)	Chol. (mg)	Sod. (mg)	Cal.
NOODLES *(cont'd)*					
Dry Noodles					
Bean Thread (Sai Fun) (1 cup)					
Ka-me (Shaffer, Clarke & Co) . . .	0.0	0.0	0	0	190
Chinese Plain Noodles (½ cup)					
Ka-me (Shaffer, Clarke & Co) . . .	0.0	0.0	0	1	200
Chinese Wide Lo Mein Noodles (½ cup)					
Ka-me (Shaffer, Clarke & Co) . . .	0.0	0.0	0	1	200
Cholesterol-Free Noodle Style Pasta (2 oz)					
Mueller's (Best Foods)	1.0	0.0	0	10	210
Curly Noodles (Chuka Soba) (2 oz)					
Ka-me (Shaffer, Clarke & Co) . . .	1.0	0.0	0	310	200
Japanese Buckwheat Noodles (Shin Shu Soba) (2 oz)					
Ka-me (Shaffer, Clarke & Co) . . .	1.0	0.0	0	80	200
Japanese Thick Noodles (Udon) (2 oz)					
Ka-me (Shaffer, Clarke & Co) . . .	1.0	0.0	0	670	190
Lasagna (2 oz)					
Most brands	**1.0**	**0.0**	**0**	**0**	**210**
Manicotti Creamette (Borden) (3 pieces)	1.0	0.0	0	0	180
Rice Sticks (Py Mai Fun) (2 oz)					
Ka-me (Shaffer, Clarke & Co) . . .	0.0	0.0	0	100	193
Somen Noodles (Tomoshiraga) (2 oz)					
Ka-me (Shaffer, Clarke & Co) . . .	1.0	0.0	0	670	190
PASTA—*see also* SPAGHETTI, page 319					
Dry Pasta					
All-American Pasta (2 oz)					
Buckeye Beans & Herbs	1.0	0.0	0	5	210
Pasta (2 oz)					
Most brands	**1.0**	**0.0**	**0**	**0**	**210**
Tri-Colored Wheels (2 oz)					
Creamette (Borden)	1.0	0.0	0	20	210
Various pasta shapes (2 oz)					
Buckeye Beans & Herbs	1.0	0.0	0	5	210

	Tot. Fat (g)	Sat. Fat (g)	Chol. (mg)	Sod. (mg)	Cal.
Pasta Mixes					
Macaroni and Cheese Sauce Alternative (⅔ cup)					
Förmagg (Galaxy Foods)	2.0	0.0	0	470	190
Penne Pasta Alfredo Alternative (⅔ cup)					
Förmagg (Galaxy Foods)	2.0	0.0	0	470	190
Penne Pasta Primavera Alternative (⅔ cup)					
Förmagg (Galaxy Foods)	2.0	0.0	0	470	190
Vegetable Pasta & Caesar Italian Garden Alternative (⅔ cup)					
Förmagg (Galaxy Foods)	2.0	0.0	0	470	190
SPAGHETTI					
Cooked Spaghetti					
Spaghetti (1 cup)					
Most brands (USDA)	**0.9**	**0.1**	**0**	**1**	**197**
Spinach spaghetti (1 cup)					
Most brands (USDA)	**1.0**	**0.0**	**0**	**20**	**183**
Spinach Fettuccini (2 oz)					
Creamette (Borden)	1.0	0.0	0	25	210
Whole wheat spaghetti, cooked (1 cup)					
Most brands (USDA)	**1.0**	**0.0**	**0**	**4**	**174**
Whole Wheat Thin Spaghetti (⅛ box)					
Pritikin (Quaker Oats Company)	1.0	0.0	0	0	190
Refrigerated Spaghetti					
Angel's Hair (2 oz)					
DiGiorno (Kraft General Foods)*	1.0	0.0	0	190	160
Fettuccine (2.5 oz)					
DiGiorno (Kraft General Foods)*	1.5	0.0	0	125	190
Herb Linguine (2.5 oz)					
DiGiorno (Kraft General Foods)*	1.5	0.0	0	125	190
Linguine (2.5 oz)					
DiGiorno (Kraft General Foods)*	1.5	0.0	0	125	190
Spinach Fettuccine (2.5 oz)					
DiGiorno (Kraft General Foods)*	1.5	0.0	0	140	190

*Tobacco company, corporate subsidiary, or parent.

	Tot. Fat (g)	Sat. Fat (g)	Chol. (mg)	Sod. (mg)	Cal.
RICE					
CANNED RICE					
Chinese Fried Rice (¾ cup)					
La Choy (Hunt-Wesson)	1.0	0.1	0	820	190
Spanish Rice (1 cup)					
Old El Paso (Pet)	1.0	<1.0	0	1340	130
Van Camp's (Quaker Oats Company)	3.0	0.5	0	1290	180
INSTANT/QUICK-COOKING RICE					
Brown Instant/Quick-Cooking Rice					
Brown Rice (½ cup dry)					
Success (Riviana Foods)	2.1	0.4	0	17	345
Instant Whole Grain Brown Rice, made without fat or salt (⅔ cup cooked)					
Minute (Kraft General Foods)*	1.5	0.0	0	10	170
White Instant/Quick-Cooking Rice					
Boil-in-Bag Rice, made without fat or salt (1 cup cooked)					
Minute (Kraft General Foods)*	0.0	0.0	0	10	190
Long Grain Enriched Parboiled Rice (¼ cup dry)					
Canilla Dorado (Producers Rice Mill)	0.0	0.0	0	0	170
Original Rice, made without fat or salt (¾ cup cooked)					
Minute (Kraft General Foods)*	0.0	0.0	0	10	170
Premium Long Grain Rice, made without fat or salt (1 cup cooked)					
Minute (Kraft General Foods)*	0.0	0.0	0	10	170
White Rice (½ cup dry)					
Success (Riviana Foods)	0.0	0.0	0	5	190
Other Instant/Quick-Cooking Rice					
Beef Oriental (½ cup dry)					
Success (Riviana Foods)	0.5	0.0	0	920	190
Broccoli & Cheese (½ cup dry)					
Success (Riviana Foods)	2.0	1.0	10	690	200

*Tobacco company, corporate subsidiary, or parent.

	Tot. Fat (g)	Sat. Fat (g)	Chol. (mg)	Sod. (mg)	Cal.
Brown & Wild Rice (½ cup dry)					
Success (Riviana Foods)	1.0	0.0	0	830	190
Classic Chicken Rice (½ cup dry)					
Success (Riviana Foods)	1.0	0.0	0	720	150
Long Grain & Wild Rice (½ cup dry)					
Success (Riviana Foods)	0.0	0.0	0	890	190
Long Grain & Wild Rice Mix, made without fat (1 cup cooked)					
Minute (Kraft General Foods)*	0.5	0.0	0	960	230
Rice Pilaf (½ cup dry)					
Success (Riviana Foods)	0.0	0.0	0	630	200
Spanish Rice (½ cup dry)					
Success (Riviana Foods)	0.5	0.0	0	780	190
REGULAR-COOKING RICE					
Brown Regular-Cooking Rice					
Extra Long Grain Brown Rice (¼ cup dry)					
Carolina (Riviana Foods)	1.0	0.0	0	0	150
Mahatma (Riviana Foods)	1.0	0.0	0	0	150
Long-grain brown rice, made without salt (1 cup cooked)					
Most brands (USDA)	**2.0**	**0.0**	**0**	**9**	**216**
Mixed Regular-Cooking Rice					
Long Grain & Wild Rice Mix (2 oz dry)					
Mahatma (Riviana Foods)	0.5	0.0	0	1240	190
White Regular-Cooking Rice					
Extra Long Grain White Rice (¼ cup dry)					
Carolina (Riviana Foods)	1.0	0.0	0	0	150
Mahatma (Riviana Foods)	0.0	0.0	0	0	150
Long Grain Rice (¼ cup dry)					
Water Maid (Riviana Foods)	0.0	0.0	0	0	160
Long-grain rice, made without fat and salt (1 cup cooked)					
Most brands (USDA)	**1.0**	**0.0**	**0**	**4**	**264**
Wild Regular-Cooking Rice					
Wild rice, made without salt (1 cup cooked)					
Most brands (USDA)	**1.0**	**0.0**	**0**	**6**	**166**

*Tobacco company, corporate subsidiary, or parent.

	Tot. Fat (g)	Sat. Fat (g)	Chol. (mg)	Sod. (mg)	Cal.
REGULAR-COOKING RICE *(cont'd)*					
Yellow Regular-Cooking Rice					
Yellow Rice Mix (2 oz dry)					
Mahatma (Riviana Foods)	0.0	0.0	0	970	190
Other Regular-Cooking Rice					
Black Beans & Rice Mix (2 oz dry)					
Mahatma (Riviana Foods)	1.5	0.0	0	850	200
Broccoli with Cheese & Long Grain Rice (2 oz dry)					
Mahatma (Riviana Foods)	1.5	0.5	5	620	200
Jambalaya Mix (2 oz dry)					
Mahatma (Riviana Foods)	1.0	0.0	0	700	190
Pilaf Rice Mix (2 oz dry)					
Mahatma (Riviana Foods)	0.0	0.0	0	820	190
Red Beans & Rice Mix (2 oz dry)					
Mahatma (Riviana Foods)	1.0	0.0	0	790	190
Sesame Chicken Rice Mix (2 oz dry)					
Mahatma (Riviana Foods)	1.5	0.0	0	970	190
Spanish Rice Mix (2 oz dry)					
Mahatma (Riviana Foods)	0.5	0.0	0	760	180

SALAD DRESSINGS AND SANDWICH SPREADS

Salad lovers will jump for joy when they see the dozens of nonfat and low-fat dressings listed on the following pages. Of course, some of the dressings and sandwich spreads we've listed are high in total fat, but they contain almost no saturated fat or cholesterol when prepared according to package directions.

Like all the other entries in this book, the salad dressings and sandwich spreads entries that follow list sodium content. The AHA does not have criteria for sodium but recommends a total of no more than 3,000 mg a day.

If you find products that were introduced after this book went to press, use the listings and the following tables to help you evaluate them.

AHA Criteria for Salad Dressings and Sandwich Spreads*

	Tot. Fat (g)	Sat. Fat (g)	Chol. (mg)
All salad dressings and sandwich spreads	**	1	<2

*Per serving.

**No criterion; these foods are naturally high in fat but low in saturated fat.

Salad Dressings You'll Want to Limit

Some salad dressings, like the examples below, are too high in fat, saturated fat, and/or cholesterol to meet AHA criteria. They aren't included in this book, and we recommend that you don't eat them often.

Compare the amounts of fat, saturated fat, cholesterol, sodium, and calories in these examples with the more healthful alternatives listed on the following pages.

Sample Salad Dressings and Sandwich Spreads to Limit

	Tot. Fat (g)	Sat. Fat (g)	Chol. (mg)	Sod. (mg)	Cal.
French dressing (2 tbsp)	12.8	3.0*	(18)*	427	134
Italian dressing (2 tbsp)	14.2	2.0*	(0)	232	137
Mayonnaise (1 tbsp)	11.0	1.6*	8*	78	99

Adapted from USDA Handbook No. 8 series.

*These values exceed AHA criteria for salad dressings and sandwich spreads.

	Tot. Fat (g)	Sat. Fat (g)	Chol. (mg)	Sod. (mg)	Cal.
BLUE CHEESE SALAD DRESSINGS					
Blue Cheese Dressing Mix (1 tbsp prepared)					
Weight Watchers (H.J. Heinz)	0.0	0.0	0	110	8
Blue Cheese Flavor Salad Dressing (2 tbsp)					
Kraft Free (Kraft General Foods)*	0.0	0.0	0	340	50
Blue Cheese Salad Dressing (2 tbsp)					
Healthy Sensation! (T.J. Lipton)	0.0	0.0	0	300	35
Light Blue Cheese Salad Dressing (2 tbsp)					
Henri's (Henri's Food Products)	2.0	0.5	0	430	60
Luscious Creamy Blue Cheese Low Fat Dressing (2 tbsp)					
Marie's (Campbell Soup Co)	2.0	0.0	0	270	45
BUTTERMILK/RANCH SALAD DRESSINGS—*see also* CUCUMBER SALAD DRESSINGS, page 326					
Buttermilk Ranch Salad Dressing (2 tbsp)					
Smart Temptations (American Specialty Brands)	0.0	0.0	0	230	20
Fat Free Ranch Salad Dressing					
Henri's (Henri's Food Products) (2 tbsp)	0.0	0.0	0	340	40
Medford Farms (Chelten House Products) (2 tbsp)	0.0	0.0	0	230	20
Seven Seas Free (Kraft General Foods)* (2 tbsp)	0.0	0.0	0	330	50
Walden Farms (WFI Corp) (2 tbsp)	0.0	0.0	0	290	25
Weight Watchers Salad Celebrations (H.J. Heinz) (2 tbsp)	0.0	0.0	0	270	35
Weight Watchers Salad Celebrations (H.J. Heinz) (single-serving pkt)	0.0	0.0	0	200	25

*Tobacco company, corporate subsidiary, or parent.

	Tot. Fat (g)	Sat. Fat (g)	Chol. (mg)	Sod. (mg)	Cal.
BUTTERMILK/RANCH SALAD DRESSINGS *(cont'd)*					
Fat Free Ranch with Sun Dried Tomato Salad Dressing (2 tbsp)					
Walden Farms (WFI Corp)	0.0	0.0	0	290	25
Luscious Zesty Ranch Low Fat Dressing (2 tbsp)					
Marie's (Campbell Soup Co) ...	2.0	0.0	0	330	45
Peppercorn Ranch Salad Dressing (2 tbsp)					
Kraft Free (Kraft General Foods)*	0.0	0.0	0	360	50
Ranch Salad Dressing (2 tbsp)					
Healthy Sensation! (T.J. Lipton) .	0.0	0.0	0	270	40
Herb Magic (Reily Foods Co) ...	0.0	0.0	0	270	15
Kraft Free (Kraft General Foods)*	0.0	0.0	0	310	50
CAESAR SALAD DRESSINGS					
Caesar Reduced Calorie Dressing (2 tbsp)					
Kraft Deliciously Right (Kraft General Foods)*	5.0	1.0	<5	560	60
Fat Free Caesar Salad Dressing					
Medford Farms (Chelten House Products) (2 tbsp)	0.0	0.0	0	200	15
Walden Farms (WFI Corp) (2 tbsp)	0.0	0.0	0	360	25
Weight Watchers Salad Celebrations (H.J. Heinz) (2 tbsp)	0.0	0.0	0	390	10
Weight Watchers Salad Celebrations (H.J. Heinz) (single-serving pkt)	0.0	0.0	0	290	5
CUCUMBER SALAD DRESSINGS—*see also* BUTTERMILK/RANCH SALAD DRESSINGS, page 325					
Creamy Cucumber Dressing (2 tbsp)					
Herb Magic (Reily Foods Co) ...	0.0	0.0	0	270	15

*Tobacco company, corporate subsidiary, or parent.

	Tot. Fat (g)	Sat. Fat (g)	Chol. (mg)	Sod. (mg)	Cal.
Cucumber Ranch Reduced Calorie Dressing (2 tbsp) Kraft Deliciously Right (Kraft General Foods)*	5.0	1.0	0	450	60
FRENCH SALAD DRESSINGS					
Catalina French Reduced Calorie Dressing (2 tbsp) Kraft Deliciously Right (Kraft General Foods)*	4.0	0.5	0	400	80
Catalina Salad Dressing (2 tbsp) Kraft Free (Kraft General Foods)*	0.0	0.0	0	360	45
Fat Free French Salad Dressing (2 tbsp) Henri's (Henri's Food Products)	0.0	0.0	0	240	45
Fat Free French Style (2 tbsp) Weight Watchers Salad Celebrations (H.J. Heinz)	0.0	0.0	0	200	40
French Reduced Calorie Dressing (2 tbsp) Kraft Deliciously Right (Kraft General Foods)*	3.0	0.5	0	260	50
French Salad Dressing (2 tbsp) Kraft Free (Kraft General Foods)*	0.0	0.0	0	300	50
French Style Dressing Mix (1 tbsp prepared) Weight Watchers (H.J. Heinz)	0.0	0.0	0	150	3
French Style Salad Dressing (2 tbsp) Pritikin (Quaker Oats Company)	0.0	0.0	0	130	35
Honey French Salad Dressing (2 tbsp) Pritikin (Quaker Oats Company)	0.0	0.0	0	135	40
Light Hearty French Salad Dressing (2 tbsp) Henri's (Henri's Food Products)	2.0	0.0	0	200	60
Light Original French Salad Dressing (2 tbsp) Henri's (Henri's Food Products)	2.0	0.0	0	280	70
Light Tas-Tee French Salad Dressing (2 tbsp) Henri's (Henri's Food Products)	2.0	0.0	0	220	60

*Tobacco company, corporate subsidiary, or parent.

	Tot. Fat (g)	Sat. Fat (g)	Chol. (mg)	Sod. (mg)	Cal.
FRENCH SALAD DRESSINGS (*cont'd*)					
Lite French Style Salad Dressing (2 tbsp)					
Wish-Bone (T.J. Lipton)	1.0	0.0	0	280	45
HERB SALAD DRESSINGS—*see also* ITALIAN SALAD DRESSINGS, page 329; VINAIGRETTE SALAD DRESSINGS, page 333					
Fat Free Creamy Dill Dressing (2 tbsp)					
Medford Farms (Chelten House Products)	0.0	0.0	0	260	20
Zesty Herb Salad Dressing Mix for Fat Free Dressing, made with vinegar and water (2 tbsp)					
Good Seasons (Kraft General Foods)*	0.0	0.0	0	260	10
HONEY DIJON/HONEY MUSTARD SALAD DRESSINGS					
Fat Free Honey Dijon (2 tbsp)					
Weight Watchers Salad Celebrations (H.J. Heinz)	0.0	0.0	0	150	45
Fat Free Honey Dijon Vinaigrette Salad Dressing (2 tbsp)					
Walden Farms (WFI Corp)	0.0	0.0	0	240	25
Fat Free Honey Mustard Salad Dressing (2 tbsp)					
Henri's (Henri's Food Products)	0.0	0.0	0	180	50
Medford Farms (Chelten House Products)	0.0	0.0	0	200	30
French Honey Dijon Salad Dressing (2 tbsp)					
Smart Temptations (American Specialty Brands)	0.0	0.0	0	250	20
Honey Dijon Salad Dressing (2 tbsp)					
Healthy Sensation! (T.J. Lipton)	0.0	0.0	0	390	45
Kraft Free (Kraft General Foods)*	0.0	0.0	0	330	50
Pritikin (Quaker Oats Company)	0.0	0.0	0	130	45

*Tobacco company, corporate subsidiary, or parent.

	Tot. Fat (g)	Sat. Fat (g)	Chol. (mg)	Sod. (mg)	Cal.
Honey Mustard Salad Dressing (2 tbsp)					
Henri's (Henri's Food Products)	6.0	1.0	0	230	100
Honey Mustard Salad Dressing Mix for Fat Free Dressing, made with vinegar and water (2 tbsp)					
Good Seasons (Kraft General Foods)*	0.0	0.0	0	280	20
HONEY MUSTARD SALAD DRESSINGS—*see* HONEY DIJON/HONEY MUSTARD SALAD DRESSINGS, above					
ITALIAN SALAD DRESSINGS—*see also* VINAIGRETTE SALAD DRESSINGS, page 333					
CREAMY ITALIAN SALAD DRESSINGS					
Creamy Italian Dressing Mix (1 tbsp)					
Weight Watchers (H.J. Heinz)	0.0	0.0	0	180	3
Creamy Italian Reduced Calorie Dressing (2 tbsp)					
Kraft Deliciously Right (Kraft General Foods)*	5.0	1.0	0	250	50
Seven Seas (Kraft General Foods)*	5.0	1.0	0	490	60
Creamy Italian Salad Dressing Mix for Fat Free Dressing, made with skim milk, vinegar, and water (2 tbsp)					
Good Seasons (Kraft General Foods)*	0.0	0.0	0	280	20
Fat Free Creamy Italian Salad Dressing (2 tbsp)					
Medford Farms (Chelten House Products)	0.0	0.0	0	230	15
Weight Watchers Salad Celebrations (H.J. Heinz)	0.0	0.0	0	360	30
Fat Free Creamy Italian with Parmesan Salad Dressing (2 tbsp)					
Walden Farms (WFI Corp)	0.0	0.0	0	360	25

*Tobacco company, corporate subsidiary, or parent.

	Tot. Fat (g)	Sat. Fat (g)	Chol. (mg)	Sod. (mg)	Cal.
CREAMY ITALIAN SALAD DRESSINGS *(cont'd)*					
Light Creamy Italian Salad Dressing (2 tbsp)					
Henri's (Henri's Food Products)	2.0	0.0	0	420	50
Luscious Creamy Italian Herb Low Fat Dressing (2 tbsp)					
Marie's (Campbell Soup Co)	2.0	0.0	0	290	40
REGULAR ITALIAN SALAD DRESSINGS					
Fat Free Italian Salad Dressing (2 tbsp)					
Henri's (Henri's Food Products)	0.0	0.0	0	320	15
Kraft Free (Kraft General Foods)*	0.0	0.0	0	290	10
Medford Farms (Chelten House Products)	0.0	0.0	0	65	10
Seven Seas Free (Kraft General Foods)*	0.0	0.0	0	480	10
Walden Farms (WFI Corp)	0.0	0.0	0	290	10
Weight Watchers Salad Celebrations (H.J. Heinz)	0.0	0.0	0	360	10
Fat Free Italian with Sun Dried Tomato Salad Dressing (2 tbsp)					
Walden Farms (WFI Corp)	0.0	0.0	0	290	15
Fat Free Sodium Free Italian Salad Dressing (2 tbsp)					
Walden Farms (WFI Corp)	0.0	0.0	0	0	10
Fat Free Sugar Free Italian Salad Dressing (2 tbsp)					
Walden Farms (WFI Corp) ..0.0	0.0	0	290	0	
Italian Dressing Mix (1 tbsp prepared)					
Weight Watchers (H.J. Heinz)	0.0	0.0	0	140	2
Italian Reduced Calorie Dressing (2 tbsp)					
Kraft Deliciously Right (Kraft General Foods)*	7.0	1.0	0	240	70
Italian Salad Dressing (2 tbsp)					
Healthy Sensation! (T.J. Lipton)	0.0	0.0	0	280	15
Herb Magic (Reily Foods Co)	0.0	0.0	0	400	10
Pritikin (Quaker Oats Company)	0.0	0.0	0	115	20

*Tobacco company, corporate subsidiary, or parent.

	Tot. Fat (g)	Sat. Fat (g)	Chol. (mg)	Sod. (mg)	Cal.
Italian Salad Dressing Mix for Fat Free Dressing, made with vinegar and water (2 tbsp)					
Good Seasons (Kraft General Foods)*	0.0	0.0	0	290	10
Italian Salad Dressing Mix for Reduced Calorie Dressing, made with vinegar, water, and oil (2 tbsp)					
Good Seasons (Kraft General Foods)*	5.0	1.0	0	280	50
Italian Salad Dressings (single-serving pkt)					
Weight Watchers (H.J. Heinz)	0.0	0.0	0	270	8
Italian with Olive Oil, Reduced Calorie Oil Blend Dressing (2 tbsp)					
Seven Seas (Kraft General Foods)*	5.0	1.0	0	450	50
Light Italian Salad Dressing (2 tbsp)					
Newman's Own	0.5	0.0	0	380	20
Wish-Bone (T.J. Lipton)	0.5	0.0	0	480	15
Oil-Free Italian Fat Free Dressing (2 tbsp)					
Kraft (Kraft General Foods)*	0.0	0.0	0	450	5
Two Cheese Italian Salad Dressing (2 tbsp)					
Seven Seas (Kraft General Foods)*	7.0	1.0	0	240	70
Viva Italian Reduced Calorie Dressing (2 tbsp)					
Seven Seas (Kraft General Foods)*	4.0	1.0	0	390	45
Zesty Italian Salad Dressing Mix for Reduced Calorie Dressing, made with vinegar, water, and oil (2 tbsp)					
Good Seasons (Kraft General Foods)*	5.0	1.0	0	260	50

*Tobacco company, corporate subsidiary, or parent.

	Tot. Fat (g)	Sat. Fat (g)	Chol. (mg)	Sod. (mg)	Cal.
MAYONNAISE/MAYONNAISE-TYPE SALAD DRESSINGS					
Canola Light Reduced Fat Mayonnaise (1 tbsp)					
Heart Beat Foods Smart Beat (GFA Brands)	3.0	0.0	0	110	35
Fat Free Mayonnaise Dressing (1 tbsp)					
Heart Beat Foods Smart Beat (GFA Brands)	0.0	0.0	0	135	10
Kraft Free (Kraft General Foods)*	0.0	0.0	0	105	10
Weight Watchers (H.J. Heinz)	0.0	0.0	0	105	10
Fat Free Whipped Dressing (1 tbsp)					
Weight Watchers (H.J. Heinz)	0.0	0.0	0	95	15
Light Dressing (1 tbsp)					
Kraft Miracle Whip (Kraft General Foods)*	3.0	0.0	0	120	40
Light Reduced Fat Mayonnaise (1 tbsp)					
Heart Beat Foods Smart Beat (GFA Brands)	3.0	0.0	0	110	35
Nonfat Dressing (1 tbsp)					
Kraft Miracle Whip Free (Kraft General Foods)*	0.0	0.0	0	120	15
Nonfat Mayonnaise Dressing (1 tbsp)					
Heart Beat Foods Smart Beat (GFA Brands)	0.0	0.0	0	130	64
Reduced Fat Cholesterol Free Mayonnaise Dressing (1 tbsp)					
Best Foods	3.0	0.5	0	120	40
Blue Plate (Reily Foods Co)	5.0	0.5	0	90	50
Hellmann's (Best Foods)	3.0	0.5	0	120	40
RANCH SALAD DRESSINGS—*see* BUTTERMILK/RANCH SALAD DRESSINGS, page 325					
RUSSIAN SALAD DRESSINGS					
Fat Free Russian Salad Dressing (2 tbsp)					
Walden Farms (WFI Corp)	0.0	0.0	5	240	30

*Tobacco company, corporate subsidiary, or parent.

	Tot. Fat (g)	Sat. Fat (g)	Chol. (mg)	Sod. (mg)	Cal.
Russian Dressing Mix (1 tbsp prepared)					
Weight Watchers (H.J. Heinz)	0.0	0.0	0	120	4
SWEET AND SOUR SALAD DRESSINGS					
Sweet-Sour Dressing (2 tbsp)					
Herb Magic (Reily Foods Co)	0.0	0.0	0	240	35
Sweet/Sour Dressing (2 tbsp)					
Old Dutch (Reily Foods Co)	0.0	0.0	0	480	50
THOUSAND ISLAND SALAD DRESSINGS					
Fat Free Thousand Island Salad Dressing (2 tbsp)					
Henri's (Henri's Food Products)	0.0	0.0	0	260	40
Thousand Island Dressing (2 tbsp)					
Herb Magic (Reily Foods Co)	0.0	0.0	0	170	15
Thousand Island Dressing Mix (1 tbsp prepared)					
Weight Watchers (H.J. Heinz)	0.0	0.0	0	140	4
Thousand Island Salad Dressing (2 tbsp)					
Healthy Sensation! (T.J. Lipton)	0.0	0.0	0	300	40
Kraft Free (Kraft General Foods)*	0.0	0.0	0	300	45
VINAIGRETTE SALAD DRESSINGS—*see also* HERB SALAD DRESSINGS, page 328; ITALIAN SALAD DRESSINGS, page 329					
Dijon Balsamic Vinaigrette Salad Dressing (2 tbsp)					
Pritikin (Quaker Oats Company)	0.0	0.0	0	125	30
Fat Free Balsamic Vinaigrette Dressing (2 tbsp)					
Medford Farms (Chelten House Products)	0.0	0.0	0	240	10
Fat Free Raspberry Vinaigrette Salad Dressing (2 tbsp)					
Walden Farms (WFI Corp)	0.0	0.0	0	290	20

*Tobacco company, corporate subsidiary, or parent.

	Tot. Fat (g)	Sat. Fat (g)	Chol. (mg)	Sod. (mg)	Cal.
VINAIGRETTE SALAD DRESSINGS *(cont'd)*					
Raspberry Vinaigrette Salad Dressing (2 tbsp)					
Pritikin (Quaker Oats Company) .	0.0	0.0	0	70	45
Red Wine Vinegar and Oil Reduced Calorie Dressing (2 tbsp)					
Seven Seas (Kraft General Foods)*	5.0	1.0	0	310	60
Red Wine Vinegar Fat Free Dressing (2 tbsp)					
Kraft Free (Kraft General Foods)*	0.0	0.0	0	400	15
Seven Seas Free (Kraft General Foods)*	0.0	0.0	0	400	15
Vinaigrette Dressing (2 tbsp)					
Herb Magic (Reily Foods Co) . . .	0.0	0.0	0	270	10
Zesty Fat Free Classic Herb Vinaigrette Dressing (2 tbsp)					
Marie's (Campbell Soup Co) . . .	0.0	0.0	0	250	30
Zesty Fat Free Honey Dijon Vinaigrette Dressing (2 tbsp)					
Marie's (Campbell Soup Co) . . .	0.0	0.0	0	125	50
Zesty Fat Free Italian Vinaigrette Dressing (2 tbsp)					
Marie's (Campbell Soup Co) . . .	0.0	0.0	0	280	35
Zesty Fat Free Raspberry Vinaigrette Dressing (2 tbsp)					
Marie's (Campbell Soup Co) . . .	0.0	0.0	0	35	35
Zesty Fat Free Red Wine Vinaigrette Dressing (2 tbsp)					
Marie's (Campbell Soup Co) . . .	0.0	0.0	0	300	40
Zesty Fat Free White Wine Vinaigrette Dressing (2 tbsp)					
Marie's (Campbell Soup Co) . . .	0.0	0.0	0	310	40
OTHER SALAD DRESSINGS					
Cilantro Lime Salad Dressing (2 tbsp)					
Smart Temptations (American Specialty Brands)	0.0	0.0	0	220	20

*Tobacco company, corporate subsidiary, or parent.

	Tot. Fat (g)	Sat. Fat (g)	Chol. (mg)	Sod. (mg)	Cal.
Cracked Coriander Salad Dressing (2 tbsp)					
Smart Temptations (American Specialty Brands)	0.0	0.0	0	220	20
Creamy Peppercorn Salad Dressing (1 tbsp)					
Weight Watchers (H.J. Heinz)	0.0	0.0	0	85	8
Lemon Peppercorn Salad Dressing (2 tbsp)					
Smart Temptations (American Specialty Brands)	0.0	0.0	0	250	20
Luscious Creamy Parmesan Low Fat Dressing (2 tbsp)					
Marie's (Campbell Soup Co)	2.0	0.0	0	270	45
Salsa Zesty Garden Salad Dressing (2 tbsp)					
Kraft (Kraft General Foods)*	6.0	1.0	0	280	70
Sun-Dried Tomato Salad Dressing (2 tbsp)					
Smart Temptations (American Specialty Brands)	0.0	0.0	0	280	20
Zesty Tomato Dressing (2 tbsp)					
Herb Magic (Reily Foods Co)	0.0	0.0	0	220	10

*Tobacco company, corporate subsidiary, or parent.

SNACK FOODS

Have the munchies? No problem! In this chapter, you'll find dozens of snack foods that are low in fat, saturated fat, and cholesterol but high in flavor. We have chips and dips, fruit snacks, granola bars, popcorn, and pretzels. Just remember that when you prepare dip mixes, use nonfat or low-fat sour cream or yogurt instead of regular sour cream.

Like all the other entries in this book, the snack foods entries that follow list sodium content. The AHA does not have criteria for sodium but recommends a total of no more than 3,000 mg a day.

Generic Listings

By far, most of the foods in this book are brand name products. However, if a product is listed without a brand name, it means that most brands of that product contain about the same amount of fat, saturated fat, and cholesterol and that these amounts are within the guidelines cited below.

If you find products that were introduced after this book went to press, use the generic listings and the following tables to help you evaluate them.

AHA Criteria for Snack Foods*

	Tot. Fat (g)	Sat. Fat (g)	Chol. (mg)
All snack foods	3	<0.5	<2

*Per serving.

Snack Foods You'll Want to Limit

Some snack foods, like the examples below, are too high in fat, saturated fat, and/or cholesterol to meet AHA criteria. They aren't included in this book, and we recommend that you don't eat them often.

Compare the amounts of fat, saturated fat, cholesterol, sodium, and calories in these examples with the more healthful alternatives listed on the following pages.

Sample Snack Foods to Limit

	Tot. Fat (g)	Sat. Fat (g)	Chol. (mg)	Sod. (mg)	Cal.
Barbecue-flavor potato chips (1 oz)	9.2*	2.3*	0	213	139
Nut and raisin granola bar, soft, uncoated (1 oz)	5.8*	2.7*	0	72	129
Popcorn, regular microwave (1 oz, or about 2½ cups popped)	8.0*	1.4*	0	251	142
Trail mix with coconut (1 oz)	8.3*	1.6*	0	65	131

Adapted from USDA Handbook No. 8 series.

*These values exceed AHA criteria for snack foods.

	Tot. Fat (g)	Sat. Fat (g)	Chol. (mg)	Sod. (mg)	Cal.
CHEESE PUFFS					
Cheese Puff Snacks (about 35 puffs)					
Pacific Grain Products No Fries (Pacific Grain Products)	2.0	0.0	0	190	120
Fat-Free Green Onion Cheese Puffs (1½ cups)					
Health Valley (Health Valley Foods)	0.0	0.0	0	260	110
Fat-Free Original Cheese Puffs (1½ cups)					
Health Valley (Health Valley Foods)	0.0	0.0	0	260	110
Fat-Free Zesty Chili Cheese Puffs (1½ cups)					
Health Valley (Health Valley Foods)	0.0	0.0	0	260	110
DIPS					
Bean Dips					
BBQ Black Bean Dip (2 tbsp)					
Guiltless Gourmet	0.0	0.0	0	120	35
BBQ Pinto Bean Dip (2 tbsp)					
Guiltless Gourmet	0.0	0.0	0	120	35
Black Bean Dip					
Guiltless Gourmet (2 tbsp)	0.0	0.0	0	100	30
The Fat Free Gourmet (Harry's Premium Snacks) (1 oz)	<1.0	0.0	0	150	30
Hot Bean Dip (2 tbsp)					
Frito-Lay	1.0	0.0	0	220	35
Mild Black Bean Dip (2 tbsp)					
Smart Temptations (American Specialty Brands)	0.0	0.0	0	150	20
Mild Garbanzo Bean Dip (2 tbsp)					
Smart Temptations (American Specialty Brands)	0.0	0.0	0	130	20
Mild Pinto Bean Dip (2 tbsp)					
Smart Temptations (American Specialty Brands)	0.0	0.0	0	130	20

	Tot. Fat (g)	Sat. Fat (g)	Chol. (mg)	Sod. (mg)	Cal.
Pinto Bean Dip					
Guiltless Gourmet (2 tbsp)	0.0	0.0	0	130	30
The Fat Free Gourmet (Harry's Premium Snacks) (1 oz)	<1.0	0.0	0	160	20
Spicy Black Bean Dip (2 tbsp)					
Smart Temptations (American Specialty Brands)	0.0	0.0	0	160	20
Spicy Garbanzo Bean Dip (2 tbsp)					
Smart Temptations (American Specialty Brands)	0.0	0.0	0	140	20
Spicy Pinto Bean Dip (2 tbsp)					
Smart Temptations (American Specialty Brands)	0.0	0.0	0	140	20
Nacho/Picante/Salsa Dips					
Fat Free Sour Cream Salsa Dip (Hot) (2 tbsp)					
Borden	0.0	0.0	0	130	25
Fat Free Sour Cream Salsa Dip (Mild) (2 tbsp)					
Borden	0.0	0.0	0	130	25
Hot Picante Dip (2 tbsp)					
Tostitos (Frito-Lay)	0.0	0.0	0	260	15
Medium Cheese 'n Salsa Dip (2 tbsp)					
Old El Paso (Pet)	3.0	1.0	<5	300	25
Medium Chunky Salsa Dip (2 tbsp)					
Old El Paso (Pet)	0.0	0.0	0	230	15
Medium Picante Dip (2 tbsp)					
Tostitos (Frito-Lay)	0.0	0.0	0	250	15
Medium Salsa Dip (2 tbsp)					
Doritos (Frito-Lay)	0.0	0.0	0	200	15
Mild Chunky Salsa Dip (2 tbsp)					
Old El Paso (Pet)	0.0	0.0	0	230	15
Mild Picante Dip (2 tbsp)					
Tostitos (Frito-Lay)	0.0	0.0	0	140	15
Mild Salsa Dip (2 tbsp)					
Doritos (Frito-Lay)	0.0	0.0	0	220	15
Nacho Dip (2 tbsp)					
Guiltless Gourmet	0.0	0.0	0	150	25

	Tot. Fat (g)	Sat. Fat (g)	Chol. (mg)	Sod. (mg)	Cal.
NACHO/PICANTE/SALSA DIPS *(cont'd)*					
Salsa Dip (2 tbsp)					
Guiltless Gourmet	0.0	0.0	0	150	10
OTHER DIPS					
Fat Free French Onion Sour Cream Dip (2 tbsp)					
Borden	0.0	0.0	0	170	25
Fat Free Sour Cream Ranch Dip (2 tbsp)					
Borden	0.0	0.0	0	150	25
Fat Free Vegetable Ranch Sour Cream Dip (2 tbsp)					
Borden	0.0	0.0	0	160	25
FRUIT SNACKS					
Apple Chips (0.75 oz)					
Weight Watchers Smart Snackers (H.J. Heinz)	0.0	0.0	0	125	70
Apple Fruit Roll (1 roll)					
Sunkist (T.J. Lipton)	0.0	0.0	0	20	70
Apple Fruit Snacks (0.5 oz)					
Weight Watchers Smart Snackers (H.J. Heinz)	0.0	0.0	0	125	50
Apricot Fruit Roll (1 roll)					
Sunkist (T.J. Lipton)	0.0	0.0	0	15	70
Cherry Fruit Roll (1 roll)					
Sunkist (T.J. Lipton)	0.0	0.0	0	15	70
Cherry Fruit Roll-Ups (2 rolls)					
General Mills	1.5	0.0	0	80	110
Cinnamon Fruit Snacks (0.5 oz)					
Weight Watchers Smart Snackers (H.J. Heinz)	0.0	0.0	0	125	50
Crazy Colors Fruit Roll-Ups (2 rolls)					
General Mills	1.0	0.0	0	80	110
Fruit Punch Fruit Roll (1 roll)					
Sunkist (T.J. Lipton)	0.0	0.0	0	25	70
Grape Fruit Roll (1 roll)					
Sunkist (T.J. Lipton)	0.0	0.0	0	35	80

	Tot. Fat (g)	Sat. Fat (g)	Chol. (mg)	Sod. (mg)	Cal.
Peach Fruit Snacks (0.5 oz) Weight Watchers Smart Snackers (H.J. Heinz)	0.0	0.0	0	125	50
Raspberry Fruit Roll (1 roll) Sunkist (T.J. Lipton)	0.0	0.0	0	20	70
Strawberry Fruit Roll (1 roll) Sunkist (T.J. Lipton)	0.0	0.0	0	20	70
Strawberry Fruit Snacks (0.5 oz) Weight Watchers Smart Snackers (H.J. Heinz)	0.0	0.0	0	125	50
GRANOLA BARS/SNACK BARS					
Apple Granola/Snack Bars					
Apple Breakfast Bars (1 bar) Health Valley (Health Valley Foods)	0.0	0.0	0	25	110
Fat-Free Apple Fruit Bar (1 bar) Health Valley (Health Valley Foods)	0.0	0.0	0	0	140
One Gram Low Fat Granola Bars, Apple Cinnamon (1 bar) Fi-Bar (Natural Nectar)	1.0	0.0	0	65	90
Apricot Granola/Snack Bars					
Apricot Breakfast Bars (1 bar) Health Valley (Health Valley Foods)	0.0	0.0	0	25	110
Fat-Free Apricot Fruit Bar (1 bar) Health Valley (Health Valley Foods)	0.0	0.0	0	5	140
Blueberry Granola/Snack Bars					
Blueberry Breakfast Bars (1 bar) Health Valley (Health Valley Foods)	0.0	0.0	0	25	110
Fat-Free Blueberry Apple Granola Fruit Bar (1 bar) Health Valley (Health Valley Foods)	0.0	0.0	0	5	140
One Gram Low Fat Blueberry (1 bar) Fi-Bar (Natural Nectar)	1.0	0.0	0	65	90

	Tot. Fat (g)	Sat. Fat (g)	Chol. (mg)	Sod. (mg)	Cal.
Cherry Granola/Snack Bars					
Cherry Breakfast Bars (1 bar)					
Health Valley (Health Valley Foods)	0.0	0.0	0	25	110
Chocolate Granola/Snack Bars					
Fat-Free Chocolate Breakfast Bar (1 bar)					
Health Valley (Health Valley Foods)	0.0	0.0	0	30	110
Fat-Free Chocolate Chip Granola Bar (1 bar)					
Health Valley (Health Valley Foods)	0.0	0.0	0	5	140
Cranberry Granola/Snack Bars					
One Gram Low Fat Cranberry Apple (1 bar)					
Fi-Bar (Natural Nectar)	1.0	0.0	0	65	90
Date Granola/Snack Bars					
Fat-Free Date Almond Granola Fruit Bar (1 bar)					
Health Valley (Health Valley Foods)	0.0	0.0	0	5	140
Fat-Free Date Fruit Bar (1 bar)					
Health Valley (Health Valley Foods)	0.0	0.0	0	5	140
Raisin Granola/Snack Bars					
Fat-Free Raisin Fruit Bar (1 bar)					
Health Valley (Health Valley Foods)	0.0	0.0	0	5	140
Fat-Free Raisin Granola Fruit Bar (1 bar)					
Health Valley (Health Valley Foods)	0.0	0.0	0	5	140
Raspberry Granola/Snack Bars					
Fat-Free Raspberry Granola Fruit Bar (1 bar)					
Health Valley (Health Valley Foods)	0.0	0.0	0	5	140

	Tot. Fat (g)	Sat. Fat (g)	Chol. (mg)	Sod. (mg)	Cal.
STRAWBERRY GRANOLA/SNACK BARS					
Fat-Free Strawberry Granola Fruit Bar (1 bar) Health Valley (Health Valley Foods)	0.0	0.0	0	5	140
Strawberry Breakfast Bars (1 bar) Health Valley (Health Valley Foods)	0.0	0.0	0	25	110
Strawberry-Apple Breakfast Bars (1 bar) Health Valley (Health Valley Foods)	0.0	0.0	0	25	110
OAT GRANOLA/SNACK BARS					
Oatmeal Raisin Lowfat Chewy Granola Bar (1 bar) Nature Valley (General Mills)	2.0	0.0	0	65	110
Oats & Honey Lowfat Bite-Sized Granola Bars (1 pouch) Nature Valley (General Mills)	2.0	0.0	0	135	120
OTHER GRANOLA/SNACK BARS					
Cinnamon Lowfat Crunchy Granola Bar (1 pouch) Nature Valley (General Mills)	2.0	0.0	0	190	140
Fat-Free Cappuccino Breakfast Bar (1 bar) Health Valley (Health Valley Foods)	0.0	0.0	0	30	110
Fruit & Fitness Bar (1 bar) Health Valley (Health Valley Foods)	0.0	0.0	0	25	110
Variety Pack Lowfat Bite-Sized Granola Bars (1 pouch) Nature Valley (General Mills)	2.0	0.0	0	110	120
Variety Pack Lowfat Chewy Granola Bars (1 bar) Nature Valley (General Mills)	2.0	0.0	0	70	110

	Tot. Fat (g)	Sat. Fat (g)	Chol. (mg)	Sod. (mg)	Cal.
POPCORN/POPCORN SNACKS—*see also* "CRACKERS," POPCORN/RICE/ OTHER GRAIN CAKES, page 114					
CARAMEL CORN					
Caramel Popcorn (0.9 oz) Weight Watchers Smart Snackers (H.J. Heinz)	1.0	0.0	0	45	100
Fat-Free Apple Cinnamon Caramel Corn Puffs (30 g) Health Valley (Health Valley Foods)	0.0	0.0	0	60	110
Fat-Free Original Caramel Corn Puffs (30 g) Health Valley (Health Valley Foods)	0.0	0.0	0	60	110
Lite N'Tasty Caramel Popcorn (1 oz) Ultra Slim-Fast (Slim-Fast Foods)	2.0	(0.4)	0	120	110
Low Fat Caramel Popcorn (⅔ cup) Greenfield Healthy Foods	2.0	0.0	0	70	120
REGULAR POPCORN					
American's Best White Pop Corn (5 cups air popped) Jolly Time (American Pop Corn)	0.5	0.0	0	0	100
American's Best Yellow Pop Corn (5 cups air popped) Jolly Time (American Pop Corn)	1.0	0.0	0	0	100
Butter Flavor Popcorn By Request (3 tbsp unpopped = 6 cups popped) Pop Secret (General Mills)	2.5	0.5	0	370	130
Gourmet Hot Air Popping Corn (3 cups popped) Orville Redenbacher's (Hunt-Wesson)	<1.0	0.0	0	0	40
Microwave Popcorn (1 oz) Weight Watchers Smart Snackers (H.J. Heinz)	1.0	0.0	0	0	90

	Tot. Fat (g)	Sat. Fat (g)	Chol. (mg)	Sod. (mg)	Cal.
Natural Flavor Popcorn By Request (3 tbsp unpopped = 6 cups popped)					
Pop Secret (General Mills)	2.5	0.5	0	370	130
Original Pop Chips (31 chips)					
Pop Secret (General Mills)	3.0	0.5	0	380	120
Popcorn (3 tbsp unpopped)					
Newman's Own	1.5	0.0	0	0	110
Popcorn, made without fat or salt (3½ cups popped)					
Most brands (USDA)	**1.4**	**0.2**	**0**	**1**	**109**
White Pop Corn (5 cups air popped)					
Jolly Time (American Pop Corn)	0.5	0.0	0	0	100
Yellow Pop Corn (5 cups air popped)					
Jolly Time (American Pop Corn)	1.0	0.0	0	0	100
OTHER POPCORN					
Fat Free Popcorn Delight (1 bar)					
Lance	0.0	0.0	0	70	100
POTATO SNACKS					
Au Gratin Potato Snacks (30 pieces)					
Pacific Grain Products No Fries (Pacific Grain Products)	2.0	0.0	0	125	120
BBQ Potato Snacks (about 22 round pieces)					
Pacific Grain Products No Fries (Pacific Grain Products)	2.0	0.0	0	140	120
Bar-B-Que Potato Snacks (30 square pieces)					
Pacific Grain Products No Fries (Pacific Grain Products)	1.5	0.0	0	140	120
Jalapeño & Cheese Flavored Potato Corns (¾ cup)					
The Fat Free Gourmet (Harry's Premium Snacks)	0.0	0.0	0	115	100
Maui Onion Fat-Free Potato Chips (1 oz)					
Louise's (ATGTBT)	0.0	0.0	0	160	100

	Tot. Fat (g)	Sat. Fat (g)	Chol. (mg)	Sod. (mg)	Cal.
POTATO SNACKS *(cont'd)*					
Nacho Flavored Baked Potato Corns (about ¾ cup)					
The Fat Free Gourmet (Harry's Premium Snacks)	0.0	0.0	0	21	90
Potato Snacks					
Pacific Grain Products No Fries (Pacific Grain Products) (about 23 round pieces)	2.0	0.0	0	200	120
Pacific Grain Products No Fries (Pacific Grain Products) (34 square pieces)	0.5	0.0	0	150	120
Sour Cream & Chives Potato Snacks (30 pieces)					
Pacific Grain Products No Fries (Pacific Grain Products)	2.0	0.0	0	105	120
PRETZELS					
NO-SALT PRETZELS					
No Salt Oat Bran Pretzels (3 pretzels)					
Keystone (Keystone Pretzel Bakery)	0.0	0.0	0	5	70
No Salt Pretzels Juniors (22 pretzels)					
Keystone (Keystone Pretzel Bakery)	0.0	0.0	0	0	90
Unsalted Sourdough Pretzels (1 oz)					
The Fat Free Gourmet (Harry's Premium Snacks)	1.0	0.0	0	60	114
REGULAR PRETZELS					
Dutch Pretzels					
Keystone (Keystone Pretzel Bakery) (3 pretzels)	1.0	0.5	0	210	90
Mike-sell's ("Mike-sell's" Potato Chip) (3 pretzels)	2.0	0.0	0	600	130
Nabisco Mister Salty (Nabisco Foods)* (2 pretzels)	1.0	0.0	0	580	120
Fat Free Pretzel Chips (16 chips)					
Nabisco Mr. Phipps (Nabisco Foods)*	0.0	0.0	0	630	100
Nabisco Mister Salty (Nabisco Foods)*	0.0	0.0	0	620	100

*Tobacco company, corporate subsidiary, or parent.

	Tot. Fat (g)	Sat. Fat (g)	Chol. (mg)	Sod. (mg)	Cal.
Fat Free Pretzel Knots (7 pretzels) Keebler (Keebler)	0.0	0.0	0	400	120
Fat Free Pretzel Sticks (about 47 sticks) Nabisco Mister Salty (Nabisco Foods)*	0.0	0.0	0	370	110
Fat Free Pretzel Twists (about 9 twists) Nabisco Mister Salty (Nabisco Foods)*	0.0	0.0	0	380	110
Fat Free Sticks (48 pretzels) Rold Gold (Frito-Lay)	0.0	0.0	0	530	110
Fat Free Thins (Less Sodium) (10 pretzels) Rold Gold (Frito-Lay)	0.0	0.0	0	340	110
Fat Free Tiny Twist (18 pretzels) Rold Gold (Frito-Lay)	0.0	0.0	0	420	100
Hard Sour Dough Pretzels (1 pretzel) Rold Gold (Frito-Lay)	1.5	0.0	0	200	90
Lite N'Tasty Pretzels (1 oz) Ultra Slim-Fast (Slim-Fast Foods)	1.0	(0.2)	0	460	100
Lower Sodium Pretzel Chips (16 chips) Nabisco Mr. Phipps (Nabisco Foods)*	2.5	0.0	0	410	120
Mini Pretzels (about 22 pretzels) Nabisco Mister Salty (Nabisco Foods)*	1.0	0.0	0	440	110
Mini Twist Pretzels (21 pretzels) Mike-sell's ("Mike-sell's" Potato Chip)	1.5	0.0	0	710	110
No Fat Pretzel Sticks (50 sticks) Keystone (Keystone Pretzel Bakery)	0.0	0.0	0	440	80
Oat Bran Pretzel Nuggets (1.5 oz) Weight Watchers Smart Snackers (H.J. Heinz)	2.5	0.0	0	250	170
Oat Bran Pretzels (3 pretzels) Keystone (Keystone Pretzel Bakery)	0.0	0.0	0	110	80

*Tobacco company, corporate subsidiary, or parent.

	Tot. Fat (g)	Sat. Fat (g)	Chol. (mg)	Sod. (mg)	Cal.
REGULAR PRETZELS *(cont'd)*					
Original Pretzel Chips					
Nabisco Mr. Phipps (Nabisco Foods)* (16 chips)	2.5	0.0	0	630	120
Rold Gold (Frito-Lay) (10 chips)	1.0	0.0	0	370	110
Party Pretzels (23 pieces)					
Delicious (Delicious Cookie Co)1.0	0.0	0	400	120	
Pretzel Chips (16 chips)					
Nabisco Mister Salty (Nabisco Foods)*	0.0	0.0	0	620	110
Pretzel Sticks					
Delicious (Delicious Cookie Co) (52 pieces)	0.0	0.0	0	560	120
Mike-sell's ("Mike-sell's" Potato Chip) (33 sticks)	1.0	0.0	0	670	110
Rold Gold (Frito-Lay) (48 pretzels)	1.0	0.0	0	430	110
Pretzel Thins (9 pretzels)					
Mike-sell's ("Mike-sell's" Potato Chip)	1.5	0.0	0	600	120
Pretzel Twists (10 pieces)					
Delicious (Delicious Cookie Co)	1.0	0.0	0	520	130
Pretzels					
Most brands (USDA) (1 oz)	**1.4**	**(0.3)**	**(0)**	**504**	**117**
California (Sunshine) (1 oz)	1.5	0.0	0	350	110
Lance (9 pretzels)	1.0	0.0	0	470	140
Sourdough Pretzels (1 oz)					
Harry's (Harry's Premium Snacks)	0.0	0.0	0	548	102
The Fat Free Gourmet (Harry's Premium Snacks)	1.0	0.0	0	560	120
Thin Twist (10 pretzels)					
Rold Gold (Frito-Lay)	1.0	0.0	0	510	110
Tiny Twist (18 pretzels)					
Rold Gold (Frito-Lay)	1.0	0.0	0	420	110
TORTILLA CHIPS					
Baked Tostitos (13 chips)					
Tostitos (Frito-Lay)	1.0	0.0	0	140	110

*Tobacco company, corporate subsidiary, or parent.

	Tot. Fat (g)	Sat. Fat (g)	Chol. (mg)	Sod. (mg)	Cal.
Cheddar Jalapeño Tortilla Snacks (30 pieces)					
Pacific Grain Products No Fries (Pacific Grain Products)	2.0	0.0	0	170	120
Nacho Flavored Baked Tortilla Chips					
Guiltless Gourmet (about 22 chips)	1.0	0.0	0	200	110
The Fat Free Gourmet (Harry's Premium Snacks) (about 15 chips)	1.0	0.0	0	224	95
Natural Flavor Baked Tortilla Chips (about 15 chips)					
The Fat Free Gourmet (Harry's Premium Snacks)	1.0	0.0	0	189	92
No Salt Baked Tortilla Chips (12 chips)					
Smart Temptations (American Specialty Brands)	1.0	0.0	0	0	120
Original Baked Tortilla Chips (12 chips)					
Smart Temptations (American Specialty Brands)	1.0	0.0	0	0	120
Original Style Baked Tortilla Chips (about 22 chips)					
Guiltless Gourmet	1.0	0.0	0	160	110
Original Style No Salt Baked Tortilla Chips (about 22 chips)					
Guiltless Gourmet	1.0	0.0	0	26	110
Ranch Tortilla Snacks (30 pieces)					
Pacific Grain Products No Fries (Pacific Grain Products)	2.0	0.0	0	190	120
Salsa & Sour Cream Tortilla Snacks (30 pieces)					
Pacific Grain Products No Fries (Pacific Grain Products)	2.0	0.0	0	170	120
Salsa Flavored Baked Tortilla Chips (about 15 chips)					
The Fat Free Gourmet (Harry's Premium Snacks)	1.0	0.0	0	224	95

	Tot. Fat (g)	Sat. Fat (g)	Chol. (mg)	Sod. (mg)	Cal.
TORTILLA CHIPS *(cont'd)*					
Tortilla Snacks (34 pieces)					
Pacific Grain Products No Fries (Pacific Grain Products)	1.0	0.0	0	55	120
Unsalted Baked Tostitos (13 chips)					
Tostitos (Frito-Lay)	1.0	0.0	0	0	110
White Corn Baked Tortilla Chips (about 22 chips)					
Guiltless Gourmet	1.0	0.0	0	140	110
OTHER SNACKS					
BBQ Flavor Bugles (1½ cups)					
General Mills	2.5	0.5	0	390	130
Barbecue Flavored Curls (0.5 oz)					
Weight Watchers Smart Snackers (H.J. Heinz)	1.5	0.0	0	110	60
Caraway Rye Cocktail Chips (9 chips)					
Rubschlager	0.5	0.0	0	240	100
Chili Corn Cocktail Chips (9 chips)					
Rubschlager	0.5	0.0	0	240	110
Fat Free Bagel Crisps (5 pieces)					
Burns & Ricker	0.0	0.0	0	280	100
Fat Free Party Mix (¾ cup)					
Burns & Ricker	0.0	0.0	0	210	120
Garlic Cocktail Chips (9 chips)					
Rubschlager	0.5	0.0	0	240	100
Pizza Cocktail Chips (9 chips)					
Rubschlager	0.5	0.0	0	240	100
Ranch-O's Snacks (about 20 pieces)					
Pacific Grain Products No Fries (Pacific Grain Products)	2.0	0.0	0	180	120

SOUPS

Nothing tastes quite as good on a blustery day as a steaming bowl of your favorite soup. And the soups listed in this chapter are low in fat, saturated fat, and cholesterol, if prepared as indicated on the package or in the listings here. If a soup recipe suggests adding milk, do your heart a favor and use skim or 1% milk.

Like all the other entries in this book, the soups entries that follow list sodium content. The AHA does not have criteria for sodium but recommends a total of no more than 3,000 mg a day.

Generic Listings

By far, most of the foods in this book are brand name products. However, if a product is listed without a brand name, it means that most brands of that product contain about the same amount of fat, saturated fat, and cholesterol and that these amounts are within the guidelines cited below.

If you find products that were introduced after this book went to press, use the generic listings and the following tables to help you evaluate them.

AHA Criteria for Soups*

	Tot. Fat (g)	Sat. Fat (g)	Chol. (mg)
All soups	3	2	20

*Per serving.

Soups You'll Want to Limit

Some soups, like the examples below, are too high in fat, saturated fat, and/or cholesterol to meet AHA criteria. They aren't included in this book, and we recommend that you don't eat them often.

Compare the amounts of fat, saturated fat, cholesterol, sodium, and calories in these examples with the more healthful alternatives listed on the following pages.

Sample Soups to Limit

	Tot. Fat (g)	Sat. Fat (g)	Chol. (mg)	Sod. (mg)	Cal.
Chicken and dumplings soup, condensed, made with water (1 cup)	5.5*	1.3	34*	861	97
Chunky beef soup, ready-to-serve (1 cup)	5.1*	2.6*	14	867	171
Cream of potato soup, condensed, made with whole milk (1 cup)	6.5*	3.8*	22	1060	148
Oyster stew, condensed, made with whole milk (1 cup)	7.9*	5.1*	32*	1040	134

Adapted from USDA Handbook No. 8 series.

*These values exceed AHA criteria for soups.

	Tot. Fat (g)	Sat. Fat (g)	Chol. (mg)	Sod. (mg)	Cal.
BEAN SOUPS					
Bean and Ham Soups					
Bean and Ham Soup (1 cup)					
Progresso (Pet)	2.0	0.5	10	870	160
Bean and Ham Soup, Ready-to-Serve					
Campbell's Home Cookin' (Campbell Soup Co) (1 cup)	2.0	1.0	5	720	180
Campbell's Home Cookin' (Campbell Soup Co) (10¾ oz)	2.0	1.0	5	890	230
Chunky Old Fashioned Bean'N Ham Soup, Ready-to-Serve					
Campbell's (Campbell Soup Co) (1 cup)	2.0	1.0	15	880	190
Campbell's (Campbell Soup Co) (11 oz)	3.0	1.0	20	1130	240
Black Bean Soups					
Black Bean Soup (1 cup)					
Health Valley (Health Valley Foods)	0.0	0.0	0	290	110
Black Bean Soup, condensed, made with water (1 cup)					
Campbell's (Campbell Soup Co)	2.0	1.0	0	1030	120
Black Bean with Bacon Soup (1 cup)					
Old El Paso (Pet)	1.5	0.5	5	960	160
Fat-Free Black Bean Vegetable Soup (1 cup)					
Health Valley (Health Valley Foods)	0.0	0.0	0	280	110
Hearty Black Bean Soup (1 cup)					
Progresso (Pet)	1.5	0.0	<5	730	170
No Salt Black Bean Soup (1 cup)					
Health Valley (Health Valley Foods)	0.0	0.0	0	45	110
Other Bean Soups					
Beef 15 Bean Soup (3 tbsp soup mix)					
N.K. Hurst (Hurst Beans)	1.0	0.0	0	360	160
Cajun 15 Bean Soup (3 tbsp soup mix)					
N.K. Hurst (Hurst Beans)	1.0	0.0	0	140	160

	Tot. Fat (g)	Sat. Fat (g)	Chol. (mg)	Sod. (mg)	Cal.
OTHER BEAN SOUPS *(cont'd)*					
Chicken 15 Bean Soup (3 tbsp soup mix) N.K. Hurst (Hurst Beans)	1.0	0.0	0	380	160
Chili 15 Bean Soup (3 tbsp soup mix) N.K. Hurst (Hurst Beans)	1.0	0.0	0	240	160
Five Bean Vegetable Soup (1 cup) Health Valley (Health Valley Foods)	0.0	0.0	0	250	140
Ham 15 Bean Soup (3 tbsp soup mix) N.K. Hurst (Hurst Beans)	1.0	0.0	0	90	160
Many Bean Soup, made with onions, canned tomatoes, and tomato sauce (1 cup) Aunt Patsy's Pantry (Buckeye Beans & Herbs)	1.3	0.0	0	816	200
Veggie Bean Soup, made with onions, canned tomatoes, and tomato sauce (1 cup) Buckeye Beans & Herbs	1.3	0.0	0	816	200
BEEF SOUPS—*see also* BROTHS/CONSOMMÉS, BEEF BROTHS/CONSOMMÉS, page 355; VEGETABLE SOUPS, ONION SOUPS, page 370; BEEF VEGETABLE SOUPS, page 364					
BEEF NOODLE SOUPS					
Beef Noodle Soup, condensed, made with water (1 cup) Campbell's (Campbell Soup Co)	3.0	1.0	15	920	70
Chunky Beef Pasta Soup, Ready-to-Serve (1 cup) Campbell's (Campbell Soup Co)	3.0	1.0	20	970	150
OTHER BEEF SOUPS					
Beefy Mushroom Soup Mix (2 tbsp soup mix) Lipton Recipe Secrets (T.J. Lipton)	0.0	0.0	0	650	35

	Tot. Fat (g)	Sat. Fat (g)	Chol. (mg)	Sod. (mg)	Cal.
Beefy Mushroom Soup, condensed, made with water (1 cup)					
Campbell's (Campbell Soup Co)	3.0	1.0	10	1000	70
Chunky Beef Pepper Soup, Ready-to-Serve (1 cup)					
Campbell's (Campbell Soup Co)	3.0	1.0	20	830	140
BROCCOLI SOUPS—see VEGETABLE SOUPS, BROCCOLI SOUPS, page 365					
BROTHS/CONSOMMÉS					
BEEF BROTHS/CONSOMMÉS					
Canned Beef Broths/Consommés					
Beef Broth (1 cup)					
College Inn (Nabisco Foods)* . .	0.0	0.0	0	1140	20
Clear Beef Broth, Ready-to-Serve (1 cup)					
Swanson (Campbell Soup Co) .	1.0	1.0	0	820	20
Consomme Beef Soup, condensed, made with water (½ cup)					
Campbell's (Campbell Soup Co)	0.0	0.0	5	820	25
Double Rich Double Strength Beef Broth, condensed, made with water (1 cup)					
Campbell's (Campbell Soup Co)	0.0	0.0	<5	900	15
Fat-Free Beef Broth (1 cup)					
Health Valley (Health Valley Foods)	0.0	0.0	0	160	20
Fat-Free No Salt Beef Broth (1 cup)					
Health Valley (Health Valley Foods)	0.0	0.0	0	70	20
Lower Sodium Beef Broth (1 cup)					
College Inn (Nabisco Foods)* . .	0.0	0.0	0	620	20
Granular/Powdered Beef Broths/Consommés					
Beef Bouillon Cubes (1 cube)					
Herb-Ox (Hormel)	0.0	0.0	0	700	10
Beef Instant Bouillon Powder (1 tsp)					
Herb-Ox (Hormel)	0.0	0.0	0	750	10

*Tobacco company, corporate subsidiary, or parent.

	Tot. Fat (g)	Sat. Fat (g)	Chol. (mg)	Sod. (mg)	Cal.
Beef Broths/Consommés *(cont'd)*					
Beef Instant Broth & Seasoning Low Sodium Packet (1 pkt)					
Herb-Ox (Hormel)	0.0	0.0	0	5	15
Beef Instant Broth & Seasoning Packet (1 pkt)					
Herb-Ox (Hormel)	0.0	0.0	0	900	10
Instant Beef Broth Mix (0.16 oz)					
Weight Watchers (H.J. Heinz)	0.0	0.0	1	820	10
Chicken Broths/Consommés					
Canned Chicken Broths/ Consommés					
Chicken Broth (1 cup)					
Health Valley (Health Valley Foods)	0.0	0.0	0	250	35
Pritikin (Quaker Oats Company)	0.0	0.0	0	290	15
Progresso (Pet)	0.5	0.0	5	860	20
Chicken Broth, Ready-to-Serve (1 cup)					
Campbell's (Campbell Soup Co)	1.0	0.0	0	820	15
Campbell's Healthy Request (Campbell Soup Co)	0.0	0.0	0	480	20
Chicken Broth Soup, condensed, made with water (1 cup)					
Campbell's (Campbell Soup Co)	2.0	1.0	<5	770	30
Clear Chicken Broth (1 cup)					
Swanson (Campbell Soup Co)	2.0	1.0	0	1000	30
Fat-Free Chicken Broth (1 cup)					
Health Valley (Health Valley Foods)	0.0	0.0	0	170	30
Low Sodium Chicken Broth, Ready-to-Serve (1 cup)					
Campbell's (Campbell Soup Co)	2.0	1.0	5	60	25
Lower Sodium Chicken Broth (1 cup)					
College Inn (Nabisco Foods)*	2.0	0.5	<5	640	25
Natural Goodness Clear Chicken Broth (1 cup)					
Swanson (Campbell Soup Co)	0.0	0.0	0	560	15
No Salt Chicken Broth (1 cup)					
Health Valley (Health Valley Foods)	0.0	0.0	0	75	35

*Tobacco company, corporate subsidiary, or parent.

	Tot. Fat (g)	Sat. Fat (g)	Chol. (mg)	Sod. (mg)	Cal.
Granular/Powdered Chicken Broths/Consommés					
Chicken Bouillon Cubes (1 cube)					
Herb-Ox (Hormel)	0.0	0.0	0	1040	10
Chicken Instant Bouillon Powder (1 tsp)					
Herb-Ox (Hormel)	0.0	0.0	0	1040	10
Chicken Instant Broth & Seasoning Low Sodium Packet (1 pkt)					
Herb-Ox (Hormel)	0.0	0.0	0	20	15
Chicken Instant Broth & Seasoning Packet (1 pkt)					
Herb-Ox (Hormel)	0.0	0.0	0	760	10
Instant Chicken Broth Mix (0.16 oz)					
Weight Watchers (H.J. Heinz)	0.0	0.0	0	900	10
VEGETABLE BROTHS/CONSOMMÉS					
Canned Vegetable Broths/ Consommés					
Vegetable Broth (1 cup)					
Pritikin (Quaker Oats Company)	0.0	0.0	0	290	10
Swanson (Campbell Soup Co)	1.0	0.0	0	1000	20
Granular/Powdered Vegetable Broths/Consommés					
Vegetable Bouillon Cubes (1 cube)					
Herb-Ox (Hormel)	0.0	0.0	0	1000	10
OTHER BROTHS/CONSOMMÉS					
Consomme Madrilene (⅔ cup)					
Pepperidge Farm (Campbell Soup Co)	1.0	0.0	0	910	50
CHICKEN SOUPS—*see also* BEAN SOUPS, OTHER BEAN SOUPS, page 353; BROTHS/ CONSOMMÉS, CHICKEN BROTHS/ CONSOMMÉS, page 356; VEGETABLE SOUPS, CHICKEN VEGETABLE SOUPS, page 365					
CHICKEN BARLEY SOUPS					
Chicken Barley Soup (1 cup)					
Progresso (Pet)	2.5	0.5	15	720	110

	Tot. Fat (g)	Sat. Fat (g)	Chol. (mg)	Sod. (mg)	Cal.
CHICKEN GUMBO SOUPS					
Chicken Gumbo Soup, condensed, made with water (1 cup)					
Campbell's (Campbell Soup Co)	2.0	1.0	10	990	60
CHICKEN NOODLE SOUPS					
Chicken Noodle Cup-A-Soup, made with water (6 fl oz)					
Lipton (T.J. Lipton)	1.0	0.5	10	570	50
Chicken Noodle Hearty Soup Mix, made with water (1 cup)					
Lipton (T.J. Lipton)	1.0	0.5	15	660	80
Chicken Noodle O's Soup, condensed, made with water (1 cup)					
Campbell's (Campbell Soup Co)	3.0	1.0	15	980	80
Chicken Noodle Soup					
Lunch Bucket (Dial Corp) (7¼ oz)	2.0	1.0	10	830	80
Progresso (Pet) (1 cup)	2.0	0.5	20	730	80
Progresso Healthy Classics (Pet) (1 cup)	2.0	0.5	20	480	80
Weight Watchers (H.J. Heinz) (7.5 oz)	1.0	0.0	15	450	80
Weight Watchers (H.J. Heinz) (10.5 oz)	1.0	0.0	10	950	80
Chicken Noodle Soup, condensed, made with water (1 cup)					
Campbell's (Campbell Soup Co)	3.0	1.0	15	950	70
Campbell's Healthy Request (Campbell Soup Co)	3.0	1.0	15	480	70
Chicken Noodle Soup, Ready-to-Serve (7¼ oz)					
Campbell's (Campbell Soup Co)	2.0	1.0	15	870	60
Chicken Noodle Soup with Chicken Soup Mix, made with water (8 fl oz)					
Lipton (T.J. Lipton)	2.5	1.0	15	650	80
Curly Noodle Soup with Chicken Broth, condensed, made with water (1 cup)					
Campbell's (Campbell Soup Co)	3.0	1.0	15	840	80

	Tot. Fat (g)	Sat. Fat (g)	Chol. (mg)	Sod. (mg)	Cal.
Double Noodle Soup in Chicken Broth, condensed, made with water (1 cup) Campbell's (Campbell Soup Co)	3.0	1.0	15	810	100
Giggle Noodle Soup Mix with Real Chicken Broth, made with water (8 fl oz) Lipton (T.J. Lipton)	2.0	1.0	15	730	80
Hearty Chicken Noodle Cup-A-Soup, made with water (6 fl oz) Lipton (T.J. Lipton)	1.0	0.5	10	540	60
Noodle Soup with Real Chicken Broth Soup Mix, made with water (8 fl oz) Lipton (T.J. Lipton)	2.0	1.0	15	710	60
Quality Chicken Noodle Soup Mix with White Meat (3 tbsp soup mix) Campbell's (Campbell Soup Co)	2.0	1.0	10	650	90
Quality Noodle Soup Mix with Real Chicken Broth (3 tbsp soup mix) Campbell's (Campbell Soup Co)	2.0	1.0	10	790	100
Ring-O-Noodle Soup Mix with Real Chicken Broth, made with water (8 fl oz) Lipton (T.J. Lipton)	2.0	1.0	10	710	70
CHICKEN WITH RICE SOUPS					
Chicken and Rice Soup (1 cup) Pritikin (Quaker Oats Company) .	1.0	0.0	5	250	80
Chicken & Wild Rice Soup (1 cup) Progresso (Pet)	2.0	0.5	20	820	100
Chicken Rice and Vegetable Soup (1 cup) Progresso (Pet)	3.0	1.0	15	750	110
Chicken Rice Soup, Ready-to-Serve (1 cup) Campbell's Home Cookin' (Campbell Soup Co)	3.0	1.0	20	770	115
Chicken Rice with Vegetables (1 cup) Progresso Healthy Classics (Pet)	1.5	0.0	10	450	90

	Tot. Fat (g)	Sat. Fat (g)	Chol. (mg)	Sod. (mg)	Cal.
CHICKEN WITH RICE SOUPS *(cont'd)*					
Chicken with Rice Soup (1 cup)					
Old El Paso (Pet)	2.5	0.5	15	680	90
Chicken with Rice Soup, condensed, made with water (1 cup)					
Campbell's (Campbell Soup Co)	3.0	1.0	<5	830	70
Campbell's Healthy Request (Campbell Soup Co)	3.0	1.0	10	480	70
Chicken with Rice Soup, Ready-to-Serve (7¼ oz)					
Campbell's (Campbell Soup Co)	2.0	1.0	5	780	50
Chicken with Wild Rice Soup, condensed, made with water (1 cup)					
Campbell's (Campbell Soup Co)	2.0	1.0	10	900	70
Hearty Chicken Rice Soup, Ready-to-Serve (1 cup)					
Campbell's Healthy Request (Campbell Soup Co)	3.0	1.0	15	480	120
Microwave Chicken Rice Soup, Ready-to-Serve (10½ oz)					
Campbell's (Campbell Soup Co)	3.0	1.0	10	1130	120
CREAM OF CHICKEN SOUPS					
Cream of Chicken Cup-A-Soup, made with water (6 fl oz)					
Lipton (T.J. Lipton)	2.5	0.5	0	650	70
Cream of Chicken Soup, condensed, made with water (1 cup)					
Campbell's Healthy Request (Campbell Soup Co)	3.0	1.0	10	480	80
OTHER CHICKEN SOUPS					
Chicken Alphabet Soup with Vegetables, condensed, made with water (1 cup)					
Campbell's (Campbell Soup Co)	2.0	1.0	10	880	80
Chicken and Stars Soup, condensed, made with water (1 cup)					
Campbell's (Campbell Soup Co)	2.0	1.0	0	1010	70

	Tot. Fat (g)	Sat. Fat (g)	Chol. (mg)	Sod. (mg)	Cal.
Chicken Corn Chowder Soup, Ready-to-Serve (1 cup) Campbell's Healthy Request (Campbell Soup Co)	3.0	1.0	15	480	140
Chicken Fiesta (7½ oz) Lunch Bucket (Dial Corp)	2.0	0.5	5	530	160
Chicken Pasta Soup (1 cup) Pritikin (Quaker Oats Company)	1.0	0.0	5	290	100
Chicken Won Ton Soup, condensed, made with water (1 cup) Campbell's (Campbell Soup Co)	1.0	0.0	15	940	45
Hearty Chicken & Rotini Soup (1 cup) Progresso (Pet)	2.0	0.5	20	860	90
Hearty Penne Pasta in Chicken Broth (1 cup) Progresso (Pet)	1.0	0.0	<5	930	70
Tortellini in Chicken Broth (1 cup) Progresso (Pet)	2.0	0.5	5	750	80
CLAM CHOWDERS					
MANHATTAN CLAM CHOWDERS					
Manhattan Clam Chowder (1 cup) Progresso (Pet)	2.0	0.0	10	710	110
Manhattan Style Clam Chowder, condensed, made with water (1 cup) Campbell's (Campbell Soup Co)	2.0	1.0	5	910	70
NEW ENGLAND CLAM CHOWDERS					
New England Clam Chowder Progresso Healthy Classics (Pet) (1 cup)	2.0	0.5	5	530	120
Weight Watchers (H.J. Heinz) (7.5 oz)	0.0	0.0	0	330	90
New England Clam Chowder Seashore Soup, condensed, made with water (1 cup) Campbell's (Campbell Soup Co)	3.0	1.0	5	970	90

CONSOMMÉS—*see* BROTHS/ CONSOMMÉS, page 355

	Tot. Fat (g)	Sat. Fat (g)	Chol. (mg)	Sod. (mg)	Cal.
LENTIL SOUPS					
Fat-Free Lentil and Carrot Soup (1 cup)					
Health Valley (Health Valley Foods)	0.0	0.0	0	220	90
Hearty Lentil Soup, Ready-to-Serve					
Campbell's Home Cookin' (Campbell Soup Co) (1 cup)	2.0	1.0	0	860	150
Campbell's Home Cookin' (Campbell Soup Co) (10¾ oz)	3.0	0.0	0	1070	190
Lentil & Shells Soup (1 cup)					
Progresso (Pet)	1.5	0.0	0	840	130
Lentil Soup					
Pritikin (Quaker Oats Company) (1 cup)	0.5	0.0	0	280	130
Progresso (Pet) (1 cup)	2.0	0.0	0	750	140
Progresso (Pet) (10.5 oz)	2.5	0.0	0	930	170
Progresso Healthy Classics (Pet) (1 cup)	1.5	0.0	0	440	130
Organic Lentil Soup (1 cup)					
Health Valley (Health Valley Foods)	0.0	0.0	0	240	90
Organic No Salt Lentil Soup (1 cup)					
Health Valley (Health Valley Foods)	0.0	0.0	0	40	90
Red Lentil Soup, made with onions and tomatoes (1 cup)					
Aunt Patsy's Pantry (Buckeye Beans & Herbs)	1.3	0.0	0	792	220
MINESTRONE					
Fat-Free Minestrone Soup (1 cup)					
Health Valley (Health Valley Foods)	0.0	0.0	0	210	80
Hearty Minestrone Soup, Ready-to-Serve (1 cup)					
Campbell's Healthy Request (Campbell Soup Co)	2.0	1.0	<5	480	120
Hearty Minestrone with Shells Soup (1 cup)					
Progresso (Pet)	1.5	0.0	0	700	120

	Tot. Fat (g)	Sat. Fat (g)	Chol. (mg)	Sod. (mg)	Cal.
Minestrone Soup (1 cup)					
Pritikin (Quaker Oats Company) .	1.0	0.0	0	290	90
Progresso (Pet)	3.0	0.5	0	850	130
Progresso Healthy Classics (Pet)	2.5	0.0	0	510	120
Minestrone Soup, condensed, made with water (1 cup)					
Campbell's (Campbell Soup Co)	2.0	1.0	0	960	100
Campbell's Healthy Request (Campbell Soup Co)	1.0	1.0	0	480	90
Minestrone Soup, Ready-to-Serve (1 cup)					
Campbell's Home Cookin' (Campbell Soup Co)	2.0	1.0	5	990	120
Organic Minestrone Soup (1 cup)					
Health Valley (Health Valley Foods)	0.0	0.0	0	190	90
Organic No Salt Minestrone Soup (1 cup)					
Health Valley (Health Valley Foods)	0.0	0.0	0	115	90

MUSHROOM SOUPS—*see* BEEF SOUPS, OTHER BEEF SOUPS, page 354; VEGETABLE SOUPS, MUSHROOM SOUPS, page 369

NOODLE SOUPS—*see also* BEEF SOUPS, BEEF NOODLE SOUPS, page 354; CHICKEN SOUPS, CHICKEN NOODLE SOUPS, page 358; OTHER CHICKEN SOUPS, page 360; TURKEY SOUPS, page 364

	Tot. Fat (g)	Sat. Fat (g)	Chol. (mg)	Sod. (mg)	Cal.
Harvest Noodle Soup Mix, made with water (8 fl oz)					
Lipton (T.J. Lipton)	1.0	0.0	15	650	70
Hearty Noodle with Vegetables Soup Mix, made with water (8 fl oz)					
Lipton (T.J. Lipton)	2.0	1.0	10	710	70
Ring Noodle Cup-A-Soup, made with water (6 fl oz)					
Lipton (T.J. Lipton)	<1.0	0.0	5	560	50

	Tot. Fat (g)	Sat. Fat (g)	Chol. (mg)	Sod. (mg)	Cal.
NOODLE SOUPS *(cont'd)*					
Teddy Bear Pasta Shapes Soup, condensed, made with water (1 cup)					
Campbell's (Campbell Soup Co)	2.0	1.0	5	840	80
ONION SOUPS—*see* VEGETABLE SOUPS, ONION SOUPS, page 370					
PEA SOUPS—*see* VEGETABLE SOUPS, PEA SOUPS, page 370					
POTATO SOUPS—*see* VEGETABLE SOUPS, POTATO SOUPS, page 371					
TOMATO SOUPS—*see* VEGETABLE SOUPS, TOMATO SOUPS, page 371					
TURKEY SOUPS					
Turkey Noodle Soup, condensed, made with water (1 cup)					
Campbell's (Campbell Soup Co)	3.0	1.0	15	970	80
Turkey Vegetable Soup, condensed, made with water (1 cup)					
Campbell's (Campbell Soup Co)	3.0	1.0	10	840	120
Turkey Vegetable with Wild Rice Soup, Ready-to-Serve (1 cup)					
Campbell's Healthy Request (Campbell Soup Co)	3.0	1.0	15	480	120
VEGETABLE SOUPS—*see also* BEAN SOUPS, page 353; BROTHS/CONSOMMÉS, VEGETABLE BROTHS/CONSOMMÉS, page 357; MINESTRONE, page 362; TURKEY SOUPS, above					
BEEF VEGETABLE SOUPS					
Beef Soup with Vegetables and Barley, condensed, made with water (1 cup)					
Campbell's (Campbell Soup Co)	2.0	1.0	15	920	80

	Tot. Fat (g)	Sat. Fat (g)	Chol. (mg)	Sod. (mg)	Cal.
Beef Vegetable Micro Cup Soups (1 cup)					
Hormel (Hormel)	1.0	0.0	10	740	90
Beef Vegetable Soup (1 cup)					
Progresso Healthy Classics (Pet)	1.5	0.5	15	410	150
Hearty Vegetable Beef Soup, Ready-to-Serve (1 cup)					
Campbell's Healthy Request (Campbell Soup Co)	3.0	1.0	20	480	140
Microwave Vegetable Beef Soup, Ready-to-Serve (7¾ oz)					
Campbell's (Campbell Soup Co)	2.0	1.0	10	780	90
Vegetable Beef Soup (7.5 oz)					
Weight Watchers (H.J. Heinz)	1.0	0.0	0	450	80
Vegetable Beef Soup, condensed, made with water (1 cup)					
Campbell's (Campbell Soup Co)	2.0	1.0	10	810	80
Campbell's Healthy Request (Campbell Soup Co)	2.0	1.0	5	480	80
Vegetable Beef Soup, Ready-to-Serve (1 cup)					
Campbell's Home Cookin' (Campbell Soup Co)	2.0	1.0	5	1010	120
BROCCOLI SOUPS					
Broccoli & Shells Soup (1 cup)					
Progresso (Pet)	1.0	0.0	<5	720	70
Cream of Broccoli Soup (1 cup)					
Progresso Healthy Classics (Pet)	3.0	0.5	<5	580	90
Cream of Broccoli Soup, condensed, made with water (1 cup)					
Campbell's Healthy Request (Campbell Soup Co)	2.0	1.0	2	480	70
Super Broccoli Carotene Soup (1 cup)					
Health Valley (Health Valley Foods)	0.0	0.0	0	240	70
CHICKEN VEGETABLE SOUPS					
Chicken Vegetable Cup-A-Soup, made with water (6 fl oz)					
Lipton (T.J. Lipton)	1.0	0.5	5	510	50

	Tot. Fat (g)	Sat. Fat (g)	Chol. (mg)	Sod. (mg)	Cal.
CHICKEN VEGETABLE SOUPS *(cont'd)*					
Chicken Vegetable Soup (1 cup)					
Old El Paso (Pet)	2.5	0.5	15	620	110
Chicken Vegetable Soup, condensed, made with water (1 cup)					
Campbell's (Campbell Soup Co)	2.0	1.0	10	940	80
Chicken, Vegetables & Penne Pasta Soup (1 cup)					
Progresso (Pet)	2.5	0.5	10	780	100
Hearty Chicken Vegetable Soup, Ready-to-Serve (1 cup)					
Campbell's Healthy Request (Campbell Soup Co)	3.0	1.0	15	480	120
Homestyle Chicken and Vegetable Soup (1 cup)					
Progresso (Pet)	2.5	0.5	15	680	100
MIXED VEGETABLE SOUPS					
Chunky Vegetable Soup, Ready-to-Serve (1 cup)					
Campbell's (Campbell Soup Co)	3.0	1.0	0	870	130
Country Vegetable Soup (7¼ oz)					
Lunch Bucket (Dial Corp)	0.5	0.0	0	750	60
Country Vegetable Soup, Ready-to-Serve					
Campbell's Home Cookin' (Campbell Soup Co) (1 cup)	1.0	0.0	5	760	110
Campbell's Home Cookin' (Campbell Soup Co) (10¾ oz)	2.0	0.0	5	940	130
Fat-Free Carotene Vegetable Power Soup (1 cup)					
Health Valley (Health Valley Foods)	0.0	0.0	0	240	70
Fat-Free Country Corn & Vegetable Soup (1 cup)					
Health Valley (Health Valley Foods)	0.0	0.0	0	135	70
Fat-Free Garden Vegetable Soup (1 cup)					
Health Valley (Health Valley Foods)	0.0	0.0	0	250	80

	Tot. Fat (g)	Sat. Fat (g)	Chol. (mg)	Sod. (mg)	Cal.
Fat-Free Italian Plus Carotene Soup (1 cup)					
Health Valley (Health Valley Foods)	0.0	0.0	0	240	80
Fat-Free Tomato Vegetable Soup (1 cup)					
Health Valley (Health Valley Foods)	0.0	0.0	0	240	80
Fat-Free Vegetable Barley Soup (1 cup)					
Health Valley (Health Valley Foods)	0.0	0.0	0	210	90
Garden Vegetable Soup (1 cup)					
Old El Paso (Pet)	2.5	0.5	<5	710	110
Gazpacho Soup (⅔ cup)					
Pepperidge Farm (Campbell Soup Co)	2.0	0.0	0	1050	70
Hearty Harvest Vegetable Cup-A-Soup, made with water (6 fl oz)					
Lipton (T.J. Lipton)	1.5	0.5	0	450	90
Hearty Vegetable Soup (1 cup)					
Pritikin (Quaker Oats Company)	0.5	0.0	0	290	90
Hearty Vegetable Soup, condensed, made with water (1 cup)					
Campbell's Healthy Request (Campbell Soup Co)	1.0	1.0	5	480	90
Hearty Vegetable Soup, Ready-to-Serve (1 cup)					
Campbell's Healthy Request (Campbell Soup Co)	1.0	0.0	0	470	100
Homestyle Vegetable Soup, condensed, made with water (1 cup)					
Campbell's (Campbell Soup Co)	2.0	1.0	0	970	70
Low Sodium Vegetable Soup, Ready-to-Serve (7¼ oz)					
Campbell's (Campbell Soup Co)	2.0	1.0	0	30	90
Microwave Vegetable Soup, Ready-to-Serve (7¾ oz)					
Campbell's (Campbell Soup Co)	2.0	1.0	0	850	100

	Tot. Fat (g)	Sat. Fat (g)	Chol. (mg)	Sod. (mg)	Cal.
Mixed Vegetable Soups ***(cont'd)***					
Old Fashioned Vegetable Soup, condensed, made with water (1 cup)					
Campbell's (Campbell Soup Co)	3.0	1.0	<5	950	70
Organic No Salt Vegetable Soup (1 cup)					
Health Valley (Health Valley Foods)	0.0	0.0	0	80	80
Organic Vegetable Soup (1 cup)					
Health Valley (Health Valley Foods)	0.0	0.0	0	230	80
Quality Vegetable Soup and Recipe Mix (2 tbsp soup mix)					
Campbell's (Campbell Soup Co)	0.0	0.0	0	650	35
Southwest Style Vegetable Soup, Ready-to-Serve (1 cup)					
Campbell's Healthy Request (Campbell Soup Co)	2.0	1.0	0	480	150
Southwestern Vegetable Soup, Ready-to-Serve (1 cup)					
Campbell's Home Cookin' (Campbell Soup Co)	3.0	1.0	0	750	130
Spring Vegetable Cup-A-Soup, made with water (6 fl oz)					
Lipton (T.J. Lipton)	1.0	0.5	<5	470	50
Tomato Garden Vegetable Soup (1 cup)					
Progresso Healthy Classics (Pet)	1.0	0.0	0	480	100
Tomato Vegetable Soup, Ready-to-Serve (1 cup)					
Campbell's Healthy Request (Campbell Soup Co)	2.0	1.0	5	480	120
Vegetable Soup Mix (3 tbsp soup mix)					
Lipton Recipe Secrets (T.J. Lipton)	0.0	0.0	0	580	30
Vegetable Soup (1 cup)					
Progresso (Pet)	2.0	0.5	<5	850	90
Progresso Healthy Classics (Pet)	1.5	0.0	5	470	80

	Tot. Fat (g)	Sat. Fat (g)	Chol. (mg)	Sod. (mg)	Cal.
Vegetable Soup, condensed, made with water (1 cup)					
Campbell's (Campbell Soup Co)	1.0	0.0	0	750	90
Campbell's Healthy Request (Campbell Soup Co)	2.0	1.0	0	480	90
Vegetable Soup, Ready-to-Serve (7¼ oz)					
Campbell's (Campbell Soup Co)	2.0	1.0	0	730	70
Vegetarian Vegetable Soup (1 cup)					
Pritikin (Quaker Oats Company) .	0.0	0.0	0	290	100
Vegetarian Vegetable Soup, condensed, made with water (1 cup)					
Campbell's (Campbell Soup Co)	1.0	0.0	0	770	70
MUSHROOM SOUPS—*see also* BEEF SOUPS, OTHER BEEF SOUPS, page 354					
Cream of Mushroom Soup (10.5 oz)					
Weight Watchers (H.J. Heinz) ..	0.5	0.0	0	1260	70
Cream of Mushroom Soup, condensed, made with water (1 cup)					
Campbell's Healthy Request (Campbell Soup Co)	3.0	1.0	10	480	70
Creamy Mushroom Cup-A-Soup, made with water (6 fl oz)					
Lipton (T.J. Lipton)	2.5	0.5	0	610	60
Golden Mushroom Soup, condensed, made with water (1 cup)					
Campbell's (Campbell Soup Co)	3.0	1.0	5	930	80
Organic Mushroom Barley Soup (1 cup)					
Health Valley (Health Valley Foods)	0.0	0.0	0	220	60
Organic No Salt Mushroom Barley Soup (1 cup)					
Health Valley (Health Valley Foods)	0.0	0.0	0	95	60

	Tot. Fat (g)	Sat. Fat (g)	Chol. (mg)	Sod. (mg)	Cal.
Onion Soups					
Beefy Onion Soup Mix (1 tbsp soup mix) Lipton Recipe Secrets (T.J. Lipton)	0.5	0.0	0	610	25
French Onion Soup made with Beef Stock (⅔ cup) Pepperidge Farm (Campbell Soup Co)	1.0	1.0	<5	1080	50
French Onion Soup made with Beef Stock, condensed, made with water (1 cup) Campbell's (Campbell Soup Co)	3.0	0.0	1	980	70
Golden Onion Soup Mix (2 tbsp soup mix) Lipton Recipe Secrets (T.J. Lipton)	1.5	0.0	0	650	60
Onion Mushroom Soup Mix (2 tbsp soup mix) Lipton Recipe Secrets (T.J. Lipton)	1.0	0.0	0	620	35
Onion Soup Mix (1 tbsp soup mix) Lipton Recipe Secrets (T.J. Lipton)	0.0	0.0	0	610	20
Onion Soup N' Recipe Mix with Chicken Broth (2 tbsp soup mix) Campbell's (Campbell Soup Co)	1.0	0.0	0	680	50
Quality Onion Soup and Recipe Mix (1 tbsp soup mix) Campbell's (Campbell Soup Co)	0.0	0.0	0	660	25
Pea Soups					
Chunky Split Pea N' Ham Soup, Ready-to-Serve (1 cup) Campbell's (Campbell Soup Co)	3.0	1.0	20	1120	190
Fat-Free Split Pea & Carrot Soup (1 cup) Health Valley (Health Valley Foods)	0.0	0.0	0	230	110
Green Pea Soup, condensed, made with water (1 cup) Campbell's (Campbell Soup Co)	3.0	1.0	5	890	180

	Tot. Fat (g)	Sat. Fat (g)	Chol. (mg)	Sod. (mg)	Cal.
Green Split Pea Soup (1 cup)					
Progresso (Pet)	3.0	1.0	5	870	170
Organic No Salt Split Pea Soup (1 cup)					
Health Valley (Health Valley Foods)	0.0	0.0	0	115	110
Organic Split Pea Soup (1 cup)					
Health Valley (Health Valley Foods)	0.0	0.0	0	160	110
Plentiful Pea Soup, made with onions (1 cup)					
Aunt Patsy's Pantry (Buckeye Beans & Herbs)	0.7	0.0	0	768	210
Split Pea Soup (1 cup)					
Pritikin (Quaker Oats Co)	0.5	0.0	0	290	140
Progresso Healthy Classics (Pet)	2.5	1.0	<5	420	180
Real Fresh	0.0	0.0	0	740	130
Split Pea with Bacon Soup (1 cup)					
Real Fresh	1.0	0.0	<5	760	140
Split Pea with Ham Soup, Ready-to-Serve					
Campbell's Healthy Request (Campbell Soup Co) (1 cup)	3.0	1.0	10	480	170
Campbell's Home Cookin' (Campbell Soup Co) (1 cup)	2.0	1.0	5	880	170
Campbell's Home Cookin' (Campbell Soup Co) (10¾ oz)	2.0	1.0	5	1100	210
POTATO SOUPS					
Organic No Salt Potato Leek Soup (1 cup)					
Health Valley (Health Valley Foods)	0.0	0.0	0	35	70
Organic Potato Leek Soup (1 cup)					
Health Valley (Health Valley Foods)	0.0	0.0	0	230	70
TOMATO SOUPS—*see also* MIXED VEGETABLE SOUPS, page 366					
Hearty Tomato and Rotini Soup (1 cup)					
Progresso (Pet)	1.0	0.0	5	820	90

	Tot. Fat (g)	Sat. Fat (g)	Chol. (mg)	Sod. (mg)	Cal.
TOMATO SOUPS *(cont'd)*					
Homestyle Cream of Tomato Soup, condensed, made with water (1 cup)					
Campbell's (Campbell Soup Co)	3.0	1.0	5	860	110
Italian Tomato with Basil and Oregano Soup, condensed, made with water (1 cup)					
Campbell's (Campbell Soup Co)	1.0	0.0	0	820	100
Old Fashioned Tomato Rice Soup, condensed, made with water (1 cup)					
Campbell's (Campbell Soup Co)	2.0	1.0	5	790	120
Organic No Salt Tomato Soup (1 cup)					
Health Valley (Health Valley Foods)	0.0	0.0	0	25	90
Organic Tomato Soup (1 cup)					
Health Valley (Health Valley Foods)	0.0	0.0	0	250	90
Tomato Cup-A-Soup, made with water (6 fl oz)					
Lipton (T.J. Lipton)	2.0	1.0	<5	490	90
Tomato Soup (1 cup)					
Progresso (Pet)	2.0	0.0	0	990	90
Tomato Soup, condensed, made with water (1 cup)					
Campbell's (Campbell Soup Co)	2.0	0.0	0	730	100
Campbell's Healthy Request (Campbell Soup Co)	2.0	1.0	0	460	90
Tomato Soup, Ready-to-Serve (7¼ oz)					
Campbell's (Campbell Soup Co)	2.0	1.0	0	790	110
VEGETABLE WITH PASTA SOUPS—*see also* NOODLE SOUPS, page 363					
Hearty Vegetable with Pasta Soup, condensed, made with water (1 cup)					
Campbell's (Campbell Soup Co)	1.0	0.0	0	830	90
Hearty Vegetable with Rotini Soup (1 cup)					
Progresso (Pet)	1.0	0.0	0	720	110

	Tot. Fat (g)	Sat. Fat (g)	Chol. (mg)	Sod. (mg)	Cal.
OTHER VEGETABLE SOUPS					
Cream of Celery Soup, condensed, made with water (1 cup)					
Campbell's Healthy Request (Campbell Soup Co)	2.0	1.0	2	480	70
Escarole in Chicken Broth (1 cup)					
Progresso (Pet)	1.0	0.0	<5	980	25
OTHER SOUPS					
Crab Soup (⅔ cup)					
Pepperidge Farm (Campbell Soup Co)	2.0	1.0	10	1150	80
Garlic & Pasta Soup (1 cup)					
Progresso Healthy Classics (Pet)	1.5	0.0	<5	450	100
Golden Herb with Lemon Soup Mix (2 tbsp soup mix)					
Lipton Recipe Secrets (T.J. Lipton)	0.5	0.0	<5	510	35
Italian Herb Soup Mix (1 tbsp soup mix)					
Lipton Recipe Secrets (T.J. Lipton)	0.0	0.0	0	520	40
Savory Herb with Garlic Soup Mix (1 tbsp soup mix)					
Lipton Recipe Secrets (T.J. Lipton)	0.5	0.0	0	460	30

SWEET TOPPINGS AND SAUCES

Chocolate topping while you're on a low-fat diet? Yes, as long as you choose a topping from our listings on the following pages. Kids from age 3 to 103 love sweet toppings—on pancakes, toast, and frozen yogurts. But remember that although these toppings may be low in fat, they're often high in calories.

Like all the other entries in this book, the sweet toppings and sauces entries that follow list sodium content. The AHA does not have criteria for sodium but recommends a total of no more than 3,000 mg a day.

Generic Listings

By far, most of the foods in this book are brand name products. However, if a product is listed without a brand name, it means that most brands of that product contain about the same amount of fat, saturated fat, and cholesterol and that these amounts are within the criteria cited below.

If you find products that were introduced after this book went to press, use the generic listings and the following tables to help you evaluate them.

AHA Criteria for Sweet Toppings and Sauces*

	Tot. Fat (g)	Sat. Fat (g)	Chol. (mg)
All sweet toppings and sauces	<0.5	<0.5	<2

*Per serving.

Sweet Toppings and Sauces You'll Want to Limit

Some sweet toppings and sauces, like the examples below, are too high in fat, saturated fat, and/or cholesterol to meet AHA criteria. They aren't included in this book, and we recommend that you don't eat them often.

Compare the amounts of fat, saturated fat, cholesterol, sodium, and calories in this example with the more healthful alternatives listed on the following pages.

Sample Sweet Topping to Limit

	Tot. Fat (g)	Sat. Fat (g)	Chol. (mg)	Sod. (mg)	Cal.
Fudge-type chocolate syrup (2 tbsp)	5.6*	2.4*	(5)*	54	146

Adapted from USDA Handbook No. 8 series.

*These values exceed AHA criteria for sweet toppings and sauces.

	Tot. Fat (g)	Sat. Fat (g)	Chol. (mg)	Sod. (mg)	Cal.
BEVERAGE SYRUPS					
Chocolate Syrup (2 tbsp)					
Hershey's (Hershey Food Co)	0.0	0.0	0	25	100
Strawberry Syrup (2 tbsp)					
Hershey's (Hershey Food Co)	0.0	0.0	0	5	110
FRUIT/VEGETABLE BUTTERS					
Apple Butter (1 tbsp)					
Smucker's Autumn Harvest (The J.M. Smucker Co)	0.0	0.0	0	42	36
Smucker's Simply Fruit (The J.M. Smucker Co)	0.0	0.0	0	0	36
Cider Apple Butter (1 tbsp)					
Smucker's (The J.M. Smucker Co)	0.0	0.0	0	0	36
Natural Apple Butter (1 tbsp)					
Smucker's (The J.M. Smucker Co)	0.0	0.0	0	0	36
Peach Butter (1 tbsp)					
Smucker's (The J.M. Smucker Co)	0.0	0.0	0	0	45
Pumpkin Butter (1 tbsp)					
Smucker's Autumn Harvest (The J.M. Smucker Co)	0.0	0.0	0	0	36
HONEY					
Honey (1 tbsp)					
Most brands (USDA)	**0.0**	**0.0**	**0**	**1**	**64**
Sue Bee (Sioux Honey Association)	0.0	0.0	0	0	60
FRUIT SPREADS (INCLUDES JAMS, JELLIES, MARMALADES, AND PRESERVES)					
Apple Jellies					
Apple Jelly (1 tbsp)					
Kraft (Kraft General Foods)*	0.0	0.0	0	10	60
Apple-Strawberry Jelly (1 tbsp)					
Kraft (Kraft General Foods)*	0.0	0.0	0	10	50
Pure Apple Jelly (1 tbsp)					
America's Choice (A & P)	0.0	0.0	0	10	60

*Tobacco company, corporate subsidiary, or parent.

	Tot. Fat (g)	Sat. Fat (g)	Chol. (mg)	Sod. (mg)	Cal.
APRICOT PRESERVES					
Apricot Preserves (1 tbsp)					
America's Choice (A & P)	0.0	0.0	0	10	50
Gedney Minnesota State Fair (M.A. Gedney Co)	0.0	0.0	0	0	50
Kraft (Kraft General Foods)*	0.0	0.0	0	10	50
BLACKBERRY FRUIT SPREADS					
Blackberry Jelly (1 tbsp)					
Kraft (Kraft General Foods)*	0.0	0.0	0	10	50
Blackberry Preserves (1 tbsp)					
Kraft (Kraft General Foods)*	0.0	0.0	0	10	50
GRAPE FRUIT SPREADS					
Grape Fruit Spread (1 tsp)					
Weight Watchers (H.J. Heinz)	0.0	0.0	0	0	8
Grape Jam (1 tbsp)					
Kraft (Kraft General Foods)*	0.0	0.0	0	10	60
Grape Jelly (1 tbsp)					
Kraft (Kraft General Foods)*	0.0	0.0	0	10	50
Grape Reduced Calorie Spread (1 tbsp)					
Kraft (Kraft General Foods)*	0.0	0.0	0	20	20
Pure Grape Jelly (1 tbsp)					
America's Choice (A & P)	0.0	0.0	0	10	60
Pure Grape Preserves (1 tbsp)					
America's Choice (A & P)	0.0	0.0	0	10	60
Jams or preserves, any flavor (1 tbsp)					
Most brands (USDA)	**0.1**	**0.0**	**0**	**0**	**48**
Jellies, any flavor (1 tbsp)					
Most brands (USDA)	**0.0**	**0.0**	**0**	**7**	**52**
Smucker's (The J.M. Smucker Co)	0.0	0.0	0	0	54
Marmalades, any flavor (1 tbsp)					
Most brands (USDA)	**0.0**	**0.0**	**0**	**11**	**49**
ORANGE MARMALADES					
Orange Marmalade (1 tbsp)					
Kraft (Kraft General Foods)*	0.0	0.0	0	10	50
Smucker's (The J.M. Smucker Co)	0.0	0.0	0	0	54
Pure Orange Marmalade (1 tbsp)					
America's Choice (A & P)	0.0	0.0	0	10	50

*Tobacco company, corporate subsidiary, or parent.

	Tot. Fat (g)	Sat. Fat (g)	Chol. (mg)	Sod. (mg)	Cal.
PEACH PRESERVES					
Peach Preserves (1 tbsp)					
Kraft (Kraft General Foods)*	0.0	0.0	0	10	50
Pure Peach Preserves (1 tbsp)					
America's Choice (A & P)	0.0	0.0	0	10	50
PINEAPPLE PRESERVES					
Pineapple Preserves (1 tbsp)					
Kraft (Kraft General Foods)*	0.0	0.0	0	10	50
Pure Pineapple Preserves (1 tbsp)					
America's Choice (A & P)	0.0	0.0	0	10	50
RASPBERRY FRUIT SPREADS					
Pure Raspberry Preserves (1 tbsp)					
America's Choice (A & P)	0.0	0.0	0	10	60
Raspberry Fruit Spread (1 tsp)					
Weight Watchers (H.J. Heinz)	0.0	0.0	0	0	8
Red Raspberry Preserves (1 tbsp)					
Gedney Minnesota State Fair (M.A. Gedney Co)	0.0	0.0	0	0	50
Kraft (Kraft General Foods)*	0.0	0.0	0	10	50
STRAWBERRY FRUIT SPREADS—*see also* APPLE JELLIES, page 376					
Pure Strawberry Preserves (1 tbsp)					
America's Choice (A & P)	0.0	0.0	0	10	50
Strawberry Fruit Spread (1 tsp)					
Weight Watchers (H.J. Heinz)	0.0	0.0	0	0	8
Strawberry Jam (1 tbsp)					
Kraft (Kraft General Foods)*	0.0	0.0	0	10	50
Strawberry Jelly (1 tbsp)					
Kraft (Kraft General Foods)*	0.0	0.0	0	10	60
Strawberry Preserves (1 tbsp)					
Gedney Minnesota State Fair (M.A. Gedney Co)	0.0	0.0	0	0	45
Kraft (Kraft General Foods)*	0.0	0.0	0	10	50
Strawberry Reduced Calorie Spread (1 tbsp)					
Kraft (Kraft General Foods)*	0.0	0.0	0	20	20
OTHER FRUIT SPREADS					
Double Berry Preserves (1 tbsp)					
Gedney Minnesota State Fair (M.A. Gedney Co)	0.0	0.0	0	0	50

*Tobacco company, corporate subsidiary, or parent.

	Tot. Fat (g)	Sat. Fat (g)	Chol. (mg)	Sod. (mg)	Cal.
Extra Fruit Spread (1 tbsp)					
Smucker's (The J.M. Smucker Co)	0.0	0.0	0	0	45
Fruit Spreads (1 tbsp)					
Smucker's Simply Fruit (The J.M. Smucker Co)	0.0	0.0	0	0	48
Guava Jelly (1 tbsp)					
Kraft (Kraft General Foods)*	0.0	0.0	0	10	50
Light Fruit Spreads (1 tbsp)					
Smucker's (The J.M. Smucker Co)	0.0	0.0	0	0	21
Low Sugar Spreads (1 tbsp)					
Smucker's (The J.M. Smucker Co)	0.0	0.0	0	<30	24
Preserves and Jams (1 tbsp)					
Smucker's (The J.M. Smucker Co)	0.0	0.0	0	0	54
Red Currant Jelly (1 tbsp)					
Kraft (Kraft General Foods)*	0.0	0.0	0	10	50
Red Plum Jam (1 tbsp)					
Kraft (Kraft General Foods)*	0.0	0.0	0	10	60
Reduced Calorie Fruit Spread (1 tbsp)					
Smucker's Slenderella (The J.M. Smucker Co)	0.0	0.0	0	0	21
MOLASSES AND OTHER SYRUPS					
CORN SYRUPS/MAPLE SYRUPS/ PANCAKE SYRUPS					
All Natural Syrup (¼ cup)					
Sunrise (Dial Corp)	0.0	0.0	0	90	210
Artificial Butter Flavor Syrup (¼ cup)					
America's Choice (A & P)	0.0	0.0	0	60	220
Butter Flavored Syrup (¼ cup)					
Log Cabin Country Kitchen (Kraft General Foods)*	0.0	0.0	0	200	200
Butter Maple Lite Microwave Syrup (¼ cup)					
Pillsbury Hungry Jack (Grand Metropolitan PLC)	0.0	0.0	0	180	100

*Tobacco company, corporate subsidiary, or parent.

	Tot. Fat (g)	Sat. Fat (g)	Chol. (mg)	Sod. (mg)	Cal.
CORN SYRUPS/MAPLE SYRUPS/ PANCAKE SYRUPS *(cont'd)*					
Butter Maple Microwave Syrup (¼ cup)					
Pillsbury Hungry Jack (Grand Metropolitan PLC)	0.0	0.0	0	90	210
Butter Rich Syrup (¼ cup)					
Aunt Jemima (Quaker Oats Co) .	0.0	0.0	0	170	210
Butterlite Syrup (¼ cup)					
Aunt Jemima (Quaker Oats Co) .	0.0	0.0	0	150	100
Dark Corn Syrup (2 tbsp)					
Karo (Best Foods)	0.0	0.0	0	45	120
Dark Syrup (¼ cup)					
Brer Rabbit (Nabisco Foods)* . .	0.0	0.0	0	5	240
Fruit Syrups (2 tbsp)					
Smucker's (The J.M. Smucker Co)	0.0	0.0	0	<10	100
Light Corn Syrup (2 tbsp)					
Karo (Best Foods)	0.0	0.0	0	35	120
Light Syrup (¼ cup)					
Brer Rabbit (Nabisco Foods)* . .	0.0	0.0	0	0	240
Lite Microwave Syrup (¼ cup)					
Pillsbury Hungry Jack (Grand Metropolitan PLC)	0.0	0.0	0	180	100
Lite Reduced Calorie Syrup (¼ cup)					
America's Choice (A & P)	0.0	0.0	0	115	100
Log Cabin (Kraft General Foods)*	0.0	0.0	0	180	100
Log Cabin Country Kitchen (Kraft General Foods)*	0.0	0.0	0	160	100
Lite Syrup (¼ cup)					
Aunt Jemima (Quaker Oats Co) .	0.0	0.0	0	160	100
Mrs. Richardson's (Quaker Oats Co)	0.0	0.0	0	160	100
Vermont Maid (Nabisco Foods)*	0.0	0.0	0	140	100
Maple syrup (¼ cup)					
Most brands (USDA)	**0.0**	**0.0**	**0**	**8**	**200**
Microwave Syrup (¼ cup)					
Pillsbury Hungry Jack (Grand Metropolitan PLC)	0.0	0.0	0	90	210

*Tobacco company, corporate subsidiary, or parent.

	Tot. Fat (g)	Sat. Fat (g)	Chol. (mg)	Sod. (mg)	Cal.
Pancake and Waffle Syrup (¼ cup)					
Aunt Jemima (Quaker Oats Co) .	0.0	0.0	0	120	210
Pancake & Waffle Syrup with 2% Real Maple Syrup (¼ cup)					
America's Choice (A & P)	0.0	0.0	0	30	210
Pancake Syrup (4 tbsp)					
Golden Griddle (Best Foods) ...	0.0	0.0	0	55	220
Karo (Best Foods)	0.0	0.0	0	130	240
Reduced Calorie Syrup (¼ cup)					
Weight Watchers (H.J. Heinz) ..	0.0	0.0	0	150	110
Strawberry Syrup (¼ cup)					
America's Choice (A & P)	0.0	0.0	0	5	110
Syrup (¼ cup)					
Log Cabin (Kraft General Foods)*	0.0	0.0	0	60	200
Log Cabin Country Kitchen (Kraft General Foods)*	0.0	0.0	0	110	200
Vermont Maid (Nabisco Foods)*	0.0	0.0	0	25	210
MOLASSES					
Blackstrap molasses (1 tbsp)					
Most brands (USDA)	**0.0**	**0.0**	**0**	**39**	**43**
Dark Molasses (1 tbsp)					
Brer Rabbit (Nabisco Foods)* ..	0.0	0.0	0	10	50
Light Molasses (1 tbsp)					
Most brands (USDA)	**0.0**	**0.0**	**0**	**3**	**50**
Brer Rabbit (Nabisco Foods)* ..	0.0	0.0	0	10	60
Medium molasses (1 tbsp)					
Most brands (USDA)	**0.0**	**0.0**	**0**	**7**	**46**
SWEET TOPPINGS					
CARAMEL TOPPINGS					
Caramel Topping (2 tbsp)					
Kraft (Kraft General Foods)*	0.0	0.0	0	90	120
CHOCOLATE TOPPINGS					
Chocolate Flavored Syrup Topping (2 tbsp)					
Smucker's (The J.M. Smucker Co)	0.0	0.0	0	35	130
Chocolate Flavored Topping (2 tbsp)					
Kraft (Kraft General Foods)*	0.0	0.0	0	30	110

*Tobacco company, corporate subsidiary, or parent.

	Tot. Fat (g)	Sat. Fat (g)	Chol. (mg)	Sod. (mg)	Cal.
CHOCOLATE TOPPINGS *(cont'd)*					
Light Hot Fudge Topping (2 tbsp)					
Smucker's (The J.M. Smucker Co)	0.0	0.0	0	35	70
FRUIT TOPPINGS					
Pineapple Topping (2 tbsp)					
Kraft (Kraft General Foods)*	0.0	0.0	0	15	110
Smucker's (The J.M. Smucker Co)	0.0	0.0	0	0	130
Strawberry Topping (2 tbsp)					
Kraft (Kraft General Foods)*	0.0	0.0	0	15	110
Smucker's (The J.M. Smucker Co)	0.0	0.0	0	0	120
MARSHMALLOW TOPPINGS					
Marshmallow Creme (2 tbsp)					
Kraft (Kraft General Foods)*	0.0	0.0	0	30	100
Marshmallow Topping (2 tbsp)					
Smucker's (The J.M. Smucker Co)	0.0	0.0	0	0	120
NUT TOPPINGS					
Pecans in Syrup Topping (2 tbsp)					
Smucker's (The J.M. Smucker Co)	1.0	(0.2)	0	0	130
Walnuts in Syrup Topping (2 tbsp)					
Smucker's (The J.M. Smucker Co)	1.0	(0.1)	0	0	130

SYRUPS—*see* BEVERAGE SYRUPS, page 376; MOLASSES AND OTHER SYRUPS, page 379

*Tobacco company, corporate subsidiary, or parent.

SWEETS

Sweets come in two styles: high fat or low fat. On these pages, we emphasize the low-fat, low-cholesterol variety. By sticking with low-fat candies, you'll make your waistline love you almost as much as your heart does. On the other hand, if you're seriously watching your weight, go easy on candy. Remember that even low-fat candies are mostly sugar—and that means calories.

We didn't include candies that contain chocolate, nuts, peanut butter, or caramel because they're high in fat and saturated fat.

Like all the other entries in this book, the sweets entries that follow list sodium content. The AHA does not have criteria for sodium but recommends a total of no more than 3,000 mg a day.

Generic Listings

By far, most of the foods in this book are brand name products. However, if a product is listed without a brand name, it means that most brands of that product contain about the same amount of fat, saturated fat, and cholesterol and that these amounts are within the criteria cited below.

If you find products that were introduced after this book went to press, use the generic listings and the following tables to help you evaluate them.

AHA Criteria for Sweets*

	Tot. Fat (g)	Sat. Fat (g)	Chol. (mg)
All sweets	<0.5	<0.5	<2

*Per serving.

Sweets You'll Want to Limit

Some sweets, like the examples below, are too high in fat, saturated fat, and/or cholesterol to meet AHA criteria. They aren't included in this book, and we recommend that you don't eat them often.

Compare the amounts of fat, saturated fat, cholesterol, sodium, and calories in these examples with the more healthful alternatives listed on the following pages.

Sample Sweets to Limit

	Tot. Fat (g)	Sat. Fat (g)	Chol. (mg)	Sod. (mg)	Cal.
Chocolate-coated peanuts (1.4 oz, or about 10 pieces)	13.4*	5.8*	4*	16	208
Fondant coated in sweet chocolate (1 patty, about 2½″ in diameter and ½″ thick)	3.2*	1.9*	0	9	128

Adapted from USDA Handbook No. 8 series.

*These values exceed AHA criteria for sweets.

	Tot. Fat (g)	Sat. Fat (g)	Chol. (mg)	Sod. (mg)	Cal.
CANDIES					
HARD CANDIES					
Dinasour Eggs, Fruit Runts, Merry Mix, Runts Mini Hearts, Wacky Wafer Bunnys (10–17 pieces)					
Willy Wonka (The Willy Wonka Candy Factory)	0.0	0.0	0	0	60
Egg Breakers, Gobstoppers, Heart Breakers (6–9 pieces)					
Willy Wonka (The Willy Wonka Candy Factory)	0.0	0.0	0	0	60
Freckled Eggs (9 pieces)					
Willy Wonka (The Willy Wonka Candy Factory)	0.0	0.0	0	0	50
Goliath—Secret Centers (1 piece)					
Willy Wonka (The Willy Wonka Candy Factory)	0.0	0.0	0	0	40
Hard candy (1½ oz)					
Most brands (USDA)	**0.5**	**0.0**	**0**	**14**	**164**
Nerds, "New" Tart'N Tinys, Sweet & Sour Hearts (1 tbsp)					
Willy Wonka (The Willy Wonka Candy Factory)	0.0	0.0	0	0	60
JELLY BEANS					
Various flavors (2 tbsp)					
Jelly Belly (Herman Geolitz)	0.0	0.0	0	0–30	150
LICORICE—*see also* SOFT CANDIES, page 386					
All Natural Licorice Bar (1 bar)					
Panda (Shaffer, Clarke & Co) . . .	0.0	0.0	0	65	110
All Natural Licorice Chews (15 pieces)					
Panda (Shaffer, Clarke & Co) . . .	0.0	0.0	0	80	135
Licorice (2 tbsp)					
Jelly Belly (Herman Geolitz)	0.0	0.0	0	10	150
MINTS					
Butter Mints (7 pieces)					
Kraft (Kraft General Foods)*	0.0	0.0	0	25	60
Mints, uncoated (1½ oz)					
Most brands (USDA)	**0.9**	**0.2**	**0**	**90**	**155**

*Tobacco company, corporate subsidiary, or parent.

	Tot. Fat (g)	Sat. Fat (g)	Chol. (mg)	Sod. (mg)	Cal.
MINTS *(cont'd)*					
Party Mints (7 pieces)					
Kraft (Kraft General Foods)*	0.0	0.0	0	35	60
SOFT CANDIES—*see also* JELLY BEANS, page 385, LICORICE, page 385, MINTS, above					
All Natural Raspberry Bar (1 bar)					
Panda (Shaffer, Clarke & Co)	0.0	0.0	0	65	115
All Natural Raspberry Chews (15 pieces)					
Panda (Shaffer, Clarke & Co)	0.0	0.0	0	80	145
Candy corn (30 pieces)					
Most brands (USDA)	**0.9**	**0.2**	**(0)**	**90**	**155**
Gumdrops (1½ oz)					
Most brands (USDA)	**0.3**	**0.0**	**0**	**15**	**147**
Gummy Bears (17 pieces)					
Amazin' Fruit (Hershey Food Co)	0.0	0.0	0	45	130
Strawberry Strings (3 pieces)					
Twizzlers (Hershey Food Co)	0.0	0.0	0	100	150
Strawberry Twists (3 pieces)					
Twizzlers (Hershey Food Co)	0.5	0.0	0	100	130
MARSHMALLOWS					
Funmallows Marshmallows (4 pieces)					
Kraft (Kraft General Foods)*	0.0	0.0	0	20	110
Funmallows Miniature Marshmallows (½ cup)					
Kraft (Kraft General Foods)*	0.0	0.0	0	20	100
Jet-Puffed Marshmallows (5 pieces)					
Kraft (Kraft General Foods)*	0.0	0.0	0	30	110
Marshmallows (4 regular-size marshmallows)					
Most brands (USDA)	**0.0**	**0.0**	**0**	**12**	**92**
Miniature Marshmallows (½ cup)					
Kraft (Kraft General Foods)*	0.0	0.0	0	30	100
Teddy Bear Cocoa-Flavored Marshmallows (½ cup)					
Kraft (Kraft General Foods)*	0.0	0.0	0	25	100

*Tobacco company, corporate subsidiary, or parent.

VEGETABLES

Here's one food group you can eat to your heart's content! Mother Nature has packed vegetables with vitamins, minerals, and fiber—but very little fat and sodium, no cholesterol, and few calories.

With veggies, your only worry is added fat. Stay away from vegetables that have been breaded and deep-fried or cooked with butter, bacon, bacon fat, or salt pork. Do your heart a favor and avoid cream sauces and whole-milk cheese.

Like all the other entries in this book, the vegetable entries that follow list sodium content. The AHA does not have criteria for sodium but recommends a total of no more than 3,000 mg a day.

Generic Listings

By far, most of the foods in this book are brand name products. However, if a product is listed without a brand name, it means that most brands of that product contain about the same amount of fat, saturated fat, and cholesterol and that these amounts are within the criteria cited below.

If you find products that were introduced after this book went to press, use the generic listings and the following tables to help you evaluate them.

AHA Criteria for Vegetables*

	Tot. Fat (g)	Sat. Fat (g)	Chol. (mg)
Candied, French fried, hash browned, mashed, or stuffed potatoes; potato pancakes; potato skins; potatoes with sauce; or vegetables with sauce	3	1	20
Chili peppers, green onions, and garnish, such as parsley and pimiento	<0.5	<0.5	<2
Plain fresh, canned, and frozen vegetables (except those listed above)	3	1	<2

*Per serving.

Vegetables You'll Want to Limit

Some vegetables, like the examples below, are too high in fat, saturated fat, and/or cholesterol to meet AHA criteria. They aren't included in this book, and we recommend that you don't eat them often.

Compare the amounts of fat, saturated fat, cholesterol, sodium, and calories in these examples with the more healthful alternatives listed on the following pages.

Sample Vegetables to Limit

	Tot. Fat (g)	Sat. Fat (g)	Chol. (mg)	Sod. (mg)	Cal.
Breaded onion rings, frozen, heated in oven (3.9 oz, or about 11 rings)	29.3*	9.4*	0	413	447
French-fried potatoes, frozen, heated in oven (2½ oz, or about 14 strips)	5.3*	0.9	0	21	140
Scalloped potatoes, made from mix with whole milk and butter (about 5 oz)	6.0*	3.7*	(17)	476	130

Adapted from USDA Handbook No. 8 series.

*These values exceed AHA criteria for vegetables.

	Tot. Fat (g)	Sat. Fat (g)	Chol. (mg)	Sod. (mg)	Cal.
ALFALFA SPROUTS					
FRESH ALFALFA SPROUTS					
Alfalfa sprouts, raw (1 cup)	0.2	0.0	0	2	10
ARTICHOKES					
CANNED/SHELF-STABLE ARTICHOKES					
Artichoke Hearts (2 pieces)					
Progresso (Pet)	0.0	0.0	0	240	35
FRESH ARTICHOKES					
Artichokes, cooked (1 medium)	0.2	0.0	0	79	53
ASPARAGUS					
CANNED/SHELF-STABLE ASPARAGUS					
Asparagus, drained (½ cup spears)					
Most brands (USDA)	**0.8**	**0.2**	**0**	**(425)**	**24**
No-salt-added asparagus, drained (½ cup)					
Most brands (USDA)	**0.8**	**0.2**	**0**	**(5)**	**24**
FRESH ASPARAGUS					
Asparagus, cooked (½ cup)	0.3	0.1	0	7	22
Asparagus, raw (4 spears)	0.1	0.0	0	1	14
FROZEN ASPARAGUS					
Asparagus (4 spears)					
Most brands (USDA)	**0.3**	**0.1**	**0**	**2**	**17**
AVOCADOS—*see* "FATS AND OILS," AVOCADOS, page 191					
BAMBOO SHOOTS					
CANNED/SHELF-STABLE BAMBOO SHOOTS					
Bamboo shoots, sliced, drained (½ cup)					
Most brands (USDA)	**1.0**	**0.1**	**0**	**5**	**13**
BEAN SPROUTS					
CANNED/SHELF-STABLE BEAN SPROUTS					
Bean Sprouts (3 oz)					
Chun King (Chun King Corp)	0.0	0.0	0	15	5

	Tot. Fat (g)	Sat. Fat (g)	Chol. (mg)	Sod. (mg)	Cal.
BEANS					
BAKED BEANS/PORK AND BEANS					
Canned/Shelf-Stable Baked Beans/Pork and Beans					
Baked Beans (½ cup) Bush's (Bush Brothers)	1.0	<0.5	<5	550	150
Baked Beans Brown Sugar & Bacon Flavored (½ cup) Campbell's (Campbell Soup Co)	3.0	1.0	5	490	170
Baked Beans with Honey (½ cup) B&M (Pet)	1.5	0.0	0	450	170
Baked Beans with Onions (½ cup) Bush's (Bush Brothers)	1.5	0.5	0	500	150
Baked beans with pork and tomato sauce (½ cup) **Most brands** (USDA)	**1.3**	**0.5**	**9**	**554**	**123**
Baked Beans (½ cup) Green Giant (Grand Metropolitan PLC)	1.5	1.0	<5	580	160
Barbecue Baked Beans (½ cup) B&M (Pet)	2.0	0.5	<5	360	170
Brick Oven Baked Beans (½ cup) B&M (Pet)	2.0	0.5	5	390	180
Brown Sugar Beans (½ cup) Van Camp's (Quaker Oats Company)	3.0	1.0	5	410	170
Deluxe Pork and Beans (½ cup) Bush's (Bush Brothers)	1.5	0.5	5	480	160
Extra Hearty Baked Beans (½ cup) B&M (Pet)	2.0	0.5	<5	450	190
Fanci Pak Pork and Beans (½ cup) Bush's (Bush Brothers)	1.5	0.5	<5	350	160
Fat Free Baked Beans (½ cup) Van Camp's (Quaker Oats Company)	0.0	0.0	0	430	130
Homestyle Beans (½ cup) Campbell's (Campbell Soup Co)	2.0	1.0	5	490	150
Iron Kettle Baked Beans (½ cup) Heartland (Pet)	1.0	0.0	<5	500	150

	Tot. Fat (g)	Sat. Fat (g)	Chol. (mg)	Sod. (mg)	Cal.
99% Fat Free Baked Beans (½ cup)					
B&M (Pet)	1.0	0.0	0	220	160
Old Fashioned Barbecue Beans (½ cup)					
Campbell's (Campbell Soup Co)	3.0	1.0	5	460	170
Old Fashioned Beans (½ cup)					
Campbell's (Campbell Soup Co)	3.0	1.0	5	460	180
Original Baked Beans (½ cup)					
Friend's (Pet)	1.0	0.0	<5	390	170
Pork and Beans					
Bush's (Bush Brothers) (½ cup)	1.5	0.5	<5	550	120
Hunt's (Hunt-Wesson) (4 oz)	1.0	0.3	1	430	135
Trappey's (Allen Canning Co) (½ cup)	1.0	0.5	0	710	110
Wagon Master (Allen Canning Co) (½ cup)	1.0	0.5	0	710	110
Pork & Beans in Tomato Sauce (½ cup)					
Campbell's (Campbell Soup Co)	2.0	1.0	5	420	130
Pork & Beans with Tomato Sauce (½ cup)					
Green Giant (Grand Metropolitan PLC)	1.0	0.0	0	490	120
Premium Baked Beans (½ cup)					
Van Camp's (Quaker Oats Company)	1.0	0.0	0	520	140
Ranchero Beans (½ cup)					
Chi-Chi's (Hormel)	0.5	0.0	0	540	100
Red Kidney Baked Beans (½ cup)					
B&M (Pet)	2.0	0.5	<5	440	170
Friend's (Pet)	1.0	0.0	<5	510	160
Tangy Barbecue Flavor Baked Beans (½ cup)					
Campbell's (Campbell Soup Co)	3.0	1.0	5	460	170
Vegetarian Beans (½ cup)					
Bush's (Bush Brothers)	1.0	0.0	0	550	140
Vegetarian Beans in Tomato Sauce (½ cup)					
Campbell's (Campbell Soup Co)	2.0	1.0	0	460	130
Van Camp's (Quaker Oats Company)	0.5	0.0	0	400	110

	Tot. Fat (g)	Sat. Fat (g)	Chol. (mg)	Sod. (mg)	Cal.
BAKED BEANS/PORK AND BEANS *(cont'd)*					
Yellow Eye Baked Beans (½ cup)					
B&M (Pet)	2.0	0.5	<5	460	170
BLACK BEANS					
Canned/Shelf-Stable Black Beans					
Black Beans (½ cup)					
Old El Paso (Pet)	1.0	0.0	0	400	100
Progresso (Pet)	1.0	0.5	0	400	100
Seasoned Black Beans (½ cup)					
Allens (Allen Canning Co)	1.5	0.5	0	410	120
Trappey's (Allen Canning Co)	1.5	0.5	0	410	120
BLACK-EYED PEAS—*see* PEAS, BLACK-EYED PEAS, page 408					
BROADBEANS					
Canned/Shelf-Stable Broadbeans					
Broadbeans (½ cup)					
Most brands (USDA)	**0.3**	**0.0**	**0**	**580**	**91**
BUTTER BEANS—*see also* LIMA BEANS, page 395					
Canned/Shelf-Stable Butter Beans					
Butterbeans (½ cup)					
Van Camp's (Quaker Oats Company)	0.5	0.0	0	430	110
Large White Butterbeans with Sausage (½ cup)					
Trappey's (Allen Canning Co)	1.0	0.0	0	300	110
CANNELLINI BEANS					
Canned/Shelf-Stable Cannellini Beans					
Cannellini Beans (½ cup)					
Progresso (Pet)	0.5	0.0	0	270	100
CHICKPEAS/GARBANZO BEANS					
Canned/Shelf-Stable Chickpeas/ Garbanzo Beans					
Chick Peas (½ cup)					
Progresso (Pet)	2.5	0.0	0	280	120

	Tot. Fat (g)	Sat. Fat (g)	Chol. (mg)	Sod. (mg)	Cal.
Garbanzo Beans (½ cup)					
Most brands (USDA)	**1.4**	**0.1**	**0**	**359**	**143**
Bush's (Bush Brothers)	2.0	0.5	0	500	130
Old El Paso (Pet)	2.5	0.0	0	280	120
CHILI/KIDNEY/RED BEANS					
Canned/Shelf-Stable Chili/ Kidney/Red Beans					
Chili Beans (4 oz)					
Hunt's (Hunt-Wesson)	<1.0	0.0	0	490	100
Chili Beans in a Zesty Sauce (½ cup)					
Campbell's (Campbell Soup Co)	3.0	1.0	5	490	130
Chili Hot Beans (½ cup)					
Bush's (Bush Brothers)	1.0	0.5	0	480	120
Kidney beans (½ cup)					
Most brands (USDA)	**0.4**	**0.1**	**0**	**445**	**104**
Light Red Kidney Beans with Jalapeño (½ cup)					
Trappey's (Allen Canning Co)	1.0	0.0	0	420	110
Mexe Beans (½ cup)					
Old El Paso (Pet)	0.5	0.0	0	630	110
Mexi-Beans with Jalapeños (½ cup)					
Trappey's (Allen Canning Co)	1.5	0.5	0	460	130
Mexican Beans with Jalapeños (½ cup)					
Brown Beauty (Allen Canning Co)	1.0	0.0	0	370	120
Mexican Chili Beans (½ cup)					
Allens (Allen Canning Co)	1.0	0.0	0	300	120
Brown Beauty (Allen Canning Co)	1.0	0.0	0	300	120
Mexican Style Chili Beans (½ cup)					
Van Camp's (Quaker Oats Company)	2.0	0.5	0	430	110
New Orleans Style Light Red Kidney Beans with Bacon (½ cup)					
Trappey's (Allen Canning Co)	1.0	0.5	0	410	110
Red Kidney Beans (½ cup)					
Progresso (Pet)	0.5	0.0	0	280	110
Red Kidney Beans with Chili Gravy (½ cup)					
Trappey's (Allen Canning Co)	1.0	0.0	0	510	110

	Tot. Fat (g)	Sat. Fat (g)	Chol. (mg)	Sod. (mg)	Cal.
CHILI/KIDNEY/RED BEANS *(cont'd)*					
Spicy Chili Beans (½ cup)					
Green Giant (Grand Metropolitan PLC)	1.0	0.0	0	490	110
Cooked from Dried Chili/Kidney/ Red Beans					
Kidney beans (½ cup)					
Most brands (USDA)	**0.4**	**0.1**	**0**	**2**	**112**
COWPEAS—*see* PEAS, BLACK-EYED PEAS, page 408					
FAVA BEANS					
Canned/Shelf-Stable Fava Beans					
Fava Beans (½ cup)					
Progresso (Pet)	0.5	0.0	0	250	110
GARBANZO BEANS—*see* CHICKPEAS/ GARBANZO BEANS, page 392					
GREAT NORTHERN BEANS					
Canned/Shelf-Stable Great Northern Beans					
Great Northern Beans with Pork (½ cup)					
Bush's (Bush Brothers)	1.5	0.5	<5	460	110
Great Northern Beans with Sausage (½ cup)					
Trappey's (Allen Canning Co)	1.0	0.5	0	460	100
Cooked from Dried Great Northern Beans					
Great Northern Beans (½ cup)					
Most brands (USDA)	**0.4**	**0.1**	**0**	**2**	**104**
GREEN/SNAP BEANS					
Canned/Shelf-Stable Green/ Snap Beans					
50% Less Salt Green Beans (½ cup)					
Del Monte	0.0	0.0	0	180	20
Green Beans with Ham Flavor (½ cup)					
Bush's (Bush Brothers)	0.0	0.0	0	500	35
Green Beans with Ham Flavor and Potatoes (½ cup)					
Bush's (Bush Brothers)	0.0	0.0	0	560	40

	Tot. Fat (g)	Sat. Fat (g)	Chol. (mg)	Sod. (mg)	Cal.
Green or snap beans, drained (½ cup)					
Most brands (USDA)	**0.1**	**0.0**	**0**	**170**	**13**
Italian Green Beans (½ cup)					
Del Monte	0.0	0.0	0	360	30
No Salt Added Green Beans (½ cup)					
Del Monte	0.0	0.0	0	10	20
No-salt-added green or snap beans, drained (½ cup)					
Most brands (USDA)	**0.1**	**0.0**	**0**	**1**	**13**
Seasoned Green Beans (½ cup)					
Del Monte	0.0	0.0	0	360	20
Fresh Green/Snap Beans					
Green or snap beans, boiled (½ cup)	0.2	0.0	0	2	22
Frozen Green/Snap Beans					
Cut Green Beans in Butter Sauce (½ cup)					
Green Giant (Grand Metropolitan PLC)	1.0	<1.0	5	230	30
Green or snap beans, boiled (½ cup)					
Most brands (USDA)	**0.1**	**0.0**	**0**	**9**	**18**
KIDNEY BEANS—*see* CHILI/KIDNEY/ RED BEANS, page 393					
LIMA BEANS—*see also* BUTTER BEANS, page 392; SUCCOTASH, page 414					
Canned/Shelf-Stable Lima Beans					
Baby Green Lima Beans with Bacon (½ cup)					
Trappey's (Allen Canning Co)	1.0	0.5	0	330	120
Baby White Lima Beans with Bacon (½ cup)					
Trappey's (Allen Canning Co)	1.5	0.5	0	350	130
Lima beans, undrained (½ cup)					
Most brands (USDA)	**0.4**	**0.1**	**0**	**309**	**93**
No-salt-added lima beans, undrained (½ cup)					
Most brands (USDA)	**0.4**	**0.1**	**0**	**5**	**93**

	Tot. Fat (g)	Sat. Fat (g)	Chol. (mg)	Sod. (mg)	Cal.
LIMA BEANS *(cont'd)*					
Frozen Lima Beans					
Baby lima beans (½ cup)					
Most brands (USDA)	**0.3**	**0.1**	**0**	**26**	**94**
Lima beans, cooked (½ cup)					
Most brands (USDA)	**0.3**	**0.1**	**0**	**26**	**94**
MIXED BEANS					
Canned/Shelf-Stable Mixed Beans					
Country Three-Bean Salad (½ cup)					
Del Monte	0.0	0.0	0	510	100
Sweet and Tangy Garden Medley (½ cup)					
Del Monte	0.5	0.0	0	520	130
Three Bean Salad (½ cup)					
Green Giant (Grand Metropolitan PLC)	0.0	0.0	0	470	70
NAVY BEANS					
Canned/Shelf-Stable Navy Beans					
Navy Beans with Bacon (½ cup)					
Trappey's (Allen Canning Co)	1.5	0.5	0	420	110
Navy Beans with Bacon and Jalapeño (½ cup)					
Trappey's (Allen Canning Co)	1.5	0.5	0	420	110
Cooked from Dried Navy Beans					
Navy beans, boiled (½ cup)					
Most brands (USDA)	**0.5**	**0.1**	**0**	**1**	**129**
NORTHERN BEANS—see GREAT NORTHERN BEANS, page 394					
PINTO BEANS					
Canned/Shelf-Stable Pinto Beans					
Cowboy Pintos (½ cup)					
Bush's (Bush Brothers)	1.0	0.5	0	360	120
Jalapinto Pinto Beans with Bacon (½ cup)					
Trappey's (Allen Canning Co)	1.0	0.5	0	540	120

	Tot. Fat (g)	Sat. Fat (g)	Chol. (mg)	Sod. (mg)	Cal.
Pinto Beans (½ cup)					
Most brands (USDA)	**0.4**	**0.1**	**0**	**499**	**93**
Old El Paso (Pet)	0.5	0.0	0	420	110
Progresso (Pet)	1.0	0.0	0	250	110
Pinto Beans with Bacon (½ cup)					
Trappey's (Allen Canning Co)	1.0	0.5	0	270	120
Pintos with Bacon (½ cup)					
Bush's (Bush Brothers)	1.0	0.5	0	540	110
Pintos with Bacon and Jalapeño (½ cup)					
Bush's (Bush Brothers)	1.5	0.5	<5	550	110
Pintos with Pork (½ cup)					
Bush's (Bush Brothers)	2.5	1.0	<5	530	120
Cooked from Dried Pinto Beans					
Pinto beans, boiled (½ cup)					
Most brands (USDA)	**0.4**	**0.1**	**0**	**1**	**117**
Pinto Beans with Spanish Seasoning (3 tbsp dry)					
N.K. Hurst (Hurst Beans)	0.5	0.0	0	350	120
Pork and Beans—see Baked Beans/Pork and Beans, page 390					
Red Beans—*see* Chili/Kidney/Red Beans, page 393					
Refried Beans					
Canned/Shelf-Stable Refried Beans					
Fat Free Refried Beans (½ cup)					
Old El Paso (Pet)	0.0	0.0	0	480	110
No Fat Refried Beans (½ cup)					
Las Palmas (Pet)	0.0	0.0	0	470	110
Refried Beans (½ cup)					
Allens (Allen Canning Co)	2.5	1.0	0	360	150
Las Palmas (Pet)	2.0	1.0	<5	500	110
Old El Paso (Pet)	2.0	1.0	<5	500	110
Ortega (Nabisco Foods)*	2.5	0.5	0	580	140
Refried Beans with Green Chilies (½ cup)					
Old El Paso (Pet)	0.5	0.0	<5	720	110

*Tobacco company, corporate subsidiary, or parent.

	Tot. Fat (g)	Sat. Fat (g)	Chol. (mg)	Sod. (mg)	Cal.
Refried Beans *(cont'd)*					
Refried Black Beans (½ cup)					
Old El Paso (Pet)	2.0	0.0	0	340	120
Vegetarian Refried Beans (½ cup)					
Old El Paso (Pet)	1.0	0.0	0	490	100
Snap Beans—*see* Green/Snap Beans, page 394					
White Beans					
Cooked from Dried White Beans					
White beans, boiled (½ cup)					
Most brands (USDA)	**0.4**	**0.1**	**0**	**7**	**153**
BEETS					
Canned/Shelf-Stable Beets					
Beets, slices, drained (½ cup)					
Most brands (USDA)	**0.1**	**0.0**	**0**	**(324)**	**27**
Harvard beets, undrained (½ cup)					
Most brands (USDA)	**0.1**	**0.0**	**0**	**199**	**89**
No-salt-added beets, slices, drained (½ cup)					
Most brands (USDA)	**0.1**	**0.0**	**0**	**(57)**	**27**
Pickled beets, slices, undrained (½ cup)					
Most brands (USDA)	**0.1**	**0.0**	**0**	**301**	**75**
Fresh Beets					
Beets, slices, cooked (½ cup)	0.0	0.0	0	42	26
Raw beets (2)	0.1	0.0	0	118	71
BROCCOLI					
Fresh Broccoli					
Broccoli, chopped, cooked (½ cup)	0.2	0.0	0	8	23
Broccoli, chopped, raw (½ cup)	0.2	0.0	0	12	12
Broccoli spears, cooked (1 spear)	0.5	0.1	0	19	53
Frozen Broccoli					
Broccoli, chopped, cooked (½ cup)					
Most brands (USDA)	**0.1**	**0.0**	**0**	**22**	**25**
Broccoli in Cheese Flavored Sauce (⅔ cup)					
Green Giant (Grand Metropolitan PLC)	2.5	1.0	<5	520	70

	Tot. Fat (g)	Sat. Fat (g)	Chol. (mg)	Sod. (mg)	Cal.
Broccoli Spears in Butter Sauce (4 oz)					
Green Giant (Grand Metropolitan PLC)	1.5	1.0	<5	330	50
BRUSSELS SPROUTS					
Fresh Brussels Sprouts					
Brussels sprouts, cooked (½ cup)	0.4	0.1	0	17	30
Brussels sprouts, raw (1 sprout)	0.1	0.0	0	5	8
Frozen Brussels Sprouts					
Brussels sprouts (½ cup)					
Most brands (USDA)	**0.3**	**0.1**	**0**	**18**	**33**
CABBAGE					
Fresh Cabbage					
Cabbage, shredded, cooked (½ cup)	0.2	0.0	0	14	16
Cabbage, shredded, raw (½ cup)	0.1	0.0	0	6	8
Chinese cabbage, shredded, cooked (½ cup)	0.1	0.0	0	29	10
Chinese cabbage, shredded, raw (½ cup)	0.1	0.0	0	23	5
Red cabbage, shredded, cooked (½ cup)	0.2	0.0	0	6	16
Red cabbage, shredded, raw (½ cup)	0.1	0.0	0	4	10
CARROTS—*see also* **PEAS AND CARROTS, page 410**					
Canned/Shelf-Stable Carrots					
Carrots, slices (½ cup)					
Most brands (USDA)	**0.1**	**0.0**	**0**	**176**	**17**
No-salt-added carrots, slices (½ cup)					
Most brands (USDA)	**0.1**	**0.0**	**0**	**31**	**17**
Fresh Carrots					
Baby carrots, raw (2¾″ long)	0.1	0.0	0	3	4
Carrots, raw (7½″ x 1″)	0.1	0.0	0	25	31
Carrots, slices, cooked (½ cup)	0.1	0.0	0	52	35

	Tot. Fat (g)	Sat. Fat (g)	Chol. (mg)	Sod. (mg)	Cal.
FROZEN CARROTS					
Carrots, slices (½ cup)					
Most brands (USDA)	**0.1**	**0.0**	**0**	**43**	**26**
CAULIFLOWER					
FRESH CAULIFLOWER					
Cauliflower, cooked, 1″ pieces (½ cup)	0.1	0.0	0	4	15
Cauliflower, raw, 1″ pieces (½ cup)	0.9	0.0	0	7	12
FROZEN CAULIFLOWER					
Cauliflower, 1″ pieces (½ cup)					
Most brands (USDA)	**0.2**	**0.0**	**0**	**16**	**17**
Cauliflower in Cheese Flavored Sauce (½ cup)					
Green Giant (Grand Metropolitan PLC)	2.5	0.5	<5	510	60
CELERY					
FRESH CELERY					
Celery, cooked (½ cup diced)	0.8	0.0	0	48	11
Celery, raw (7½″ x 1″ stalk)	0.1	0.0	0	35	6
CHAYOTE					
FRESH CHAYOTE					
Chayote, cooked, 1″ pieces (½ cup)	0.4	0.0	0	1	19
Chayote, raw, 1″ pieces (½ cup)	0.2	0.0	0	3	16
CHIVES					
FREEZE-DRIED CHIVES					
Freeze-dried chives (1 tbsp)					
Most brands (USDA)	**0.0**	**0.0**	**0**	**(0)**	**1**
FRESH CHIVES					
Fresh chives, chopped (1 tbsp)	0.0	0.0	0	0	1
CILANTRO					
FRESH CILANTRO					
Cilantro (¼ cup)	0.1	0.0	0	1	1
CORIANDER LEAF—see CILANTRO, above					

	Tot. Fat (g)	Sat. Fat (g)	Chol. (mg)	Sod. (mg)	Cal.
CORN—*see also* **HOMINY, page 403; SUCCOTASH, page 414**					
CANNED/SHELF-STABLE CORN					
Baby Corn (½ cup)					
Ka-me (Shaffer, Clarke & Co) . . .	0.0	0.0	0	10	20
Corn, drained (½ cup)					
Most brands (USDA)	**0.8**	**0.1**	**0**	**(286)**	**66**
Cream-style corn (½ cup)					
Most brands (USDA)	**0.5**	**0.1**	**0**	**365**	**93**
Cream Style White Corn (½ cup)					
Del Monte	0.0	0.0	0	360	100
50% Less Salt Cream Style Golden Corn (½ cup)					
Del Monte	0.5	0.0	0	180	90
50% Less Salt Whole Kernel Corn (½ cup)					
Del Monte	1.0	0.0	0	130	60
Mexicorn (⅓ cup)					
Green Giant (Grand Metropolitan PLC)	0.0	0.0	0	430	60
No-salt-added corn, drained (½ cup)					
Most brands (USDA)	**0.8**	**0.1**	**0**	**(3)**	**66**
No Salt Added Cream Style Corn (½ cup)					
Most brands (USDA)	**1.0**	**0.1**	**0**	**4**	**93**
Del Monte	0.5	0.0	0	10	90
No Salt Added Whole Kernel Golden Corn (½ cup)					
Del Monte	1.0	0.0	0	10	60
Stir-Fry Corn (pre-cut) (½ cup)					
Ka-me (Shaffer, Clarke & Co) . . .	0.0	0.0	0	10	20
Whole Kernel White Corn (½ cup)					
Del Monte	0.0	0.0	0	360	80
FRESH CORN					
Corn, sweet, raw (½ cup)	0.9	0.1	0	12	66
Corn, sweet, cooked (½ cup)	1.1	0.2	0	14	89

	Tot. Fat (g)	Sat. Fat (g)	Chol. (mg)	Sod. (mg)	Cal.
FROZEN CORN					
Cob Corn (1 ear)					
Ore-Ida (H.J. Heinz)	2.5	0.0	0	5	180
Corn (½ cup)					
Most brands (USDA)	**0.1**	**0.0**	**0**	**4**	**67**
Mini-Gold Cob Corn (1 ear)					
Ore-Ida (H.J. Heinz)	1.0	0.0	0	0	90
Shoepeg White Corn in Butter Sauce (½ cup)					
Green Giant (Grand Metropolitan PLC)	2.0	<1.0	5	280	100
CUCUMBERS					
FRESH CUCUMBERS					
Cucumbers, raw (½ cup slices)	0.1	0.0	0	1	7
EGGPLANT					
FRESH EGGPLANT					
Eggplant, cooked (½ cup cubes)	0.1	0.0	0	2	13
ENDIVE					
FRESH ENDIVE					
Endive, chopped, raw (½ cup)	0.1	0.0	0	6	4
GARLIC					
FRESH GARLIC					
Garlic (1 clove)	0.0	0.0	0	1	4
GINGERROOT					
CANDIED GINGERROOT					
Ginger Root, slices, crystallized (5 pieces)					
Ka-me (Shaffer, Clarke & Co)	0.0	0.0	0	23	100
CANNED/SHELF-STABLE GINGERROOT					
Ginger Root, slices (20 pieces)					
Ka-me (Shaffer, Clarke & Co)	0.0	0.0	0	70	0
FRESH GINGERROOT					
Gingerroot, raw (5 pieces, ⅛″ × 1″)	0.1	0.0	0	1	8

	Tot. Fat (g)	Sat. Fat (g)	Chol. (mg)	Sod. (mg)	Cal.
GREENS					
BEET GREENS					
Fresh Beet Greens					
Beet greens, pieces, cooked (½ cup)	0.1	0.0	0	173	20
DANDELION GREENS					
Fresh Dandelion Greens					
Dandelion greens, chopped, cooked (½ cup)	0.3	0.0	0	23	17
KALE					
Fresh Kale					
Kale, chopped, cooked (½ cup)	0.3	0.0	0	15	21
Kale, chopped, raw (½ cup)	0.2	0.0	0	15	17
MUSTARD GREENS					
Fresh Mustard Greens					
Mustard greens, chopped, cooked (½ cup)	0.2	0.0	0	11	11
Frozen Mustard Greens					
Mustard greens (½ cup)					
Most brands (USDA)	**0.2**	**0.0**	**0**	**19**	**14**
TURNIP GREENS					
Canned/Shelf-Stable Turnip Greens					
Turnip greens, undrained (½ cup)	0.4	0.1	0	325	17
Fresh Turnip Greens					
Turnip greens, chopped, cooked (½ cup)	0.2	0.0	0	21	15
Turnip greens, chopped, raw (½ cup)	0.1	0.0	0	11	7
Frozen Turnip Greens					
Turnip greens (½ cup)					
Most brands (USDA)	**0.4**	**0.1**	**0**	**12**	**24**
HOMINY					
CANNED/SHELF-STABLE HOMINY					
Golden Hominy with Peppers (½ cup)					
Bush's (Bush Brothers)	1.0	0.0	0	570	70

	Tot. Fat (g)	Sat. Fat (g)	Chol. (mg)	Sod. (mg)	Cal.
CANNED/SHELF-STABLE HOMINY *(cont'd)*					
White Hominy with Peppers (½ cup)					
Bush's (Bush Brothers)	1.0	0.0	0	500	80
JICAMA					
FRESH JICAMA					
Jicama (yam bean), slices (1 cup)	0.1	0.0	0	5	46
KOHLRABI					
FRESH KOHLRABI					
Kohlrabi, slices, cooked (½ cup)	0.1	0.0	0	17	24
Kohlrabi, slices, raw (½ cup)	0.1	0.0	0	14	19
LEEKS					
FRESH LEEKS					
Leeks, chopped, cooked (¼ cup)	0.1	0.0	0	3	8
Leeks, chopped, raw (¼ cup)	0.1	0.0	0	5	16
LEGUMES—*see* BEANS, page 390; PEAS, page 408					
LENTILS					
COOKED FROM DRIED LENTILS					
Lentils, boiled (½ cup)					
Most brands (USDA)	**0.4**	**0.1**	**0**	**2**	**115**
LETTUCE					
FRESH LETTUCE					
Iceberg lettuce (¼ head)	0.3	0.0	0	12	18
MIXED VEGETABLES—*see also* PEAS AND CARROTS, page 410; PEAS AND ONIONS, page 410; SUCCOTASH, page 414					
CANNED/SHELF-STABLE MIXED VEGETABLES					
Cantonese Classic Vegetables & Sauce (½ cup)					
House of Tsang (Hormel)	1.0	0.0	0	930	70
Chop Suey Vegetables (½ cup)					
La Choy (Hunt-Wesson)	<1.0	0.0	0	320	10

	Tot. Fat (g)	Sat. Fat (g)	Chol. (mg)	Sod. (mg)	Cal.
Chow Mein Vegetables (3 oz)					
Chun King (Chun King Corp) . . .	0.0	0.0	0	15	10
Creole Okra Gumbo (½ cup)					
Trappey's (Allen Canning Co) . . .	0.5	0.0	0	290	35
Fancy Mix Vegetables (½ cup)					
La Choy (Hunt-Wesson)	<1.0	0.0	0	30	12
Garden Medley (½ cup)					
Green Giant (Grand Metropolitan PLC)	0.0	0.0	0	360	40
Hong Kong Sweet & Sour Vegetables & Sauce (½ cup)					
House of Tsang (Hormel)	0.0	0.0	0	580	160
Mixed vegetables, drained (½ cup)					
Most brands (USDA)	**0.4**	**0.0**	**0**	**122**	**39**
Mixed Vegetables with Corn (½ cup)					
Del Monte	0.0	0.0	0	360	40
Okra, Tomatoes and Corn (½ cup)					
Allens (Allen Canning Co)	0.0	0.0	0	280	30
Trappey's (Allen Canning Co) . . .	0.0	0.0	0	280	30
Saucy Fiesta Vegetables (½ cup)					
Del Monte	0.0	0.0	0	480	80
Savory Italian Medley (½ cup)					
Del Monte	0.0	0.0	0	510	60
Stir-Fry Vegetables (½ cup)					
Ka-me (Shaffer, Clarke & Co) . . .	0.0	0.0	0	10	20
Sweet and Sour Oriental Vegetables (½ cup)					
Del Monte	0.0	0.0	0	370	70
Szechuan Hot & Spicy Vegetables & Sauce (½ cup)					
House of Tsang (Hormel)	1.0	0.0	0	1090	70
Tokyo Teriyaki Vegetables & Sauce (½ cup)					
House of Tsang (Hormel)	0.0	0.0	0	1240	100
FROZEN MIXED VEGETABLES					
California Style Vegetables (¾ cup)					
Green Giant American Mixtures (Grand Metropolitan PLC)	0.0	0.0	0	15	25

	Tot. Fat (g)	Sat. Fat (g)	Chol. (mg)	Sod. (mg)	Cal.
Frozen Mixed Vegetables *(cont'd)*					
Heartland Style Vegetables (1 cup)					
Green Giant American Mixtures (Grand Metropolitan PLC)	0.0	0.0	0	35	30
Japanese Style Teriyaki Vegetables (4 oz)					
Green Giant International Mixtures (Grand Metropolitan PLC)	0.0	0.0	0	400	50
Lo Mein Stir Fry Vegetables (vegetables only) (2⅓ cups)					
Green Giant Create A Meal! (Grand Metropolitan PLC)	0.5	0.0	0	1070	160
Manhattan Style Vegetables (1 cup)					
Green Giant American Mixtures (Grand Metropolitan PLC)	0.0	0.0	0	15	25
Mixed vegetables (½ cup)					
Most brands (USDA)	**0.1**	**0.0**	**0**	**32**	**54**
Mixed Vegetables in Butter Sauce (¾ cup)					
Green Giant (Grand Metropolitan PLC)	2.0	1.0	<5	240	70
New England Style Vegetables (⅔ cup)					
Green Giant American Mixtures (Grand Metropolitan PLC)	1.5	0.0	0	70	70
Oriental Style Rice Vegetables (8 oz)					
Green Giant International Mixtures (Grand Metropolitan PLC)	0.5	0.0	0	980	180
San Francisco Style Vegetables (¾ cup)					
Green Giant American Mixtures (Grand Metropolitan PLC)	0.0	0.0	0	20	30
Santa Fe Style Vegetables (¾ cup)					
Green Giant American Mixtures (Grand Metropolitan PLC)	0.0	0.0	0	10	6
Seattle Style Vegetables (¾ cup)					
Green Giant American Mixtures (Grand Metropolitan PLC)	0.0	0.0	0	15	25

	Tot. Fat (g)	Sat. Fat (g)	Chol. (mg)	Sod. (mg)	Cal.
Stew Vegetables (⅔ cup)					
Ore-Ida (H.J. Heinz)	0.0	0.0	0	50	50
Sweet & Sour Stir Fry Vegetables (vegetables only) (2⅓ cups) Green Giant Create A Meal! (Grand Metropolitan PLC)	0.0	0.0	0	390	130
Teriyaki Stir Fry Vegetables (vegetables only) (1¾ cups) Green Giant Create A Meal! (Grand Metropolitan PLC)	0.0	0.0	0	870	100
Western Style Vegetables (¾ cup) Green Giant American Mixtures (Grand Metropolitan PLC)	1.5	0.0	0	10	50
MUSHROOMS					
CANNED/SHELF-STABLE MUSHROOMS					
Mushroom pieces, drained (½ cup)					
Most brands (USDA)	**0.2**	**0.0**	**0**	**(330)**	**19**
Mushrooms Broiled in Butter, Pieces & Stems (3 oz) BinB (Grand Metropolitan PLC)	0.0	0.0	0	460	30
Mushrooms Broiled in Butter, Sliced (3 oz) BinB (Grand Metropolitan PLC)	0.0	0.0	0	460	30
Mushrooms Broiled in Butter, Sliced with Garlic (3 oz) BinB (Grand Metropolitan PLC)	0.0	0.0	0	410	35
Mushrooms Broiled in Butter, Whole (3 oz) BinB (Grand Metropolitan PLC)	0.0	0.0	0	460	30
Stir-Fry Mushrooms (½ cup) Ka-me (Shaffer, Clarke & Co)	0.0	0.0	0	380	20
Straw Mushrooms, whole, peeled (½ cup) Ka-me (Shaffer, Clarke & Co)	0.0	0.0	0	380	20
FRESH MUSHROOMS					
Mushrooms, pieces, cooked (½ cup)	0.4	0.1	0	2	21
Mushrooms, pieces, raw (½ cup)	0.2	0.0	0	1	9
Mushrooms, whole, raw (1)	0.1	0.0	0	1	5

	Tot. Fat (g)	Sat. Fat (g)	Chol. (mg)	Sod. (mg)	Cal.
OKRA					
FRESH OKRA					
Okra, slices, cooked (½ cup)	0.1	0.0	0	4	25
Okra, slices, raw (½ cup)	0.1	0.0	0	4	19
FROZEN OKRA					
Okra (½ cup)					
Most brands (USDA)	**0.3**	**0.1**	**0**	**3**	**34**
ONIONS—*see also* PEAS AND ONIONS, page 410					
FRESH ONIONS					
Onions, chopped, cooked (½ cup) . .	0.2	0.0	0	8	29
Onions, chopped, raw (½ cup)	0.2	0.0	0	2	27
FROZEN ONIONS					
Chopped Onions (¾ cup)					
Ore-Ida (H.J. Heinz)	0.0	0.0	0	20	25
PARSLEY					
FREEZE-DRIED PARSLEY					
Freeze-dried parsley (¼ cup)					
Most brands (USDA)	**0.1**	**0.0**	**0**	**5**	**4**
FRESH PARSLEY					
Fresh parsley, chopped (½ cup)	0.2	0.0	0	17	11
PARSNIPS					
FRESH PARSNIPS					
Parsnips, slices, cooked (½ cup) . . .	0.2	0.0	0	8	63
Parsnips, slices, raw (½ cup)	0.4	0.0	0	7	50
PEAS—*see also* SNOW PEAS, page 410; PEAS AND CARROTS, page 410; PEAS AND ONIONS, page 410					
BLACK-EYED PEAS—*see also* COWPEAS, page 409					
Canned/Shelf-Stable Black-Eyed Peas					
Blackeye Peas with Bacon (½ cup)					
Bush's (Bush Brothers)	1.0	0.5	<5	630	110
Trappey's (Allen Canning Co) . . .	2.0	0.5	0	350	120

	Tot. Fat (g)	Sat. Fat (g)	Chol. (mg)	Sod. (mg)	Cal.
Blackeye Peas with Bacon and Jalapeño (½ cup)					
Bush's (Bush Brothers)	2.5	1.0	<5	660	120
Trappey's (Allen Canning Co)	1.5	0.5	0	470	110
Blackeye Peas with Snap Beans (½ cup)					
Bush's (Bush Brothers)	0.5	0.0	0	550	110
CHICKPEAS—*see* BEANS, CHICKPEAS/GARBANZO BEANS, page 392					
COWPEAS—*see also* BLACK-EYED PEAS, page 408					
Cooked from Dried Cowpeas					
Cowpeas, cooked (½ cup)					
Most brands (USDA)	**0.7**	**0.2**	**0**	**4**	**89**
CROWDER PEAS					
Canned/Shelf-Stable Crowder Peas					
Crowder Peas (½ cup)					
Bush's (Bush Brothers)	1.0	0.0	0	500	110
FIELD PEAS					
Canned/Shelf-Stable Field Peas					
Field Peas with Bacon (½ cup)					
Trappey's (Allen Canning Co)	1.0	0.5	0	380	90
Field Peas with Snaps and Bacon (½ cup)					
Trappey's (Allen Canning Co)	1.0	0.5	0	380	110
GREEN PEAS					
Canned/Shelf-Stable Green Peas					
50% Less Salt Peas (½ cup)					
Del Monte	0.0	0.0	0	180	60
Green peas, drained (½ cup)					
Most brands (USDA)	**0.3**	**0.1**	**0**	**186**	**59**
No-salt-added green peas, drained (½ cup)					
Most brands (USDA)	**0.3**	**0.1**	**0**	**2**	**59**
No-Salt-Added peas (½ cup)					
Del Monte	0.0	0.0	0	10	60
Fresh Green Peas					
Green peas, cooked (½ cup)	0.2	0.0	0	2	67
Green peas, raw (½ cup)	0.3	0.1	0	4	63

	Tot. Fat (g)	Sat. Fat (g)	Chol. (mg)	Sod. (mg)	Cal.
GREEN PEAS *(cont'd)*					
Frozen Green Peas					
Green peas (½ cup)					
Most brands (USDA)	**0.2**	**0.0**	**0**	**70**	**63**
SNOW PEAS					
Fresh Snow Peas					
Snow peas, cooked (½ cup)	0.2	0.0	0	3	34
Snow peas, raw (½ cup)	0.1	0.0	0	3	30
Frozen Snow Peas					
Snow peas (½ cup)					
Most brands (USDA)	**0.3**	**0.1**	**0**	**4**	**42**
OTHER PEAS					
Other Canned/Shelf Stable Peas					
Cowboy Peas (½ cup)					
Bush's (Bush Brothers)	1.0	0.0	0	500	120
PEAS AND CARROTS					
CANNED/SHELF-STABLE PEAS AND CARROTS					
No-salt-added peas and carrots, undrained (½ cup)					
Most brands (USDA)	**0.4**	**0.1**	**0**	**5**	**48**
Peas and carrots, undrained (½ cup)					
Most brands (USDA)	**0.4**	**0.1**	**0**	**332**	**48**
FROZEN PEAS AND CARROTS					
Peas and carrots (½ cup)					
Most brands (USDA)	**0.3**	**0.1**	**0**	**55**	**38**
PEAS AND ONIONS					
CANNED/SHELF-STABLE PEAS AND ONIONS					
Peas and onions, undrained (½ cup)					
Most brands (USDA)	**0.2**	**0.0**	**0**	**265**	**30**
FROZEN PEAS AND ONIONS					
Peas and onions (½ cup)					
Most brands (USDA)	**0.2**	**0.0**	**0**	**(78)**	**40**

	Tot. Fat (g)	Sat. Fat (g)	Chol. (mg)	Sod. (mg)	Cal.
PEPPERS, HOT					
CANNED/SHELF-STABLE HOT PEPPERS					
Chopped Green Chilies (2 tbsp)					
Old El Paso (Pet)	0.0	0.0	0	110	5
Diced Green Chiles (2 tbsp)					
Pancho Villa (Pet)	0.0	0.0	0	110	5
Chi-Chi's (Hormel)	0.0	0.0	0	5	10
Ortega (Nabisco Foods)*	0.0	0.0	0	20	10
Diced Jalapeño Peppers (2 tbsp)					
Ortega (Nabisco Foods)*	0.0	0.0	0	25	10
Whole Green Chilies					
Chi-Chi's (Hormel) (¾ pepper)	0.0	0.0	0	5	10
Old El Paso (Pet) (1 pepper)	0.0	0.0	0	230	10
Ortega (Nabisco Foods)* (1 pepper)	0.0	0.0	0	30	15
Whole Jalapeño Peppers (2 peppers)					
Ortega (Nabisco Foods)*	0.0	0.0	0	25	10
FRESH HOT PEPPERS					
Hot chili peppers, raw (1)	0.1	0.0	0	3	18
PEPPERS, SWEET					
CANNED/SHELF-STABLE SWEET PEPPERS					
Roasted Peppers (½ piece)					
Progresso (Pet)	0.0	0.0	0	60	10
FRESH SWEET PEPPERS					
Sweet green or red bell peppers, chopped, raw (½ cup)	0.2	0.0	0	2	12
Sweet green or red bell peppers, chopped, cooked (½ cup)	0.2	0.0	0	1	12
Sweet yellow bell peppers, raw (10 strips)	0.1	0.0	0	1	14
POTATOES—*see also* SWEET POTATOES/YAMS, page 414					
CANNED/SHELF-STABLE POTATOES					
Potatoes, whole, drained (½ cup)					
Most brands (USDA)	**0.2**	**0.0**	**0**	**(452)**	**54**

*Tobacco company, corporate subsidiary, or parent.

	Tot. Fat (g)	Sat. Fat (g)	Chol. (mg)	Sod. (mg)	Cal.
Fresh Potatoes					
Potato with skin, baked (4¾″ x 2⅓″)	0.2	0.1	0	16	220
Potato with skin, boiled (½ cup)	0.1	0.0	0	3	68
Frozen Potatoes					
Country Style Dinner Fries, baked (about 8 fries)					
Ore-Ida (H.J. Heinz)	3.0	1.0	0	20	110
Country Style Hash Browns, baked (1 cup)					
Ore-Ida (H.J. Heinz)	0.0	0.0	0	10	60
Potato Wedges with Skin, baked (about 9 fries)					
Ore-Ida (H.J. Heinz)	2.5	1.0	0	15	110
Potatoes O'Brien, baked (¾ cup)					
Ore-Ida (H.J. Heinz)	0.0	0.0	0	15	60
Shredded Hash Browns, baked (1 patty)					
Ore-Ida (H.J. Heinz)	0.0	0.0	0	25	70
Southern Style Hash Browns, baked (¾ cup)					
Ore-Ida (H.J. Heinz)	0.0	0.0	0	25	70
PUMPKIN					
Canned/Shelf-Stable Pumpkin					
Solid Pack Pumpkin (½ cup)					
Libby's (Nestlé Food Company) .	0.5	0.0	0	5	60
Fresh Pumpkin					
Pumpkin (½ cup)	0.3	0.0	0	6	41
Pumpkin, cooked, mashed (½ cup) .	0.9	0.1	0	2	24
RADICCHIO					
Fresh Radicchio					
Radicchio, raw, shredded (½ cup) ..	0.1	0.0	0	4	5
RADISHES					
Fresh Radishes					
Radishes, raw (10 1″ diam)	0.2	0.0	0	11	7
RUTABAGAS					
Fresh Rutabagas					
Rutabaga, cubed, cooked (½ cup) ..	0.2	0.0	0	15	29
Rutabagas, cubed, raw (½ cup)	0.1	0.0	0	14	25

	Tot. Fat (g)	Sat. Fat (g)	Chol. (mg)	Sod. (mg)	Cal.
SAUERKRAUT					
CANNED/SHELF-STABLE SAUERKRAUT					
Bavarian Kraut (½ cup)					
Bush's (Bush Brothers)	0.5	0.0	0	470	60
Sauerkraut, undrained (½ cup)					
Most brands (USDA)	**0.2**	**0.0**	**0**	**780**	**22**
REFRIGERATED SAUERKRAUT					
Sauerkraut (¼ cup)					
Claussen (Claussen Pickle Co)*	0.0	0.0	0	210	5
SHALLOTS					
FRESH SHALLOTS					
Shallots, chopped, raw (1 tbsp)	0.0	0.0	0	1	7
SPINACH					
CANNED/SHELF-STABLE SPINACH					
50% Less Salt Spinach (½ cup)					
Del Monte	0.0	0.0	0	180	30
No Salt Added Spinach (½ cup)					
Del Monte	0.0	0.0	0	85	30
No-salt-added spinach, drained (½ cup)					
Most brands (USDA)	**0.5**	**0.1**	**0**	**29**	**25**
Spinach, drained (½ cup)					
Most brands (USDA)	**0.5**	**0.1**	**0**	**(269)**	**25**
FRESH SPINACH					
Spinach, chopped, raw (½ cup)	0.1	0.0	0	22	6
Spinach, cooked (½ cup)	0.2	0.0	0	63	21
FROZEN SPINACH					
Cut Leaf Spinach in Butter Sauce (½ cup)					
Green Giant (Grand Metropolitan PLC)	1.5	1.0	<5	280	40
Spinach (½ cup)					
Most brands (USDA)	**0.2**	**0.0**	**0**	**82**	**27**
SQUASH					
SUMMER SQUASH					
Fresh Summer Squash					
Summer squash, all varieties, slices, cooked (½ cup)	0.3	0.1	0	1	18

*Tobacco company, corporate subsidiary, or parent.

	Tot. Fat (g)	Sat. Fat (g)	Chol. (mg)	Sod. (mg)	Cal.
SUMMER SQUASH *(cont'd)*					
Summer squash, all varieties, slices, raw (½ cup)	0.1	0.0	0	1	13
WINTER SQUASH					
Fresh Winter Squash					
Winter squash, all varieties, cubed, cooked (½ cup)	0.6	<1.0	0	1	39
Winter squash, all varieties, cubed, raw (½ cup)	0.1	0.0	0	2	21
ZUCCHINI					
Canned/Shelf-Stable Zucchini					
Italian Style Zucchini (½ cup)					
Progresso (Pet)	2.0	0.0	0	400	40
Italian-style zucchini, undrained (½ cup)					
Most brands (USDA)	**0.1**	**0.0**	**0**	**427**	**33**
Zesty Italian Zucchini (½ cup)					
Del Monte	0.0	0.0	0	520	40
Zucchini in Tomato Sauce (½ cup)					
Del Monte	0.0	0.0	0	490	30
Fresh Zucchini					
Zucchini, sliced, boiled (½ cup)	0.1	0.0	0	2	14
SUCCOTASH					
CANNED/SHELF-STABLE SUCCOTASH					
Succotash with corn (½ cup)					
Most brands (USDA)	**0.6**	**0.1**	**0**	**283**	**81**
Succotash with cream-style corn (½ cup)					
Most brands (USDA)	**0.7**	**0.1**	**0**	**325**	**102**
FRESH SUCCOTASH					
Succotash, cooked (½ cup)	0.8	0.1	0	16	111
FROZEN SUCCOTASH					
Succotash (½ cup)					
Most brands (USDA)	**0.8**	**0.1**	**0**	**38**	**79**
SWEET POTATOES/YAMS					
CANNED/SHELF-STABLE SWEET POTATOES/YAMS					
Candied Sweet Potatoes (½ cup)					
Royal Prince (Allen Canning Co)	0.5	0.0	0	30	210

	Tot. Fat (g)	Sat. Fat (g)	Chol. (mg)	Sod. (mg)	Cal.
Orange-Pineapple Sweet Potatoes (½ cup)					
Royal Prince (Allen Canning Co)	0.5	0.0	0	30	210
Sweet potatoes in syrup, drained (½ cup)					
Most brands (USDA)	**0.3**	**0.1**	**0**	**38**	**106**
Sweet potatoes, mashed (½ cup)					
Most brands (USDA)	**0.3**	**0.1**	**0**	**96**	**129**
FRESH SWEET POTATOES/YAMS					
Sweet potatoes, cooked, mashed (½ cup)	0.1	0.0	0	10	103
Sweet potatoes, raw (½ cup)	0.2	0.0	0	9	72
Yam, cubed, cooked (½ cup)	0.1	0.0	0	6	79
FROZEN SWEET POTATOES/YAMS					
Candied Sweet Potatoes (5 oz)					
Mrs. Paul's (Campbell Soup Co)	1.0	1.0	0	130	330
Candied Sweet Potatoes'N Apples (1 cup)					
Mrs. Paul's (Campbell Soup Co)	0.0	0.0	5	90	270
Sweet potatoes, cubed (½ cup)					
Most brands (USDA)	**0.1**	**0.0**	**0**	**7**	**88**
TARO					
FRESH TARO					
Taro, slices, cooked (½ cup)	0.1	0.0	0	10	94
Taro, slices, raw (½ cup)	0.1	0.0	0	6	56
TOMATOES					
CANNED/SHELF-STABLE TOMATOES					
Angela Mia Crushed Tomatoes (4 oz)					
Hunt's (Hunt-Wesson)	<1.0	0.0	0	260	35
Cajun Style Stewed Tomatoes (½ cup)					
Del Monte	0.0	0.0	0	460	35
Chunky Chili Style Stewed Tomatoes (½ cup)					
Del Monte	0.0	0.0	0	600	30
Chunky Pasta Style Stewed Tomatoes (½ cup)					
Del Monte	0.0	0.0	0	560	45

	Tot. Fat (g)	Sat. Fat (g)	Chol. (mg)	Sod. (mg)	Cal.
CANNED/SHELF-STABLE TOMATOES *(cont'd)*					
Classic Recipe Stewed Tomatoes (½ cup)					
Green Giant (Grand Metropolitan PLC)	0.0	0.0	0	360	35
Crushed Tomatoes in Puree with Basil (¼ cup)					
America's Choice (A & P)	0.0	0.0	0	170	25
Diced Tomatoes & Green Chilies (¼ cup)					
Chi-Chi's (Hormel)	0.0	0.0	0	340	20
Imported Peeled Tomatoes with Basil (½ cup)					
Progresso (Pet)	0.0	0.0	0	200	25
Italian Diced Tomatoes (½ cup)					
America's Choice (A & P)	2.0	0.0	0	270	50
Italian Flavored Crushed Tomatoes (4 oz)					
Hunt's (Hunt-Wesson)	<1.0	0.0	0	460	40
Italian Flavored Stewed Tomatoes (4 oz)					
Hunt's (Hunt-Wesson)	<1.0	0.0	0	370	40
Italian Flavored Whole Tomatoes (4 oz)					
Hunt's (Hunt-Wesson)	<1.0	0.0	0	420	25
Italian Recipe Stewed Tomatoes (½ cup)					
Green Giant (Grand Metropolitan PLC)	0.0	0.0	0	360	30
Italian Stewed Tomatoes (½ cup)					
America's Choice (A & P)	0.0	0.0	0	270	35
Italian Style Pear Shaped Tomatoes (4 oz)					
Hunt's (Hunt-Wesson)	<1.0	0.0	0	320	20
Italian Style Pear Tomatoes (½ cup)					
Contadina (Nestlé Food Company)	0.0	0.0	0	220	25

	Tot. Fat (g)	Sat. Fat (g)	Chol. (mg)	Sod. (mg)	Cal.
Italian Style Stewed Tomatoes (½ cup)					
America's Choice (A & P)	0.0	0.0	0	270	35
Contadina (Nestlé Food Company)	0.0	0.0	0	260	40
Del Monte	0.0	0.0	0	420	30
Mexican Recipe Stewed Tomatoes (½ cup)					
Green Giant (Grand Metropolitan PLC)	0.0	0.0	0	400	35
Mexican Style Stewed Tomatoes (½ cup)					
America's Choice (A & P)	0.0	0.0	0	270	35
Contadina (Nestlé Food Company)	0.0	0.0	0	220	40
Del Monte	0.0	0.0	0	400	35
No-salt-added red tomatoes, whole (½ cup)					
Most brands (USDA)	**0.3**	**0.0**	**0**	**16**	**24**
No Salt Added Stewed Tomatoes (½ cup)					
Del Monte	0.0	0.0	0	50	35
Organic Crushed Tomatoes with Basil (¼ cup)					
Muir Glen	0.0	0.0	0	85	25
Organic Diced Tomatoes (½ cup)					
Muir Glen	0.0	0.0	0	190	25
Organic Ground Peeled Tomatoes (¼ cup)					
Muir Glen	0.0	0.0	0	100	10
Organic Stewed Tomatoes (½ cup)					
Muir Glen	0.0	0.0	0	190	25
Organic Whole Peeled Tomatoes (½ cup)					
Muir Glen	0.0	0.0	0	260	30
Peeled Tomatoes with Basil (½ cup)					
Progresso (Pet)	0.0	0.0	0	220	25
Pizza Style Stewed Tomatoes (½ cup)					
Del Monte	0.0	0.0	0	670	35

	Tot. Fat (g)	Sat. Fat (g)	Chol. (mg)	Sod. (mg)	Cal.
CANNED/SHELF-STABLE TOMATOES *(cont'd)*					
Recipe Ready Tomatoes (½ cup)					
Contadina (Nestlé Food Company)	0.0	0.0	0	200	25
Red tomatoes, stewed (½ cup)					
Most brands (USDA)	**0.2**	**0.0**	**0**	**325**	**34**
Red tomatoes, whole (½ cup)					
Most brands (USDA)	**0.3**	**0.0**	**0**	**195**	**24**
Red tomatoes with green chilies (½ cup)					
Most brands (USDA)	**0.0**	**0.0**	**0**	**481**	**18**
Salsa Style Chunky Tomatoes (½ cup)					
Del Monte	0.0	0.0	0	560	35
Tomato Wedges (½ cup)					
Del Monte	0.0	0.0	0	380	35
Tomatoes (½ cup)					
Contadina Pasta Ready (Nestlé Food Company)	2.0	0.0	0	550	50
Tomatoes Primavera (½ cup)					
Contadina Pasta Ready (Nestlé Food Company)	1.5	0.5	0	600	50
Tomatoes with Crushed Red Pepper (½ cup)					
Contadina Pasta Ready (Nestlé Food Company)	3.0	0.5	0	690	60
Tomatoes with Mushrooms (½ cup)					
Contadina Pasta Ready (Nestlé Food Company)	1.5	0.5	0	640	50
Tomatoes with Olives (½ cup)					
Contadina Pasta Ready (Nestlé Food Company)	3.0	0.5	0	640	60
FRESH TOMATOES					
Green tomatoes, raw (1 2⅗″ diam)	0.3	0.0	0	16	30
Red tomatoes, cooked (½ cup)	0.3	0.0	0	13	30
Red tomatoes, raw (1 2⅗″ diam)	0.3	0.0	0	10	24
Tomatillos, raw (1 ⅝″ diam)	0.4	0.0	0	0	11

	Tot. Fat (g)	Sat. Fat (g)	Chol. (mg)	Sod. (mg)	Cal.
DRIED TOMATOES					
Sun-dried tomatoes (1 tbsp)					
Most brands (USDA)	**0.1**	**0.0**	**0**	**71**	**9**
TURNIPS					
FRESH TURNIPS					
Turnips, cubed, cooked (½ cup) . . .	0.1	0.0	0	39	14
Turnips, cubed, raw (½ cup)	0.1	0.0	0	44	18
WATER CHESTNUTS					
CANNED/SHELF-STABLE WATER CHESTNUTS					
Water chestnuts, sliced, undrained (½ cup)					
Most brands (USDA)	**0.0**	**0.0**	**0**	**6**	**35**
FRESH WATER CHESTNUTS					
Water chestnuts, raw (½ cup)	0.1	0.0	0	9	66
WATERCRESS					
FRESH WATERCRESS					
Watercress, chopped (½ cup)	0.0	0.0	0	7	2

YAM BEANS—*see* JICAMA, page 404

YAMS—*see* SWEET POTATOES/ YAMS, page 414

USDA Handbook No. 8 Series

Series No.	Food Group Issued	Year
8–1	Dairy and Egg Products	1976
8–2	Spices and Herbs	1977
8–4	Fats and Oils	1979
8–5	Poultry Products	1979
8–6	Soups, Sauces and Gravies	1980
8–7	Sausages and Luncheon Meats	1980
8–8	Breakfast Cereals	1982
8–9	Fruits and Fruit Juices	1982
8–10	Pork Products	1992
8–11	Vegetables and Vegetable Products	1984
8–12	Nut and Seed Products	1984
8–13	Beef Products	1990
8–14	Beverages	1986
8–15	Finfish and Shellfish Products	1987
8–16	Legumes and Legume Products	1986
8–17	Lamb, Veal and Game Products	1989
8–18	Baked Products	1992
8–19	Snacks and Sweets	1991
8–20	Cereal, Grains and Pasta	1989
8–21	Fast Foods	1988

USDA Handbook No. 456, 1975.

USDA Provisional Table on the Fatty Acids and Cholesterol Content of Selected Foods, 1984.

The Living Heart Brand Name Shopper's Guide—Revised and Updated.

TRADEMARK PRODUCTS

The following list shows some of the trademarked or registered products appearing in this book.

Allen® Canning Company: Allens®, Royal Prince®, TRAPPEY'S®
American Pop Corn Company: Jolly Time®
Beatrice Cheese, Inc.: HEALTHY CHOICE®
Best Foods/CPC International: Arnold®, Bakery Light™, Best Foods®, Bran'nola®, Brick Oven®, Brownberry®, Golden Griddle®, Hellmann's®, Karo®, Mazola®, Mueller's®, No Stick™, Sahara®, Thomas'®
Bremner Biscuit Company: BREMNER®
Buckeye Beans & Herbs: BUCKEYE BEANS & HERBS®
Cabot Creamery: CABOT®
Campbell Soup Company: Beach Haven, Campbell's, Campbell's Simmer Chef, Campbell's Kitchen, Chunky, Double Noodle, Franco-American, Garfield, Healthy Request, Healthy Treasures, Home Cookin', Marie's, Mrs. Paul's, Natural Goodness, Open Pit, Prego, SpaghettiO's, Swanson, Tomato Del Mar, V8, V8 Picante
Chelten House Products Inc.: Chelten House, Dockside, Medford Farms
Citrus World, Inc.: FLORIDA'S NATURAL®
Coca-Cola Foods: Minute Maid®, FIVE ALIVE®, Hi-C®
Coca-Cola USA: Coca-Cola®, Coca-Cola Classic®, Coke®, Fanta®, Fresca®, Mello Yello®, Minute Maid®, Mr. Pibb®, PowerAde™, Ramblin'®, Tab®
ConAgra Frozen Foods: HEALTHY CHOICE®
Eden Foods, Inc.: EDENBLEND®, EDENRICE®, EDENSOY®
Frito-Lay, Inc.: DORITOS®, FRITO-LAY®, ROLD GOLD®, TOSTITOS®

Frozfruit Corporation: FROZFRUIT®
Gerber Cheese Co., Inc.: SWISS KNIGHT®
Golden Jersey Products, Inc.: Golden Jersey
Guiltless Gourmet, Inc.: GUILTLESS GOURMET®
Hansen Beverage Company: HANSEN'S® Natural
Health Valley Foods: Health Valley®
Hershey Foods Corporation: HERSHEY®, SPECIAL DARK®, TWIZZLERS®
Hormel Foods Corporation: CHI-CHI'S™, CHI-CHI'S®, HERB-OX®, HONG KONG™, HORMEL™, HORMEL®, HOUSE OF TSANG™, HOUSE OF TSANG®, KOREAN™, MANDARIN™, NOT-SO-SLOPPY-JOE®
Hunt-Wesson, Inc.: LA CHOY®
International Trading Company: Hafnia®
Keebler Company: Cinnamon Crisp®, Elfin Delights®, Graham Selects®, Keebler®, Toasteds®, Zesta®
Kellogg Company: Kellogg's®, All-Bran®, Apple Cinnamon Rice Krispies™, Apple Cinnamon Squares®, Apple Jacks®, Apple Raisin Crisp®, Blueberry Squares™, Bran Buds®, Cocoa Krispies®, Complete® Bran Flakes, Corn Pops®, Crispix®, Double Dip Crunch®, Froot Loops®, Frosted Krispies®, Frosted Mini-Wheats®, Fruitful Bran®, Fruity Marshmallow Krispies®, Healthy Choice™ from Kellogg's®, Just Right®, Kellogg's Corn Flakes®, Kellogg's Frosted Bran®, Kellogg's Frosted Flakes®, Kenmei® Rice Bran, Müeslix®, Nut & Honey Crunch®, Nut & Honey Crunch O's®, Nutri-Grain®, Product 19®, Raisin Squares®, Rice Krispies®, Rice Krispies Treats® Cereal, Smacks®, Special K®, Strawberry Squares®
Kraft General Foods USA: ALPHA-BITS, BREAKSTONE'S, BREAKSTONE'S FREE, BREYERS, CAPRI SUN, CATALINA, CHEEZ WHIZ LIGHT, CHIFFON, COUNTRY TIME, COUNTRY KITCHEN, COUNTRY KITCHEN LITE, CRANBERRY BREEZE, CRYSTAL LIGHT, DI GIORNO, DI GIORNO LIGHT VARIETIES, DREAM WHIP, D-ZERTA, ENTENMANN'S, FROSTED WHEAT BITES, FRUIT WHEATS, FRUIT & FIBRE, FUNMALLOWS, GOLDEN CRISP, GOOD SEASONS, GRAPE-NUTS, GREAT BLUEDINI, HONEY BUNCHES OF OATS, HONEYCOMB, IN-

CREDIBERRY, JELL-O, JELL-O AMERICANA, JELL-O Brand FREE, KNUDSEN, KNUDSEN CAL 70, KNUDSEN FREE, KNUDSEN LIGHT, KOOL-AID, KOOL-AID BURSTS, KRAFT, KRAFT DELICIOUSLY RIGHT, KRAFT FREE, KRAFT HANDI-SNACKS, KRAFT HEALTHY FAVORITES, KRAFT THICK'N SPICY, KRAFT TOUCH OF BUTTER, KRAFT JET-PUFFED, LIGHT N' LIVELY, LIGHT N' LIVELY FREE, LIGHT N' LIVELY FREE 50 CALORIES, LIGHT N' LIVELY FREE 70 CALORIES, LOG CABIN, LOG CABIN LITE, MAUI PUNCH, MINUTE, MIRACLE WHIP, MIRACLE WHIP FREE, MIRACLE WHIP LIGHT, MOUNTAIN COOLER, MR. FREEZE, NABISCO, OVEN FRY, PACIFIC COOLER, PARKAY, PHILADELPHIA BRAND FREE, PINK SWIMMINGO, POST, POST TOASTIES, POSTUM, PURPLESAURUS REX, ROCK-A-DILE RED, SAFARI PUNCH, SALSA, SAUCEWORKS, SEALTEST, SEALTEST FREE, SEALTEST LIGHT, SEVEN SEAS, SEVEN SEAS FREE, SEVEN SEAS VIVA, SHAKE'N BAKE, SHAKE'N BAKE PERFECT POTATOES, SHREDDED WHEAT'N BRAN, SPOON SIZE, STRAWBERRY COOLER, SURFER COOLER, TANG, TEAM, THE BUDGET GOURMET, TOMBSTONE, TOMBSTONE LIGHT, VELVEETA LIGHT, YO YOGI BERRY

Lady J, Inc.: LADY J™

Lance Inc.: LANCE, SESAME TWINS

Lawry's Foods, Inc.: Lawry's®

Lifeline Food Company, Inc.: Lifetime®, Healthy Farms®

M. A. Gedney Company: GEDNEY®, STATE FAIR™

Mama Tish's Italian Specialties, Inc.: Mama Tish's®, Original Italian Ices®

Mazzone Enterprises, Inc.: Mazzone's®

Miceli Dairy Products Company: Miceli's®

"Mike-sells" Potato Chip Co: Mike-sell's®

Muir Glen Organic Tomato Products: MUIR GLEN®

Natural Nectar Corporation: FI-BAR®

Ocean Spray Cranberries, Inc.: CITRUS REFRESHERS™ Juice Drinks, CRANAPPLE®, CRAN-BLUEBERRY®, CRAN-CHERRY™, CRAN-GRAPE®, CRANICOT®, CRAN-

RASPBERRY®, CRAN-STRAWBERRY™, CRANTASTIC® Fruit Punch, ISLAND GUAVA™, LIGHTSTYLE®, MANGO-MANGO™, MAUNA LA'I®, OCEAN SPRAY®, PARADISE PASSION™

Pepperidge Farm, Incorporated: Pepperidge Farm

Pet Incorporated: B&M, DOWNYFLAKE, FRIEND'S, HEARTLAND, LAS PALMAS, OLD EL PASO, PANCHO VILLA, PET, PROGRESSO, SEGO, VAN DE KAMP'S

Riviana Foods Inc.: Carolina, Mahatma, Success, Water Maid

Rubschlager Baking Corporation: RUBSCHLAGER®

Rymer Foods Inc.: MENU MAKER®

The Willy Wonka Candy Factory: DINASOUR EGGS®, Everlasting GOBSTOPPER®, FRECKLED EGGS®, Fruit RUNTS®, Heart Breakers®, NERDS®, RUNTS Merry Mix®, Sweet N Sour Hearts®, TART n TINYS®, WACKY WAFER Bunnys®

U.S. Mills, Inc.: Apple Stroodles, Aztec, Banana-O's, Barley Plus, Erewhon, Galaxy Grahams

Yarnell's® Ice Cream: GUILT FREE®

YZ Enterprises, Inc.: ALMONDINA®

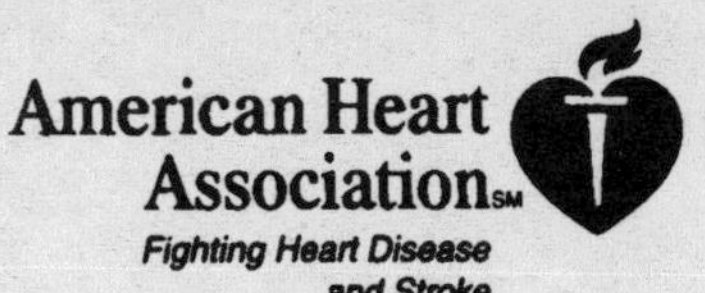
American Heart
Association
SM
Fighting Heart Disease
and Stroke